ENGINE
D0078448

Second Edition

Biomedical Signal and Image Processing

Second Edition

Biomedical Signal and Image Processing

Kayvan Najarian
Robert Splinter

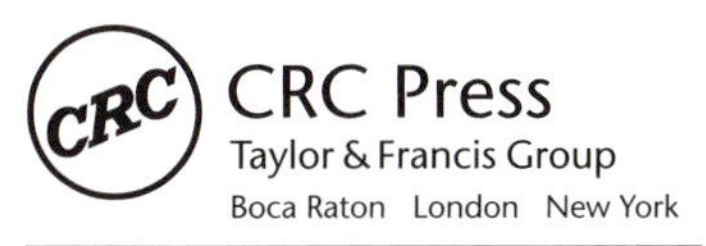

CRC Press is an imprint of the
Taylor & Francis Group, an **informa** business

CRC Press
Taylor & Francis Group
6000 Broken Sound Parkway NW, Suite 300
Boca Raton, FL 33487-2742

Printed in the United States of America on acid-free paper
Version Date: 20120330

International Standard Book Number: 978-1-4398-7033-4 (Hardback)

Visit the Taylor & Francis Web site at
http://www.taylorandfrancis.com

and the CRC Press Web site at
http://www.crcpress.com

I dedicate this book to my wife, Roya,
and my sons, Cyrus and Daniel, who have always
been the source of inspiration and love for me.

Kayvan Najarian

Contents

PART II Processing of Biomedical Signals

PART III Processing of Biomedical Images

Preface

The first edition of the book *Biomedical Signal and Image Processing* was published by CRC Press in 2005. It was used by many universities and educational institutions as a textbook for upper undergraduate level and first-year graduate level courses in signal and image processing. It was also used by a number of companies and research institutions as a reference book for their research projects. This highly encouraging impact of the first edition motivated me to look into ways to improve the book and create a second edition.

The following improvements have been made to the second edition:

- A number of editorial corrections have been made to address the typos, grammatical errors, and ambiguities in some mathematical equations.
- Many examples have been added to almost all chapters, of which the majority are MATLAB® examples, further illustrating the concepts described in the text.
- Further explanations and justifications have been provided for some signal and image processing concepts that may have needed more illustration.

Finally, I would like to thank all the people who contacted me and my coauthor, Dr. Robert Splinter, and shared with us their thoughts and ideas regarding this book. I hope that you find the second edition even more useful than the first one!

Kayvan Najarian
Virginia Commonwealth University
Richmond, Virginia

For MATLAB® and Simulink® product information, please contact:

The MathWorks, Inc.
3 Apple Hill Drive
Natick, MA, 01760-2098 USA
Tel: 508-647-7000
Fax: 508-647-7001
E-mail: info@mathworks.com
Web: www.mathworks.com

WEB DOWNLOADS

Additional materials such as data files are available from the CRC Web site: www.crcpress.com

Under the menu Electronic Products (located on the left side of the screen), click on Downloads & Updates. A list of books in alphabetical order with web downloads will appear. Locate this book by a search, or scroll down to it. After clicking on the book title, a brief summary of the book will appear. Go to the bottom of this screen and click on the hyperlinked "Download" that is in a zip file.

Or you can go directly to the web download site, which is www.crcpress.com/e_products/downloads/default.asp

Acknowledgments

Dr. Najarian thanks Dr. Joo Heon Shin for his invaluable and detailed feedback, which contained a long list of corrections addressed in this edition of the book. Above all, Dr. Najarian would like to thank Dr. Abed Al Raoof Bsoul, his former PhD student, who not only provided him with invaluable feedback on all chapters of the book, but also helped him with forming some of the additional examples included in the second edition. Raoof's diligence and deep insight into signal and image processing were instrumental in forming this edition, and Dr. Najarian cannot thank him enough for his help. Dr. Najarian also thanks Paul Junor at the Department of Electronic Engineering, La Trobe University, Australia, whose editorial corrections helped improve the presentation of this textbook.

We thank Dr. Sharam Shirani from McMaster University for sharing some of his image processing teaching ideas and slides with us and for providing us his feedback on Chapters 3 and 4. We would also like to thank Alireza Darvish and Jerry James Zacharias for providing us with their invaluable feedback on several chapters of this book. The detailed feedback from these individuals helped us improve the signal and image processing chapters of this book.

Moreover, we would like to thank all hospitals, clinics, industrial units, and individuals who shared with us their biomedical and nonbiomedical images and signals. In each chapter, the sources of all contributed images and signals are mentioned, and the contribution of the people or agencies that provided the data is acknowledged.

Introduction

I.1 PROCESSING OF BIOMEDICAL DATA

Processing of biological and medical information has long been a dynamic field of life science. Before the widespread use of digital computers, however, almost all processing was performed by human experts directly. For instance, in processing and analysis of the vital signs (such as blood pressure), physicians had to rely entirely on their hearing and visual and heuristic experience. The accuracy and reliability of such "manual" diagnostic processes are limited by a number of factors, including limitations of humans in extracting and detecting certain features from signals. Moreover, such manual analysis of medical data suffers from other factors such as human errors due to fatigue and subjectiveness of the decision-making processes. In the last few decades, advancements of the emerging biomedical sensing and imaging technologies such as magnetic resonance imaging (MRI), x-ray computed tomography (CT) imaging, and ultrasound imaging have provided us with very large amounts of biomedical data that can never be processed by medical practitioners within a finite time span.

Biomedical information processing comprises the techniques that apply mathematical tools to extract important diagnostic information from biomedical and biological data. Due to the size and complexity of such data, computers are put to the task of processing, visualizing, and even classifying samples. The main steps of a typical biomedical measurement and processing system are shown in Figure I.1. As can be seen, the first step is to identify the relevant physical properties of the biomedical system that can be measured using suitable sensors. For example, electrocardiogram (ECG) is a signal that records the electrical activities of the heart muscles and is used to evaluate many functional characteristics of the heart.

Once a biomedical signal is recorded by a sensor, it has to be preprocessed and filtered. This is necessary because the measured signal often contains some undesirable noise that is combined with the relevant biomedical signal. The usual sources of noise include the activities of other biological systems that interfere with the desirable signal and the variations due to sensor imperfections. In the ECG example, the electrical signals caused by the respiratory system are the main sources of noise and interference.

The next step is to process the filtered signal and extract features that represent or describe the status and conditions of the biomedical system under study. Such biomedical features (measures) are expected to distinguish between healthy and deviating cases. A group of extracted features are defined based on the medical characteristics of the biomedical system (such as the heart rate calculated from ECG). These features are often defined by physicians and biologists, and the task of biomedical engineers is to create algorithms to extract these features from biomedical signals. Another group of extracted features is the ones defined using signal and image processing procedures. Even though the direct biological interpretation

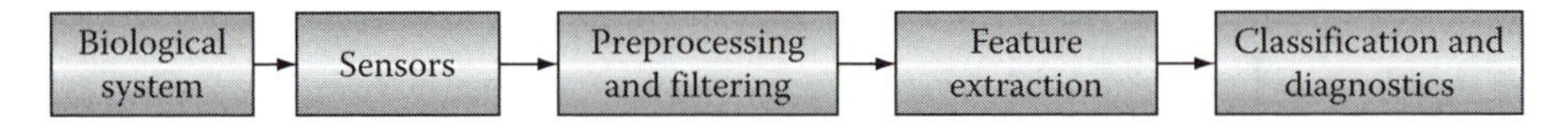

FIGURE I.1 Block diagram of a typical biomedical signal/image processing system.

of such features may not be well understood, these features are instrumental in the classification and diagnosis of biomedical systems. In the ECG example, the physiological interpretation of measures such as the fractal dimension of a filtered version of the signal or the energy of the wavelet coefficients in a certain band may not necessarily be known or understood. However, these measures are known to contain informative signal processing–based features that significantly facilitate the classification of biomedical signals.

The last step is classification and diagnostics. In this step, all the extracted features are submitted to a classifier that distinguishes among different classes of samples, e.g., normal and abnormal. These classes are defined based on the biomedical knowledge specific to the signal that is being processed. In the ECG example, these classes might include normal, myocardial infarction, flutter, different types of tachycardia, and so on. The way a classifier is designed is very application specific. In some systems, the features needed to classify samples to each respective class are well known. Therefore, the classifier can be easily designed using the direct implementation of the available knowledge base and features. In other cases, where no clear rules are available (or the existing rules are not sufficient), the classifier must be built and trained using the known examples of each class.

In some applications, other steps and features are added to the block diagram outlines in Figure I.1. For instance, in almost all biomedical imaging systems, there is an essential part of the system that helps visualize the results. This is because human users (e.g., physicians) often rely on the visualization of the two-dimensional (or three-dimensional) structure of the biomedical objects that are being scanned. In other words, visualization is an essential step and the main objective of many imaging systems. This need calls for the use of a variety of visualization and image processing techniques to modify images and to make them more understandable and more useful for human users.

A useful feature of many biomedical information processing systems is a user interface that allows interaction between the user and the processing elements. This interaction allows modification of the processing techniques based on the user's feedback. In the ECG example, the user may decide to change the filters to focus on certain frequency components of the ECG signal and extract the frequencies that are more important for a certain disease. In many image processing systems, the user may decide to focus on certain areas of an image and perform particular operations (such as image enhancement) on the selected regions of interest.

I.2 ABOUT THE BOOK

This book is designed to be used as either a senior level undergraduate course or as a first-year graduate level course. The main background needed to understand and use the book is college level calculus and some familiarity with complex variables.

Knowledge of linear algebra would also be helpful in understanding the concepts. The book describes the mathematical concepts in signal and image processing techniques in great detail and, as a result, no prior knowledge of fundamental processing techniques (such as Fourier transform) is required. At the same time, for readers who are already familiar with the main signal processing concepts, the chapters dedicated to signal and image processing techniques can serve as a detailed review of this field.

Part I provides a detailed description of the main signal processing, image processing, and pattern recognition techniques. The chapters in this part also cover the main computational methods in other fields of study such as information theory and stochastic processes. The combination of all these mathematical techniques provides the computational skills needed to analyze biomedical signal and images. Readers who have previously taken courses in all related areas, such as digital signal, image processing, information theory, and pattern recognition, are also recommended to read through Part II to familiarize themselves with the notation and practice applying their computational skills to biomedical data.

Even though the authors emphasize the importance of mathematical concepts covered in the book, they strongly believe that the best method of learning the math concepts is through doing real examples. As a result, each chapter contains several programming examples written in MATLAB® that process real biomedical signals/images using the respective mathematical methods. These examples are designed to help the reader better understand the math concepts. Even though the book is not intended to teach MATLAB, the increasing level of difficulty in the MATLAB examples allows the reader to gradually improve his or her MATLAB programming skills.

Each chapter also contains a number of exercises in the Problems section that give students the chance to practice the introduced techniques. Some of the problems are designed to help students improve their knowledge of the mathematical concepts, while the rest are practical problems defined using real data from biomedical systems (appearing on the companion website to the book). Specifically, while some of the problems are mainly mathematical problems to be done manually, the vast majority of the problems in all chapters are programming problems designed to help the readers obtain hands-on experience in dealing with real-world problems. Virtually all these problems apply the methods introduced in the previous chapters to real problems in biomedical signal and image processing applications.

Part II introduces the major one-dimensional biomedical signals. In each chapter, at first the biological origin and importance of the signal are explained, followed by a description of the main computational methods commonly used for processing the signal. Assuming that readers have acquired the signal/image processing skills in Part I, the main focus of Part II is on the physiology and diagnostic applications of the biomedical signals. Almost all examples and exercises in these chapters use real biomedical data for real biomedical signal processing applications.

The last part, Part III, deals with the main biomedical image modalities. It first covers the physical and philological principles of imaging modalities and subsequently describes the main applications of the introduced imaging modalities in biomedical diagnostics. In each chapter, the main computational methods used to process these images are also reviewed.

I.3 BRIEF DESCRIPTION OF CHAPTERS

As mentioned previously, the book is divided into three parts. Part I gives an introduction to digital signal and image processing techniques. Chapter 1 explains the main fundamental concepts of signal processing in simple conceptual language. This chapter introduces the main signal processing concepts and tools in nonmathematical terms to prepare the readers for a more rigorous description of these concepts in the following chapters. Chapter 2 describes the definition and applications of continuous and digital Fourier transform. All concepts and definitions in this chapter are explained using a number of examples to ensure that the reader is not overwhelmed by the mathematical formulae. More specifically, as demonstrated in Chapter 2 as well as in subsequent chapters, the authors feel strongly that the description of the mathematical formulation of various signal and image processing methods must be accompanied by elaborate conceptual explanations.

Chapter 3 discusses different techniques for filtering, enhancement, and restoration of images. Even though the techniques are described mainly for images, the applications of some of these techniques in the processing of one-dimensional signals are also described. In Chapter 4, different techniques for edge detection and segmentation of digital images are discussed. Chapter 5 is devoted to wavelet transforms and their main signal and image processing applications. Other advanced signal and image processing techniques, including the basic concepts of stochastic processes and information theory, are discussed in Chapter 6. Chapter 7, the last chapter in Part I, provides an introduction to pattern recognition methods, including classification and clustering techniques.

Part II describes the main one-dimensional biomedical signals and the processing techniques applied to analyze these signals. Chapter 8 provides a concise review of the electrical activities of the cell. Since all electrical signals of the human body are somehow created by action potential, this chapter acts as an introduction to the rest of the chapters in Part II.

Chapters 9 through 11 are devoted to analysis and processing of the main biomedical signals, i.e., electrocardiogram (ECG), electroencephalogram (EEG), and electromyogram (EMG). In each case, the biological origins of the signal, together with its main applications in biomedical diagnostics, are described. Then, different techniques to process each signal and extract important features from it are discussed. In addition, the main diseases that are often detected and diagnosed using each of the signals are briefly introduced, and the computational techniques applied to detect such diseases from the signals are described. In Chapter 12, other biomedical signals (including blood pressure, electrooculogram, and magnetoencephalogram) are discussed. All the chapters in this part have practical examples and exercises (with biomedical data) to help students gain hands-on experience in analyzing biomedical signals.

In Part III, the physical and physiological principles, formation, and importance of the main biomedical imaging modalities are discussed. The various processing techniques applied to analyze different types of biomedical images are also covered in this part. In Chapter 13, the principal ideas and formulations of computed tomography (CT) are presented. These techniques are essential in understanding many biomedical imaging systems and technologies such as x-ray CT, MRI, PET, and ultrasound.

Chapter 14 is devoted to the regular x-ray imaging, x-ray computed tomography, and the computational techniques used to create and process these images. Chapter 15 introduces magnetic resonance imaging (MRI). It covers the physical principles of magnetic resonance and describes the processing techniques pertinent to MRI. Functional MRI (*f*MRI) and its applications are also addressed in this chapter. Chapter 16 describes different types of ultrasound imaging technologies and the processing techniques applied to produce and analyze these images. Such techniques include the tomographic methods used in time-of-flight tomography, attenuation tomography, and reflection tomography. Positron emission tomography (PET) is discussed in Chapter 17. Chapter 18 is devoted to other types of biomedical images, including optical microscopy, confocal microscopy, electric impedance imaging, and infrared imaging.

The book is accompanied by a website maintained by CRC Press that contains the data used for examples and exercises given in the book. The site also includes the images used in the chapters. This allows forming lecture notes slides that can be used both as a teaching aid material for classroom instruction or as a brief review/overview of the contents for students and other readers.

The contents of this book are specialized for processing of biomedical signals and images. However, in order to make the book usable for readers interested in other applications of signal and image processing, the description of the introduced methods is kept general and applicable to other fields of science and technology. Moreover, throughout the book, the authors have used some nonbiomedical examples to exhibit the applicability of the introduced methods to other fields of study such as astronomy.

ADDITIONAL READINGS

Costaridou, L. (2005) *Applied Medical Image Analysis Methods*, CRC Press, Boca Raton, FL.

Jan, J. (2006) *Medical Image Processing, Reconstruction, and Restoration: Concepts and Methods*, CRC Press, Boca Raton, FL.

Murdy, K.M., Plonsey, R., and Bronzino, J.D. (2003) *Biomedical Imaging*, CRC Press, Boca Raton, FL.

Suri, J.S. and Laxminarayan, S. (2003) *Angiography and Plaque Imaging: Advanced Segmentation Techniques*, CRC Press, Boca Raton, FL.

Part I

Introduction to Digital Signal and Image Processing

1 Signals and Biomedical Signal Processing

1.1 INTRODUCTION AND OVERVIEW

The most fundamental concept that is frequently used in this book is a "signal." It is imperative to clearly define this concept and to illustrate different types of signals encountered in signal and image processing. In this chapter, different types of signals are defined, and the fundamental concepts of signal transformation and processing are presented while avoiding detailed mathematical formulations.

1.2 WHAT IS A "SIGNAL"?

The definition of a signal plays an important role in understanding the capabilities of signal processing. We start this chapter with the definition of one-dimensional (1-D) signals. A 1-D signal is an ordered sequence of numbers that describes the trends and variations of a quantity. The consecutive measurements of a physical quantity taken at different times create a typical signal encountered in science and engineering. The order of the numbers in a signal is often determined by the order of measurements (or events) in "time." A sequence of body temperature recordings collected in consecutive days forms an example of a 1-D signal in time. The characteristics of a signal lie in the order of the numbers as well as the amplitude of the recorded numbers, and the main task of all signal processing tools is to analyze the signal in order to extract important knowledge that may not be clearly visible to the human eyes.

We have to emphasize the point that not all 1-D signals are necessarily ordered in time. As an example, consider the signal formed by the recordings of the temperature simultaneously measured at different points along a metal rod where the distance from one end of the rod defines the order of the sequence. In such a signal, the points that are closer to the origin (one end of the metal rod) appear earlier in the sequence, and, as a result, the concept that orders the sequence is "distance in space" as opposed to time. However, due to abundance of time signals in many areas of science, in the literature of signal processing, the word "time" is often used to describe the axis that identifies order. In this book, without losing the generality of the results or concepts, we use the concept of time as the ordering axis, knowing that, in some signals, time should be replaced by other concepts such as space.

Many examples of biological 1-D signals are heavily used in medicine and biology. Recording of the electrical activities of the heart muscles, called electrocardiogram (ECG), is widely considered as the main diagnostic signal in assessment of the cardiovascular system. Electroencephalogram (EEG) is a signal that records the electrical activities of the brain and is heavily used in diagnostics of the central nervous system (CNS).

Multidimensional signals are simply extensions of the 1-D signals mentioned earlier, i.e., a multidimensional signal is a multidimensional sequence of numbers ordered in all dimensions. For example, an image is a two-dimensional (2-D) sequence of data where numbers are ordered in both dimensions. In almost all images, the numbers are ordered in space (for both dimensions). In a gray-scale image, the value of the signal for a given set of coordinates (x, y), i.e., $g(x, y)$, identifies the image brightness level at those coordinates. There are several important types of image modalities that are heavily used for clinical diagnostics among which magnetic resonance imaging (MRI), computed tomography (CT), ultrasonic images, and positron emission tomography (PET) are the most commonly used ones. These imaging systems will be introduced in separate chapters dedicated to each image modality.

1.3 ANALOG, DISCRETE, AND DIGITAL SIGNALS

Based on the continuity of a signal in time and amplitude axes, the following three types of signals can be recognized:

1.3.1 Analog Signals

These signals are continuous both in time and amplitude. This means that both time and amplitude axes are continuous axes and can take any real number. In other words, at any given real values of time "t" the amplitude value "$g(t)$" can take any number belonging to a continuous interval of real numbers. An example of such a signal is the body temperature readings acquired using an analog mercury thermometer over a certain period of time. In such a thermometer, the temperature is measured at all times and the temperature value (i.e., the height of the mercury column) belongs to a continuous interval of numbers. An example of such a signal is shown in Figure 1.1. The signal illustrates the readings of the body temperature measured continuously for 6000 s (or equivalently 100 min).

1.3.2 Discrete Signals

In discrete signals, the amplitude axis is continuous but the time axis is discrete. This means that, unlike in analog signals, the measurements of the quantity are available only at certain specific times. In order to see why discrete signals are often preferred over analog signals in many practical applications, consider the example given earlier for analog signals. It is very unlikely that the body temperature may change every second, or even every few minutes, and, therefore, in order to monitor the temperature over a period of time, one can easily measure and sample the temperature only at certain times (as opposed to continuously monitoring the temperature as in the analog signal described earlier). The times at which the temperature

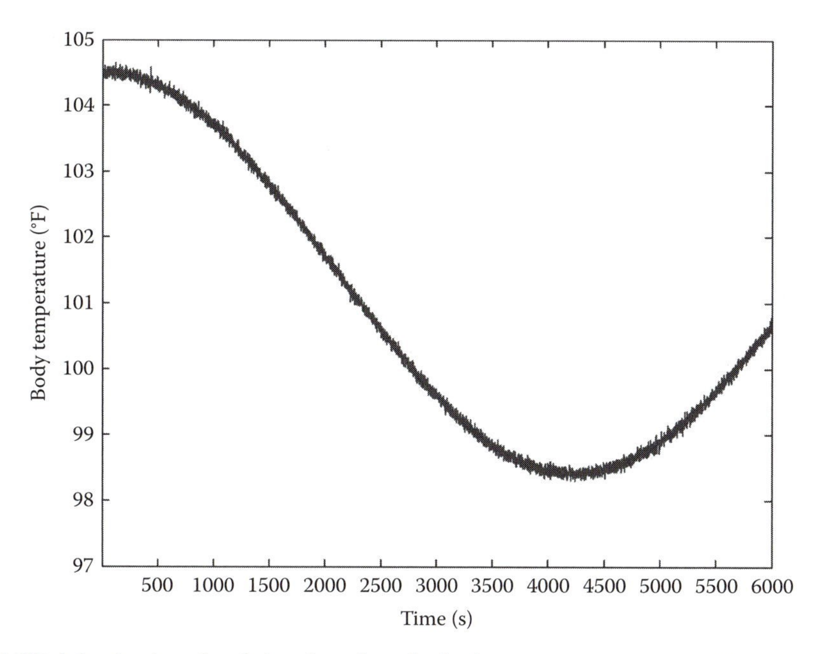

FIGURE 1.1 Analog signal that describes the body temperature measured by an analog mercury thermometer.

is sampled are often multiples of a certain sampling period "T_S." It is important to note that as long as T_S is small enough, all information in the analog signal is also contained in the discrete signal. Later in this book, an important theorem called Nyquist theorem is described that gives a limit on the size of the sampling period T_S. This size limit guarantees that the sampled signal (i.e., discrete signal) contains all information of the original analog signal.

Figure 1.2 illustrates a discrete temperature signal that is the sampled version of the analog signal in Figure 1.1. More specifically, the discrete signal (i.e., $g(nT_S)$) has sampled the analog signal every $T_S = 300$ s. As can be seen from Figure 1.2, even though the discrete signal $g(nT_S)$ is defined only at times $t = nT_S$, where $n = 0, 1, 2, \ldots$, the main characteristic and variations of the analog signal are detectable in the discrete signal too.

Another preference of digital signals over analog signals is the space required to store a signal. In the aforementioned example, the discrete signal has only 20 points and therefore can be easily stored while the analog signal needs a large amount of storage space. It is also evident that signals with smaller size are easier to process. This suggests that by sampling an analog signal with the largest possible T_S (while ensuring that all the information in the analog signal is entirely reflected in the resulting discrete signal), one can create a discrete representation of the original analog signal that has fewer points and is therefore much easier to store and process.

The shorter notation $g(n)$ is often used to represent $g(nT_S)$ in the literature and is adopted in this book.

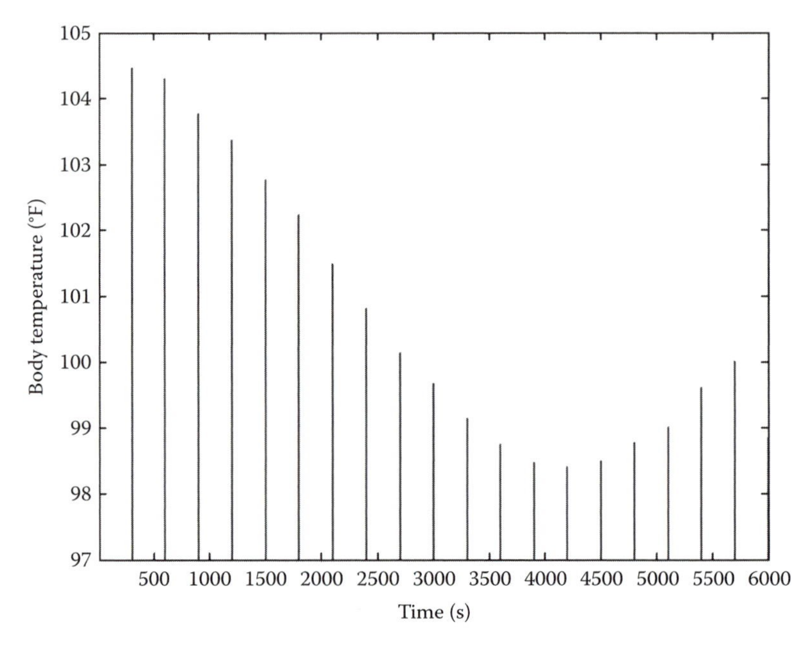

FIGURE 1.2 Discrete signal that describes the body temperature measured at every 300 s (5 min).

1.3.3 Digital Signals

In digital signals, both time and amplitude axes are discrete, i.e., a digital signal is defined only at certain times and the amplitude of the signal at each sample can only be one of a fixed finite set of values. In order to better understand this concept, consider measuring the body temperature using a digital thermometer. Such thermometers present values with certain accuracy rather than on a continuous range of amplitudes. For example, if the true temperature is 98.634562 and there are no decimal representations on the digital thermometer, the reading will be 97 (which is the closest allowed level), and the decimal digits are simply ignored. This of course causes some quantization error, but, in reality, the remaining decimals are not very important for physicians and this error can be easily disregarded. What is gained by creating a digital signal is the ease of using digital computers to store and process the data. Figure 1.3 shows the digital signal taken from the discrete signal depicted in Figure 1.2 that is rounded up to the closest integer. It is important to note that almost all techniques discussed in this book and used in digital signal processing are truly dealing with "discrete signals" and not "digital signals" as the name might suggest. The reason why these techniques are called digital signal processing is that when the algebraic operations are performed inside a digital computer, all the variables are automatically quantized and converted into digital numbers. These digital numbers have a finite but very large number of decimals, and, as a result, even though digital in nature, they are often treated as discrete numbers.

The majority of signals measured and processed in biomedical engineering are discrete signals. Consequently, even though the processing techniques for

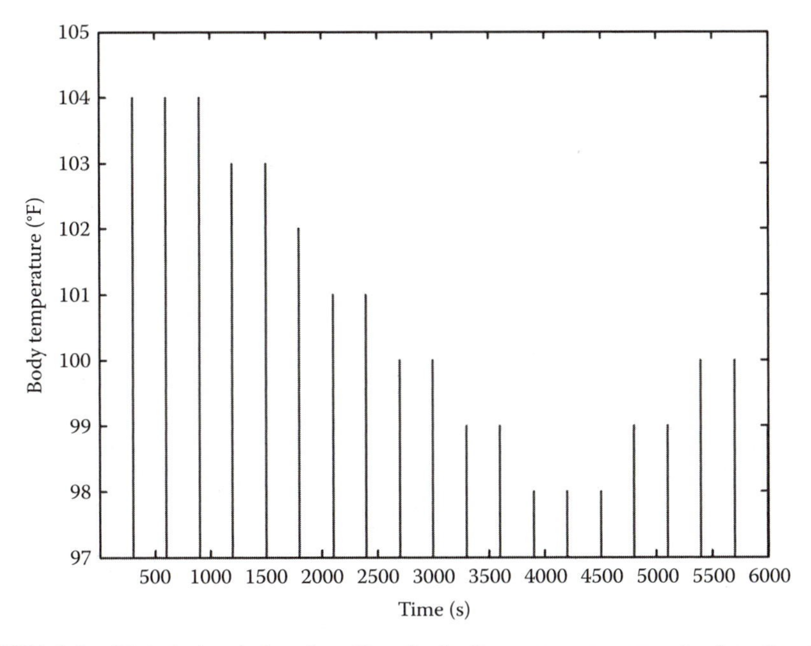

FIGURE 1.3 Digital signal that describes the body temperature quantized to the closet integer.

analog signals are briefly described in this book, the emphasis is given to processing techniques for digital signals.

1.4 PROCESSING AND TRANSFORMATION OF SIGNALS

A signal can be analyzed or processed in many different ways depending on the objectives of the signal analysis. Each of these processing technique attempts to extract, highlight, and emphasize certain properties of a signal. For example, in order to see the number of cold days during a given year, one can easily count the number of days when the temperature signal falls below a threshold value that identifies cold weather. Thresholding is only one example of many different processing techniques and transformations that can manipulate a signal to highlight some of its properties. Some transformations express and evaluate the signal in time domain, while other transformations focus on other "domains" among which frequency domain is an important one. In this section, we describe the importance and usefulness of some signal processing transformations without getting into their mathematical details. This would encourage the readers to pay a closer attention to the conceptual meanings of these transformations whose mathematical descriptions will be given in the next few chapters.

In order to see the performance of the frequency domain in highlighting certain useful information in signals, consider a signal that records the occurrence of a failure in a certain machine. For such a signal, some of the most informative measures to evaluate the performance of the machine are the answers to the following questions: "On average, how often can a failure occur?" and "Is there any visible periodicity in the failure pattern?" If we identify a specific frequency at which machine failures often occur, we can simply schedule regular periodic checkups before the expected time for possible machine failures. This can also help us identify potential reasons and causes for periodic failures and therefore associate failures to some physical events such as the regular weariness of a belt in the machine. Fourier transform (FT) is a transformation designed to describe a signal in frequency domain and highlight the important knowledge in the frequency variations of the signal. The usefulness of the knowledge contained in frequency domain explains the importance of FT. Other transformations commonly used in signal and image processing literature (such as wavelet transform) describe a signal in other domains that are often a combination of time and frequency.

It has to be emphasized that the information contained in a signal is exactly the same in all domains, regardless of the specific domain definition. This means that different transformations do not add/delete any information to/from a signal, and the same exact information can be discovered from a signal in each of these domains. The key point to realize the popularity of different types of transformations in signal processing is the fact that each transform can highlight a certain type of information (which is different from adding new knowledge to it). For example, the frequency information is much more visible in Fourier domain than in time domain, while the exact same information is also contained in the time signal. In other words, while the frequency information is entirely contained in the time signal, such information might be more difficult to notice or more computationally intensive to extract in time domain. The reason for this clarification is the answers often students give to the following tricky question: "Assume a signal is given in both time and Fourier domains. Which domain does give more information about the signal?" The authors have asked this question to their students, and almost always half of the students identify the time domain as the more informative domain while the remaining half go with the Fourier domain, and almost never does anyone realize that the answer to this tricky question is simply "neither!" The choice of the domain only affects the visibility, representation, and highlighting of certain characteristics, while the information contained in the signal remains the same in all domains. It is important for the readers to keep this fact in mind when we discuss different transformations in the following chapters.

1.5 SIGNAL PROCESSING FOR FEATURE EXTRACTION

Once certain characteristics of a signal are identified using appropriate transformations, these characteristics or features are used to evaluate the signal and the system producing the signal. As an example, once using image processing techniques, a region of a CT image is highlighted and identified as a tumor, then one can easily perform some measurements over the region (such as measuring the size of the tumor) and identify the malignancy of the tumor. As mentioned in the Preface, one of the main functions of biomedical signal and image processing is to define and extract measures that are vital for diagnostics of biomedical systems.

1.6 SOME CHARACTERISTICS OF DIGITAL IMAGES

Digital images (i.e., 2-D digital signals) are important types of data used in many fields of science and technology. The importance of imaging systems (such as MRI) in medical sciences cannot be overestimated. In this section, some general characteristics of images together with some simple operations for elementary analysis of digital images are discussed.

1.6.1 Image Capturing

Unlike photographic images in which cameras are used to capture the light intensity and/or color of objects, each medical technology uses a different set of physical properties of living tissues to generate an image. For example, while MRI is based on the magnetic prosperities of a tissue, CT scan relies on the interaction between the x-ray beams and the biological tissues to form an image. In other words, in medical imaging sensors of different physical properties of materials (including light intensity and color) are employed to record anatomical and functional information about the tissue under study.

1.6.2 Image Representation

Even though different sensor technologies are used to generate biomedical images, when it comes to the representation image, they are all visually represented as digital images. These images are either gray-level images or color images. In a gray-level image, the light intensity or brightness of an object shown at coordinates (x, y) of the image is represented by a number called "gray level." The higher the gray-level number, the brighter the image will be at the coordinate point (x, y). The maximum value on the range of gray level represents a completely bright point, while a point with the gray level of zero is a completely dark point. The gray points that are partially bright and partially dark get a gray-level value that is between 0 and the maximum value of brightness. The most popular ranges of gray level used in typical images are 0–255, 0–511, 0–1023, and so on. The gray levels are almost always set to be nonnegative integer numbers (as opposed to real numbers). This saves a lot of digital storage space (e.g., disk space) and expedites the processing of images significantly.

One can see that the wider the range of the gray level becomes, the better resolution is achieved. In order to see this more clearly, we present an example.

Example 1.1

Consider the image shown in Figure 1.4. Image (a) has the gray-level range of 0–255. In order to see how the image resolution is affected by the gray-level range, we reduce the range to smaller ranges. In order to generate the image with gray level 0–255, we divide every gray level of every point by two and round up the number to the closest integer. As can be seen in image (b), which has only 64 levels in it, the resolution of the image is not significantly affected by the gray-level reduction. However, if we continue this process, the degradation in resolution and quality becomes more visible (as shown in (c) which has only two levels of gray and dark in it). Image (c) that allows only two gray levels (0 and 1) is called a binary image.

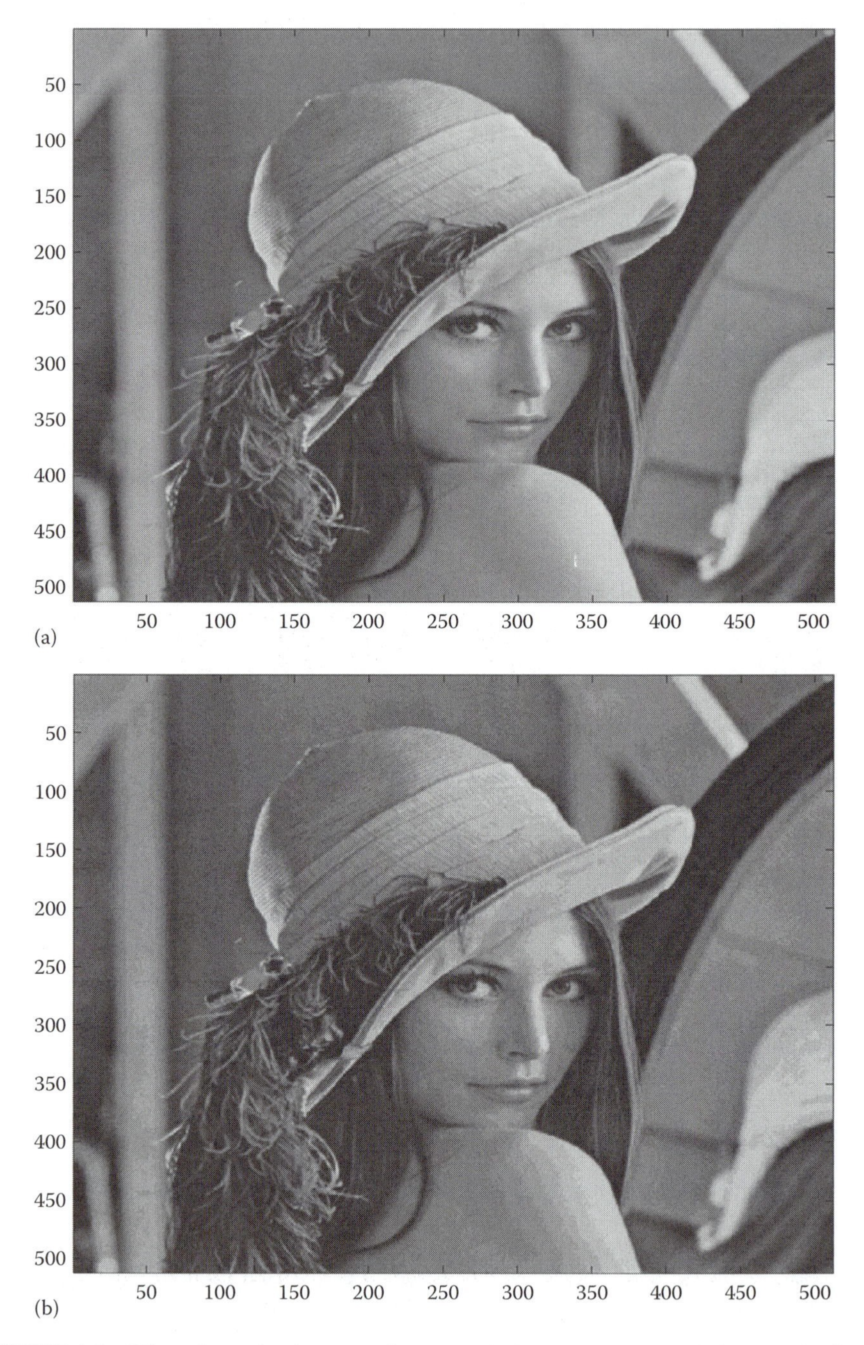

FIGURE 1.4 Effect of gray-level range on image resolution. (a) Range 0–255, (b) range 0–63.

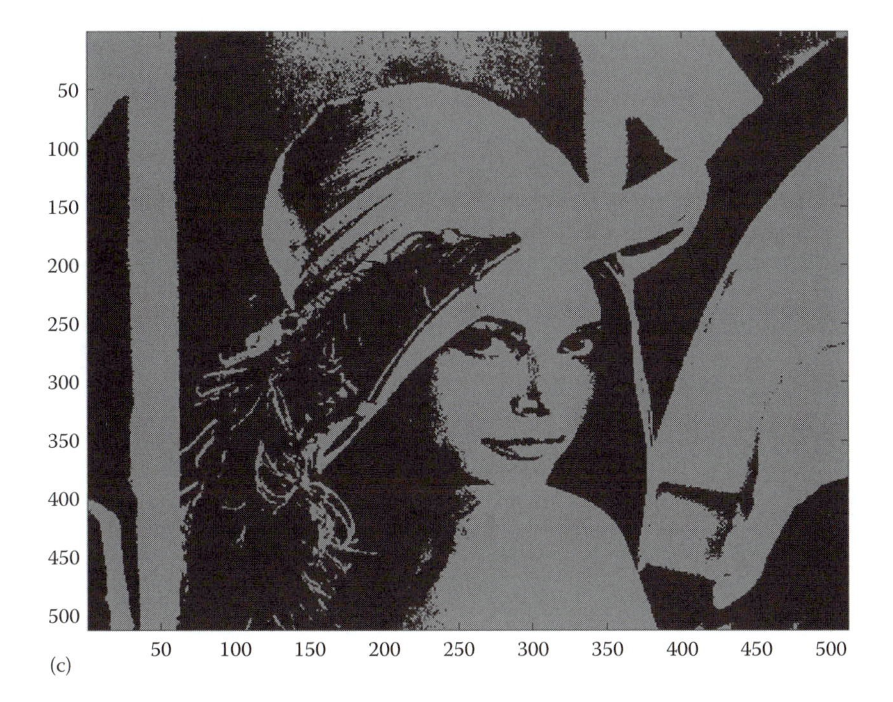

FIGURE 1.4 (continued) (c) range 0–1.

Color images are also used in medical imaging. While there are many standards for color images, here we discuss only "red green blue" or "RGB" standard. RGB is formed based on the philosophy that each color is a combination of the three primary colors: red, green, and blue. This means that if we combine the right intensity of these three colors, we can create the sense of any desired color for the human eyes. As an example, for a purple object we would have a high density of red and blue but a low intensity of green. As a result, in RGB representation of a color image, the screen (such as a monitor) provides three dots for every pixel (point): one red dot, one green dot, and one blue dot. The intensity of each of these dots is identified by the share of the corresponding primary color in forming the color of the pixel. This means that in color images for every coordinate (x, y), three numbers are provided. This in turn means that the image itself is represented by three 2-D signals, $g_R(x, y)$, $g_G(x, y)$, and $g_B(x, y)$, each representing the intensity of one primary color. As a result, every one of the 2-D signals (for one color) can be treated as one separate image and processed by the same image processing methods designed for gray-level images.

1.6.3 Image Histogram

An important statistical characteristic of an image is the histogram. Here, we define this concept and illustrate it using a simple example. Assume that the gray level of all pixels in an image belong to the interval $[0, G - 1]$, where G is an integer. Consequently, if "r" represents the gray level of a pixel of the image, then $0 \leq r \leq G - 1$, where r is an integer. Now, for all values of r, calculate the normalized frequencies, $p(r)$. In order to do so, for a given gray-level value r, we count the number of pixels in the image whose gray level equals r and name it as $n(r)$. Then, we divide that number by the total number of points in the image n, i.e.,

$$p(r) = \frac{n(r)}{n} \tag{1.1}$$

The reason for using $p(r)$ to represent these normalized frequencies is due to the fact that in limit these frequencies approach the true probabilities of gray levels. Then, histogram is defined as the graph of $p(r)$ versus r. The definition of this concept is illustrated in the following examples.

Example 1.2

Consider a test image shown in Figure 1.5. As can be seen, this image has three gray levels $r = 0$, 1, and 2, which means $G = 3$. The darkest gray level corresponds to level 0, and the brightest level is represented by level 2.

Next, we calculate the $p(r)$ for different values of r. One can see that

$$p(0) = \frac{3}{9}$$

$$p(1) = \frac{5}{9}$$

$$p(2) = \frac{1}{9}$$

The histogram for this image is shown in Figure 1.6.

The concept of image histogram will be further defined and illustrated in the following chapters.

Now that we understand the main concepts such as 1-D and 2-D signals, we can progress to the next chapter that introduces the most important image transformation, i.e., FT.

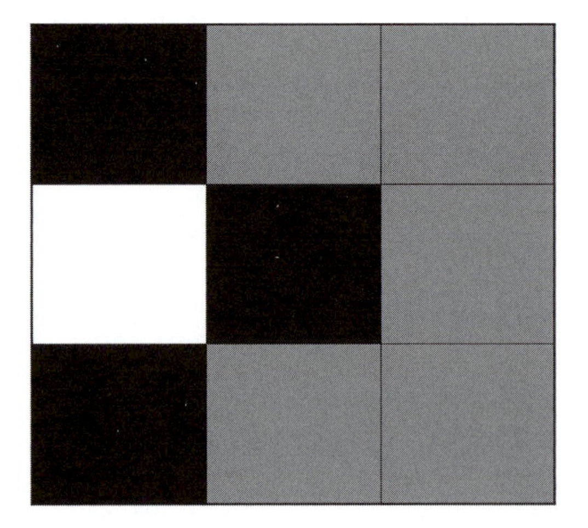

FIGURE 1.5 Test gray-level image with three levels.

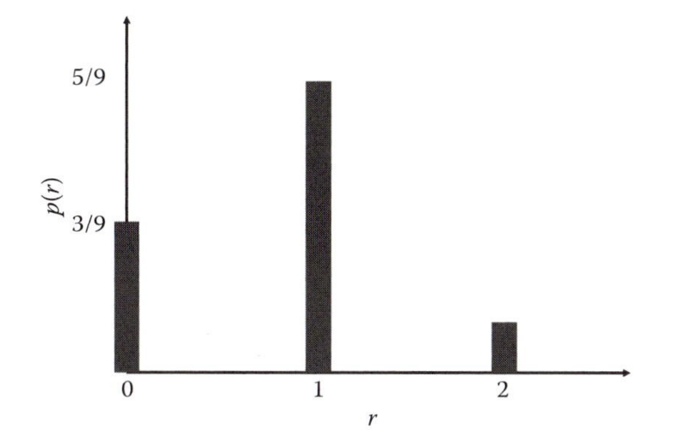

FIGURE 1.6 Histogram of image shown in Figure 1.5.

1.7 SUMMARY

A signal is a sequence of ordered numbers (often in time). Even though many signals are analog signal in nature, in order to analyze such signals in digital computers, they are often sampled and then processed using digital signal processing techniques. Such techniques and transformations often highlight certain characteristics of a signal, for example, FT emphasizes the frequency information contained in a signal. When all informative characteristics of a signal are extracted, the resulting features are presented to a classifier that evaluates the performance of the system generating the signal. In this chapter, we also defined some fundamental characteristics of digital images such as histogram.

PROBLEMS

1.1 Assume that an analog signal $x(t)$ for $t \geq 0$ is defined as

$$x(t) = e^{-2t} \tag{1.2}$$

a. Using MATLAB®, plot $x(t)$ for $0 \leq t \leq 10$.
b. Sample $x(t)$ with $T_S = 0.1$ s to form $x_{d1}(t)$ and plot the resulting discrete signal.
c. Increase the sampling period to $T_S = 1$ s to form $x_{d2}(t)$ and plot the resulting discrete signal.
d. Increase the sampling period to $T_S = 4$ s to form $x_{d3}(t)$ and plot the resulting discrete signal.
e. Compare the three discrete signals in the previous parts and intuitively decide which sampling period creates the best discrete version of the original analog signal, i.e., identify the sampling period that is small enough to preserve the waveform of the original signal $x(t)$ and at the same time reduces the number of the sampled points.

1.2 From the CD

a. Using MATLAB, load the file "p_1_2.mat," i.e., type

```
load p_1_2.mat;
```

b. Using MATLAB, get a list of variables in the file, i.e.,

```
whos
```

c. Using MATLAB, plot $x_1(t)$. i.e.,

```
plot(x1);
```

d. Disregarding the noise-like variations, the signal has clear periodicity in it. Manually measure the time of one complete period of oscillation (i.e., period T). Knowing that frequency is defined as the reciprocal of the period, i.e., $f = 1/T$, calculate the dominant frequency of the variations. In practical applications, manual frequency analysis becomes impossible. Signal processing techniques to extract the dominant frequencies of a signal (mainly using Fourier analysis) are heavily used in signal processing and will be covered in Chapter 2.
e. Using MATLAB, plot $x_2(t)$ and $x_3(t)$. Then, manually calculate the average slope of each of the signals. For each signal, identify if the slope exceeds 5. Calculation of slopes is a fundamental operation commonly used in signal and image processing, for example, a sharp slope of pixel intensity in any direction often identifies the border between two parts of an image representing two separate regions or objects. Efficient techniques for slope and gradient analysis are discussed in the following chapters.

2 Fourier Transform

2.1 INTRODUCTION AND OVERVIEW

Among all transforms used in signal and image processing, Fourier transform (FT) is probably the most commonly used transform. In this chapter, we first describe the definition as well as the concepts of FT and then discuss some of the properties of FT that are commonly used in signal processing. The emphasis of this chapter is on the conceptual interpretations as well as the applications of one-dimensional (1-D) and two-dimensional (2-D) continuous and discrete FT as opposed to mathematical formulation.

2.2 ONE-DIMENSIONAL CONTINUOUS FOURIER TRANSFORM

As mentioned in Chapter 1, a signal can be expressed in many different domains among which time is probably the most intuitive domain. Time signals can answer questions regarding "when" events happen, whereas FT domain addresses questions starting with "how often" (this is why FT domain is also called frequency domain).

As an example, assume that you are to study the shopping habits of members in a community by preparing a questionnaire. You will obtain some useful information when you ask questions such as "What days do you normally go shopping?" or "What time of the day you never go shopping?" This information helps you understand and visualize the "time" elements of people's shopping habits. Also, if you prepare a time signal that shows the number of people shopping at every instance of time (i.e., a graph of number of people shopping vs. time), you can acquire answers to all the aforementioned questions. Now, consider a different set of questions such as "How often do you go shopping?" or "What percentages of people go shopping twice a week?" Answers to these questions form the frequency domain, which in signal processing is formed by FT. Let us remind ourselves that the information in time and frequency are exactly the same, i.e., neither of the domains are more informative than the other and one can acquire all information on one domain from the other. However, considering the computation size and the visibility of certain information to humans, one domain can be preferred over the other, as discussed in Chapter 1.

Now, we give a formal definition for 1-D continuous FT. Consider $g(t)$ as a continuous signal in time. The FT of this signal, shown as $G(f)$, is defined as follows:

$$G(f) = FT\{g(t)\} = \int_{-\infty}^{+\infty} g(t)e^{-j2\pi ft}\,dt \tag{2.1}$$

where

f is the frequency variable (which is often expressed in units such as Hz, kHz, MHz, and so on)

j is the imaginary number (i.e., $j^2 = -1$)

Note that in Equation 2.1 (which is also known as the analysis equation), the integration is taking place over time and therefore the resulting function, i.e., $G(f)$, is no longer a function of time. Also, note that $G(f)$ is a complex function of f. This means that one can describe $G(f)$ as follows:

$$G(f) = |G(f)|e^{j\angle G(f)} \tag{2.2}$$

where
$|G(f)|$ is the magnitude of $G(f)$
$\angle G(f)$ represents the phase of $G(f)$

A closer look at the value of $|G(f)|$ at a given frequency reveals the main advantages of expressing a signal in the Fourier domain. Continuing our example on people's shopping habits, let us assume that $g(t)$ is the number of people shopping at time t, where time is measured in seconds. Then, in order to see how many people would go shopping once a day (i.e., once every 86,400 s), all we need to do is to calculate $|G(f)|$ for $f = 1/86{,}400$ Hz. Note that one could have obtained the same information from the time signal, but the FT provides a much easier approach to frequency-related questions such as the one we explored earlier.

If one can calculate the FT for a time signal, he or she should also be able to calculate the time signal from a frequency signal in the FT domain. Such a transformation is called the inverse FT (or the synthesis transform) that accepts $G(f)$ as input and calculates $g(t)$ as follows:

$$g(t) = IFT\{G(f)\} = \int_{-\infty}^{+\infty} G(f)e^{j2\pi ft}\,df \tag{2.3}$$

Next, we practice calculating the FT using some useful functions that are heavily used in signal processing.

Example 2.1

Consider an exponentially decaying signal $g(t) = e^{-t}$, $t \geq 0$. Then,

$$\begin{aligned}
G(f) &= \int_{-\infty}^{+\infty} g(t)e^{-j2\pi ft}dt \\
&= \int_{0}^{+\infty} e^{-t}e^{-j2\pi ft}dt \\
&= \left[-\frac{1}{1+j2\pi u}e^{-(1+j2\pi f)t}\right]_{t=0}^{t=+\infty} \\
&= (0) - \left(-\frac{1}{1+j2\pi f}\right) \\
&= \frac{1}{1+j2\pi f}
\end{aligned} \tag{2.4}$$

Also, we can calculate the magnitude and phase of $G(f)$ as follows:

$$|G(f)| = \frac{1}{|1 + j2\pi f|} = \frac{1}{\sqrt{1 + (2\pi f)^2}} \tag{2.5}$$

and

$$\angle G(f) = -\angle(1 + j2\pi f) = -\tan^{-1}(2\pi f) \tag{2.6}$$

Example 2.2

Impulse function $\delta(t)$ (also known as Dirac function) plays an important role in many areas of science and engineering such as physics, differential equations, and signal processing. Before describing the mathematical definition of the impulse function and calculating the FT of this function, we focus on the concept of the impulse function and the need for such a mathematical entity.

Impulse function is a mathematical function that describes very fast bursts of energy that are observed in some physical phenomena. As an example of such burst pulses, consider the effect of smashing the ball in a volleyball game. Volleyball players are not allowed to hold the ball in their hands; rather, they are supposed to hit the ball. When smashing the ball, players apply a significant amount of energy in a very short time. Such an impulse force applied to the ball creates the most effective move in a volleyball game. The effects of such an action can be modeled using an impulse function.

Impulse function plays an important role in the identification of unknown systems. This role can be described through a simple example. Suppose you are given a black box and you are asked to discover what is in the box. One quick way of guessing the contents of the box is tapping on it and listening to the echoes. In a more scientific world, you would apply some fast pressure impulses on the surface of the box and observe the response of the contents in the box with respect to the impulse functions you applied. If the box contains coins, you will hear a jingling sound, and if the box is full of water, an entirely different sound and echo will be sensed. This type of identifying unknown systems is a fundamental technique in a field of science called "system identification," which focuses on modeling and describing unknown systems.

Now, we slowly approach a mathematical formulation of the impulse function. The burst-like concept of the impulse function implies that the mathematical model must be zero for all points in time except for an infinitely small time interval (as discussed earlier). In a more mathematical manner, assuming that the impulse is applied at time $t = 0$, the mathematical representation of the impulse function must be zero everywhere except for a small neighborhood around the origin. If the impulse is assumed to be nonzeros for a very short period of time, then the amplitude of impulse during this very short interval of time must be infinitely large; otherwise, the total energy of the signal would become zero. In order to see this more clearly, we focus on a mathematical model of the impulse function. Consider function $\delta_\Delta(t)$ shown in Figure 2.1. Note that the energy of this signal

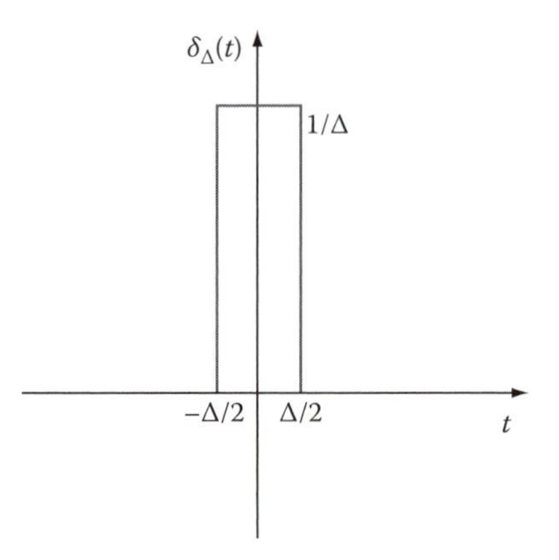

FIGURE 2.1 $\delta_\Delta(t)$ function.

(i.e., the area under the curve) is the duration (i.e., Δ) multiplied by the height of the pulse (i.e., 1/Δ). This shows that the energy of the signal is always one regardless of the value of Δ, i.e., the area (energy) independent of Δ.

Now we can define the impulse function as follows:

$$\delta(t) = \lim_{\Delta \to 0} \delta_\Delta(t) \tag{2.7}$$

The previous definition implies that even though the impulse function is nonzero only between 0^- and 0^+, the energy of the signal is still one, i.e.,

$$\int_{-\infty}^{+\infty} \delta(t)dt = \int_{0^-}^{0^+} \delta(t)dt = 1 \tag{2.8}$$

In order to have a meaningful visual representation for the impulse function emphasizing the fact that the amplitude of the impulse function is 0 everywhere except at the origin in which the amplitude approaches infinity, an arrow pointed toward infinity is used to show the impulse function (Figure 2.2).

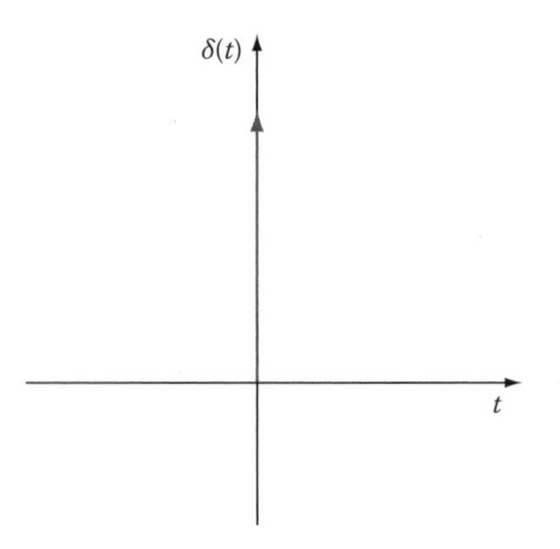

FIGURE 2.2 Visual representation of an impulse function.

Other useful properties of the impulse function include the sampling capability of the impulse function, i.e., for any signal $g(t)$,

$$\int_{-\infty}^{+\infty} \delta(t)g(t)dt = \int_{0^-}^{0^+} \delta(t)g(t)dt = g(0) \tag{2.9}$$

Equation 2.9 describes how integration with impulse function can sample the signal at the origin. One can also imagine a shifted version of an impulse function centered at t_0 as opposed to the origin (i.e., $\delta(t - t_0)$ shown in Figure 2.3). For this function,

$$\int_{-\infty}^{+\infty} \delta(t-t_0)dt = \int_{t^-}^{t^+} \delta(t-t_0)dt = 1 \tag{2.10}$$

Using a shifted impulse function, one can sample a function at any time t_0, i.e.,

$$\int_{-\infty}^{+\infty} \delta(t-t_0)g(t)dt = \int_{t^-}^{t^+} \delta(t-t_0)g(t)dt = g(t_0) \tag{2.11}$$

Knowing the good properties of the impulse function, next we use Equation 2.11 to calculate the FT of the impulse function:

$$\begin{aligned} FT\{\delta(t)\} &= \int_{-\infty}^{+\infty} \delta(t)e^{-j2\pi ft}dt \\ &= e^{-j2\pi f\times 0} \\ &= 1 \end{aligned} \tag{2.12}$$

This unique property of the impulse function indicates that the frequency spectrum of an impulse is completely flat. We will discuss the interpretation of this result later on.

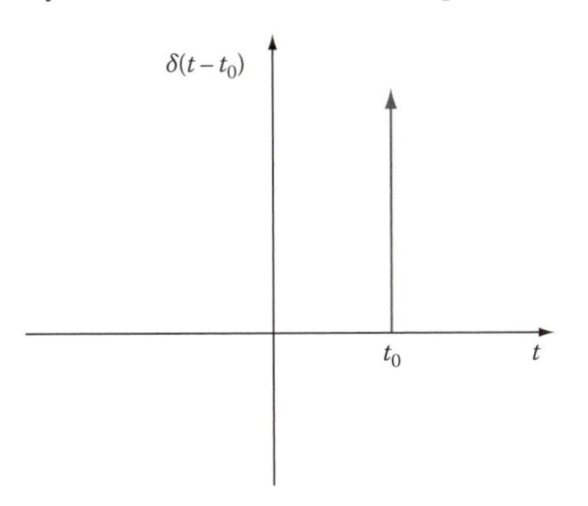

FIGURE 2.3 Shifted impulse function.

Example 2.3

Another useful function in signal processing is the unit pulse $p_\Pi(t)$ as shown in Figure 2.4.

Calculating the FT of the unit pulse function, we have

$$
\begin{aligned}
P_\Pi(f) &= \int_{-\infty}^{+\infty} p_\Pi(t) e^{-j2\pi ft} dt \\
&= \int_0^T A e^{-j2\pi ft} dt \\
&= \left[-\frac{A}{j2\pi f} e^{-j2\pi ft} \right]_{t=0}^{t=T} \\
&= -\frac{A}{j2\pi f} \left[e^{-j2\pi fT} - 1 \right] \\
&= -\frac{A}{j2\pi f} \left[e^{-j\pi fT} - e^{j\pi fT} \right] e^{-j\pi fT} \\
&= \frac{A}{\pi f} \left[\frac{e^{j\pi fT} - e^{-j\pi fT}}{2j} \right] e^{-j\pi fT} \\
&= \frac{A}{\pi f} \sin(\pi fT) e^{-j\pi fT}
\end{aligned}
\tag{2.13}
$$

which means

$$
\begin{aligned}
|P_\Pi(f)| &= AT \left| \frac{\sin(\pi ft)}{\pi fT} \right| \\
&= AT\operatorname{sinc}(\pi fT)
\end{aligned}
\tag{2.14}
$$

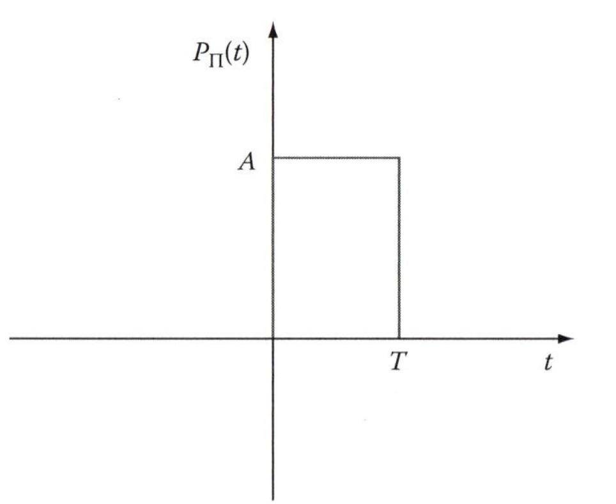

FIGURE 2.4 Unit pulse function.

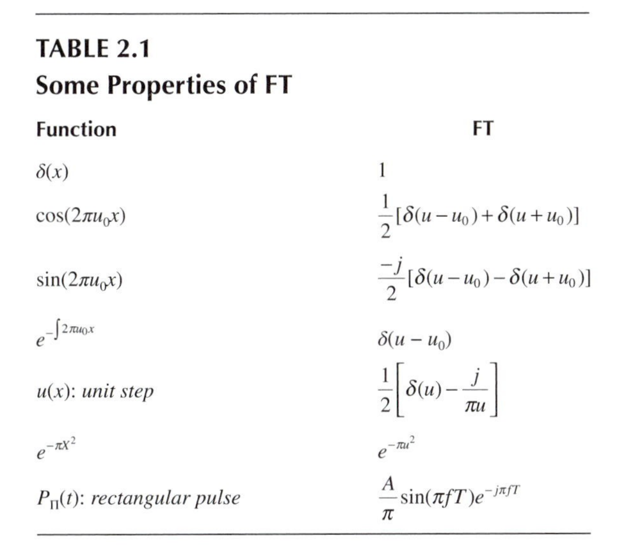

TABLE 2.1
Some Properties of FT

Function	FT
$\delta(x)$	1
$\cos(2\pi u_0 x)$	$\frac{1}{2}[\delta(u-u_0)+\delta(u+u_0)]$
$\sin(2\pi u_0 x)$	$\frac{-j}{2}[\delta(u-u_0)-\delta(u+u_0)]$
$e^{-\int 2\pi u_0 x}$	$\delta(u-u_0)$
$u(x)$: *unit step*	$\frac{1}{2}\left[\delta(u)-\frac{j}{\pi u}\right]$
$e^{-\pi x^2}$	$e^{-\pi u^2}$
$P_{\Pi}(t)$: *rectangular pulse*	$\frac{A}{\pi}\sin(\pi f T)e^{-j\pi f T}$

Table 2.1 gives the FT of some other important functions in time. The derivation of the FT for some of these functions has been left as exercises for the reader, and here we discuss the practical interpretation of some of the entries in the table. The unit step function (i.e., $u(t)$) is a function defined as $u(t) = 1$ for all $t > 0$ and $u(t) = 0$ for $t \leq 0$.

The first interesting observation is the FT of a Gaussian time signal (i.e., $e^{-\pi t^2}$). As can be seen from the table, the FT of this function also has a Gaussian form. This observation plays a vital role in applications such creating nondiffracting ultrasonic waves.

Another observation from Table 2.1 deals with the FT of sinusoidal functions. According to the table, the magnitude of the FT of a cosine function with frequency f_0 is a couple of frequency impulses centered at f_0 and $-f_0$. In analyzing many phenomena in science and engineering, it is desirable to discover any periodicity and sinusoidal variations in signals. Even though one can observe periodicity in a signal from its time domain representation, the aforementioned property of the FT makes it a perfect tool for quantitative analysis of any periodicity by naming the exact sinusoidal components forming the signal. In order to see this more clearly, here are a few simple examples.

Example 2.4

Consider the time signal given in Figure 2.5. From the time signal, it is rather easy to say that the signal is indeed periodic. However, it may be rather difficult to develop a mathematical expression for the signal to be represented as a summation of some sinusoidal components.

Now consider the magnitude of the FT shown in Figure 2.6. As you may have noticed, the graph is symmetric around the vertical axis, and when focusing on the positive f-axis, there are two impulses at frequencies 0.25 and 0.5 Hz. This tells us that the signal is composed of two sinusoidal components at these frequencies.

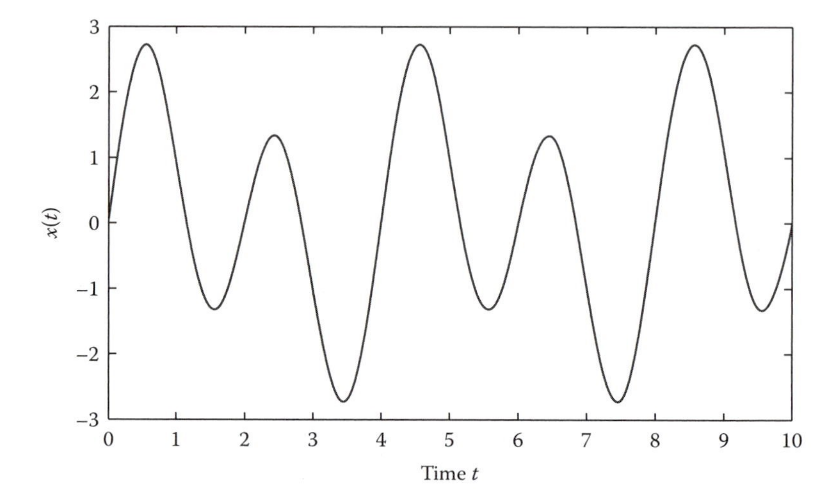

FIGURE 2.5 A given time signal.

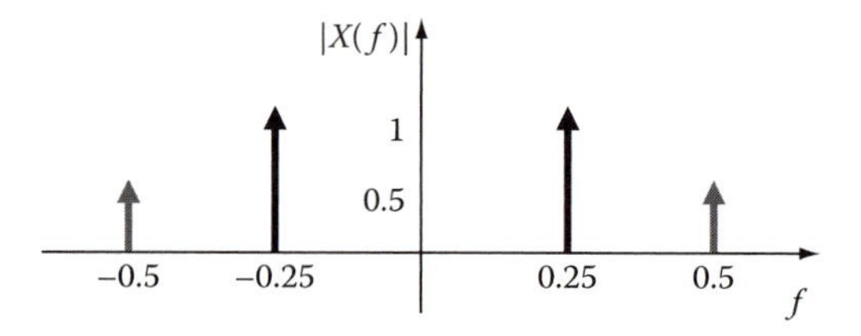

FIGURE 2.6 FT of the time signal in Figure 2.5.

Therefore, if we write the time equation of the signal, there will be two sinusoidal terms: $\sin(2\pi t \times 0.5)$ and $\sin(2\pi t \times 0.25)$. We can even identify the amplitude of the sinusoids and develop an exact mathematical formula for the signal from the FT graph given in Figure 2.6. The sinusoidal at 0.25 Hz has the height of 1 in the FT graph, which means that the amplitude of this component in time should be 2. Similarly, one can observe that the amplitude of the other sinusoidal term with frequency 0.5 Hz is 1. This means that the mathematical expression of the time signal can be written as follows:

$$g(t) = \sin(\pi t) + 2\sin(0.5\pi t) \tag{2.15}$$

The previous example shows us that sometimes it is much easier to express and analyze periodic signals in the FT domain than in time domain. The FT can even help us find mathematical expressions of signals in time (as in the previous example).

2.2.1 Properties of One-Dimensional Fourier Transform

FT has some very interesting general properties that are helpful not only in calculating the FT of a wide range of time signals but also in understanding the main concepts of this transform. Here, we will review some of the properties listed in Table 2.2.

The main properties shown in the table are discussed in the following sections.

TABLE 2.2
Properties of 1-D FT

Time Function	FT
$\frac{dg(t)}{dt}$	$(j2\pi f)G(f)$
$g(t-t_0)$	$e^{2\pi f t_0}G(f)$
$e^{j2\pi f_0 t}g(t)$	$G(f-f_0)$
$g_1(t)\times g_2(t)$	$G_1(f)\times G_2(f)$
$g_1(t)\times g_2(t)$	$G_1(f)\times G_2(f)$
$tg(t)$	$\frac{j}{2\pi}\frac{dG(f)}{df}$
$\int_{-\infty}^{+\infty}\lvert g(t)\rvert^2\,dt$	$\int_{-\infty}^{+\infty}\lvert G(f)\rvert^2\,df$
$ag_1(t)+bg_2(t)$	$aG_1(f)+bG_2(f)$

2.2.1.1 Signal Shift

According to this property, if a signal is shifted in time, the magnitude of the FT remains the same (for all frequencies). Specifically, for a signal $g(t)$ and an arbitrary time shift t_0,

$$FT\{g(t-t_0)\}=e^{j2\pi f t_0}G(f) \tag{2.16}$$

Since the magnitude of the complex exponential in Equation 2.16 evaluates to 1, it is evident that the magnitude of the FT is independent of the time shift t_0 shift in $g(t)$.

This observation matches our intuition. For example, you can listen to a piece of music once today and once tomorrow, and then if you were to listen to the same music a few days or some time later, would the music sound different to your ears? No! Though the time or day might be different (time shift) the music will always correlate with the first day! To understand this concept better, let us consider another analogy with respect to the 2-D world. Assume you are analyzing a slide under your microscope. If you were to move the slide a little to the left or right, does the original image under the microscope ever change? The response should lead you to the following conclusion: time shift of a signal in the time domain does not change the magnitudes of the FT.

As can be seen in the table of FT properties, a time shift simply introduces a "phase shift" in the FT of the time signal. A change in phase simply states that the signal has started at a different time (which is evident from the time signal).

2.2.1.2 Convolution

Convolution is a fundamental operation in the world of linear analysis and plays a central role in signal and image processing. As can be seen from Table 2.2, convolution operation between two signals, $g_1(t)$ and $g_2(t)$ (shown as $g_1(t)*g_2(t)$), is defined as follows:

$$g_1(t)*g_2(t)=\int_{-\infty}^{+\infty}g_1(t)g_2(t-\tau)d\tau=\int_{-\infty}^{+\infty}g_1(t-\tau)g_2(t)d\tau \tag{2.17}$$

Direct calculation of convolution operations involves many complicated and time-consuming mathematical computations. However, it is comforting to know that the FT creates an alternative method of calculating the convolution that is much less computationally intensive. The property described in Table 2.2 says that, in order to calculate $g_1(t) * g_2(t)$ (convolution of $g_1(t)$ and $g_2(t)$), one must identify the involved signals and calculate the FT of the respected signals (i.e., find $G_1(f)$ and $G_2(f)$), then multiply the two (i.e., find $G_1(f) \cdot G_2(f)$), and then find the inverse Fourier transform (IFT) of the result. This would compute $g_1(t) * g_2(t)$ without the long and tedious integration or math involved in the true definition of convolution. Understanding the concept of traversing from time domain to frequency domain and vice versa can save a significant amount of calculation time. The property of convolution is extremely important for analyzing linear systems, as discussed in the following. The proof for this property is left as an exercise and will be discussed further in Problems section.

2.2.1.3 Linear Systems Analysis

Before discussing the main usage of the FT in linear systems, we briefly discuss the concept of linear systems that play an important role in signal and image processing. Consider a system where an "input" stimulation of the system causes an "output" response from the system. For example, consider a cart on an open area such a parking lot. If you push the cart with a certain input power, the cart will travel an output distance. Linear systems are the systems in which the output linearly depends on the input, i.e., the amplitude of the output is linearly proportional to the amplitude of the input. Using the example mentioned earlier, if one pushes a cart with twice the original force or power, the cart will travel twice the original distance. In a more mathematical context, if a push with power $p(t)$ causes the cart to travel for $q(t)$ meters, then a push for $\alpha \cdot p(t)$ will cause the cart to travel for $\alpha \cdot q(t)$ (where α is a constant).

Linear systems have another property that deals with the response of a system to two or more inputs that are applied to the system simultaneously. This property (which is also referred to as "superposition") states that the response of a linear system to simultaneous inputs is the summation of the responses of the system to every individual input. Continuing our previous example, assume that if one person pushes the cart with power $p_1(t)$, the cart will move for $q_1(t)$, and if another person pushes the cart with $p_2(t)$, the cart will move for $q_2(t)$. Now, if both these people push the cart at the same time, i.e., with power $p_1(t) + p_2(t)$, the cart will travel for $q_1(t) + q_2(t)$ meters, i.e., a distance that is the summation of the distances the cart travels for each push.

In order to better understand the concept of linear systems, let us focus on the contrast between linear and nonlinear systems. Nonlinear systems (as the name suggests) are systems in which the relation between input and output is either not proportional or not superpositional. For example, in our previous example of pushing carts in a parking lot, let us assume that there are some obstacles (such as cars and other carts) parked in the lot. In that case, a small push can make a cart to travel for a certain distance, but a proportionally larger push may cause the cart to collide with other objects and therefore fail to produce a proportionally large distance. This is a typical example of a nonlinear system in which the complexity of the system prevents simple and well-behaved characteristics such as proportionality and superposition. Nonlinear systems are therefore much more difficult to model and analyze.

Now, let us ask ourselves a couple of good questions: "Where can we find linear systems?" and "Why linear systems are so important for us?" The answer to the first question is that in nature we almost never encounter a truly linear system! In other words, almost everything in nature and everything in man-made systems are nonlinear. In addition, we now know that the nonlinear nature of these systems makes them so flexible, dynamic, and interesting. Having such an answer for the first question, the second question becomes more relevant. If there are not many linear systems in nature, why should we spend a lot of time studying linear systems? The answer is twofold. First, many nonlinear systems, under certain conditions, can be approximated with linear models. This means that if we make sure that certain conditions are satisfied, instead of dealing with complex and difficult nonlinear mathematics, we can still use our straightforward linear math. Second, even in cases where linear models may not be the best approximates of a truly nonlinear system, considering our lack of knowledge on the type and nature of the involved nonlinearities, linear models might still be all we can do. For example, in our model of pushing a cart in crowded parking lot, even though the system is a nonlinear one, we can still model the system as a linear system if we restrict the power of the applied push.

Now we get back to the facilities FT provides for analysis of linear systems. In order to see the impact of the FT on linear systems, it suffices to describe the relationship between the input $p(t)$, output $q(t)$, and the internal characteristics of a linear system $h(t)$. The output is nothing but the convolution between the input and the internal characteristics of the model, i.e.,

$$q(t) = p(t) \times h(t) \tag{2.18}$$

As discussed previously, convolution is a rather complicated process, but FT can be used to easily calculate the output of linear systems, i.e., in linear systems, we have

$$Q(f) = P(f) \times H(f) \tag{2.19}$$

Before concluding our discussion on linear systems, it is insightful to relate the concept of $h(t)$ (or equivalently $H(f)$) to the impulse function. Let us rewrite Equation 2.19 as follows:

$$H(f) = \frac{Q(f)}{P(f)} \tag{2.20}$$

Now, assume that the input is an impulse, i.e., $p(t) = \delta(t)$. Then from Equation 2.19, we acquire

$$H(f) = \frac{Q(f)}{1} = Q(f) \tag{2.21}$$

or equivalently, $h(t) = q(t)$. This means that in order to find the internal characteristics of a linear system, one can simply apply an impulse input to the system and record the output.

This property of the impulse function is used in system identification and signal processing. Due to this observation, $h(t)$ is often called "the impulse response function."

2.2.1.4 Differentiation

Another interesting property of the FT is the conversion of derivative in time domain into a simple multiplication process in the frequency domain. This property is used to convert differential equations in time into a set of simple linear equations in frequency domain and solve multidimensional differential equations using simple linear algebra.

2.2.1.5 Scaling Property

An extremely useful property of the FT is the way time and frequency domains are inversely scaled. Specifically, assume that the FT of a signal $g(t)$ is given as $G(f)$. The scaling property states that, for a signal defined as $g_1(t) = g(\alpha t)$ with $\alpha > 1$, we can easily calculate the FT using $G(f)$ as follows:

$$FT\{g_1(t)\} = G_1(f) = \frac{1}{\alpha}G\left(\frac{f}{\alpha}\right) \tag{2.22}$$

The previous equation asserts that once a function is compressed in time, the function in frequency domain expands with the same rate. This means that once the width of a signal in time domain approaches zero, its width in frequency domain approaches infinity. This observation further explains why the FT of an impulse function must be infinitely flat.

2.3 SAMPLING AND NYQUIST RATE

The technological advancements of the Internet and other digital media, digital computers, digital communication systems, and other digital machines and systems makes the processing of digital signals and images a valued technique. In addition, the existence of very fast digital signal processors that are tailored to process digital signals with amazing high speeds, supports the processing of signals in a digital form. However, knowing that almost all signals collected from nature (including biomedical signals) are continuous in nature, we would need to "digitize" continuous signals to form digital (or discrete) signals to be processed with digital signal processors.

Next, let us discuss two important questions that require answers before any attempts to sample the continuous signals can be made: "Is it possible to form a digital signal from a continuous signal while maintaining all information in the continuous signal?" And if the answer to the first question is yes, then "How fast are we supposed to sample a continuous signal such that all information of the continuous signal is preserved in the resulting sampled (discrete) signal?" The answer to the first question is "Yes!" This answer may be to some degree counterintuitive. The reason why it may be counterintuitive is because once the continuous signal is sampled, apparently there is no guarantee that one can recover the exact values of the signal between the samples. In other words, if we can reconstruct the continuous signal from the discrete signal, then we could claim that no information has been lost from the continuous signal. However, it seems impossible to reconstruct the exact values between the sampled values since there might be several possible options for each intermediate point. The key issue to address lies on "How fast can a continuous signal be sampled?"

A theorem called Nyquist or Shannon theorem addresses our problem. The mathematical details and proof of the theorem will not be given here. However, the practical procedure introduced by the theorem for sampling a continuous signal while maintaining all information in the resulting discrete signal is described in the following steps:

Step 1: Calculate FT of the continuous signal.
Step 2: Find maximum frequency of the signal, i.e., maximum frequency at which the FT of the signal is nonzero. Call this frequency f_M.
Step 3: Sample the continuous signal with a sampling frequency f_S, which is at least twice of f_M, i.e., $f_S \geq 2f_M$. In other words, take samples of the continuous signal every $T_S \leq 1/2f_M$ s, i.e., sample the continuous signal with a period that is slower than $1/2f_M$ s.

The rate $2f_M$ that landmarks the slowest sampling rate allowed is called "Nyquist rate." The aforementioned theorem states that, if the sampling rate is faster than Nyquist rate (as indicated in the previous procedure), then the exact continuous signal can be reconstructed from the discrete signal, and, therefore, the resulting discrete signal will contain all details of the continuous signal.

2.4 ONE-DIMENSIONAL DISCRETE FOURIER TRANSFORM

Now that we know how to intelligently sample a continuous signal to preserve all the information in it, it is time to describe the discrete equivalent of the continuous FT, called discrete Fourier transform (DFT). Consider a discrete signal $g(n)$, where $n = 0, 1,\ldots, N$. The DFT of such a signal is defined as follows:

$$G(k) = \sum_{n=0}^{N-1} g(n) e^{-j\frac{2\pi knT}{N}}, \quad k = 0,\ldots, N-1 \tag{2.23}$$

The preceeding equation is also called analysis equation (since it decomposes the signal into its discrete frequencies). As can be seen, the number of samples in the frequency domain is the same as the number of points in time domain, i.e., N. The inverse of this transform, i.e., inverse discrete Fourier transform (IDFT), is calculated using the following equation (called synthesis or IDFT equation):

$$g(n) = \frac{1}{N} \sum_{k=0}^{N-1} G(k) e^{j\frac{2\pi knT}{N}}, \quad n = 0,\ldots, N-1 \tag{2.24}$$

Just like in continuous signals, there is a significant amount of similarity among the DFT and IDFT equations. This similarity causes the dual characteristics among the signal in the discrete time and frequency domains. Other properties of the DFT are very similar to the continuous FT except that in all cases integrals are replaced by summations. Most of the properties of DFT are very similar to those of continuous FT and are explored in Problems section. Some other properties of DFT that are unique to DFT are explored here.

2.4.1 Properties of DFT

Some unique properties of DFT revolve around shift, repeat, and stretch of the signal and the way these operations relate to convolution operation. These properties are explored in this section. First, we specify circular shift, repeat, and stretch operations.

As shown in Figure 2.7, the circular shift transforms a discrete signal in such a way that the time points in the far right-hand side are shifted to the beginning of the signal in the left-hand side, and the rest of the time points are simply shifted toward the right-hand side. The number of shift points is often shown as the index of the operation, for example, a shift for two time points is shown as SHIFT_2.

The stretch operation, shown in Figure 2.8, allows stretching a signal by inserting zeros between consecutive time points in the signal. As in shift operation, the number of stretch points is often shown as the index of the operation, for example, a stretch for two time points is shown as STRETCH_2. This operation is sometimes referred to as zero-insertion operation.

Figure 2.9 represents another useful operation called repeat operation and represents repeating of a signal over an entire period. As in other operations, the number of repeats is often shown as the index of the operation, for example, one complete repeat is shown as REPEAT_2.

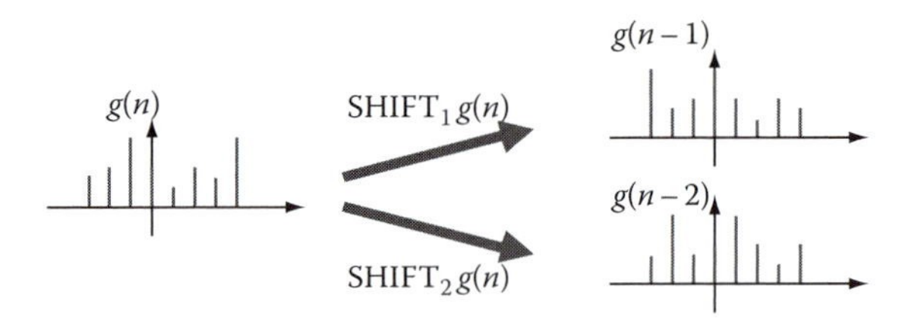

FIGURE 2.7 Circular shift of a signal $g(n)$.

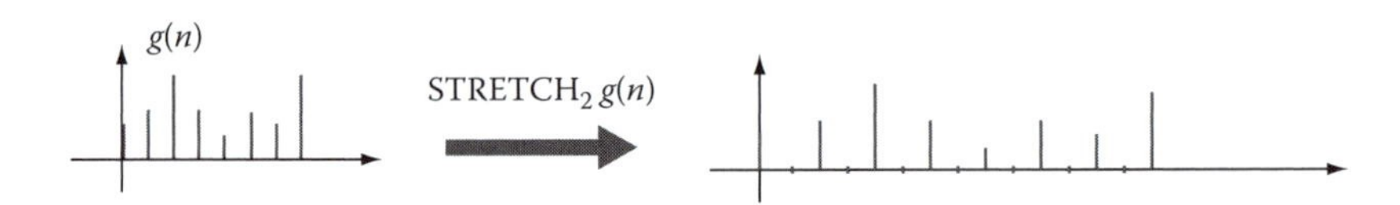

FIGURE 2.8 Stretch of a signal.

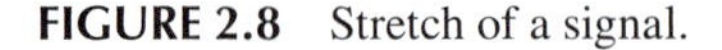

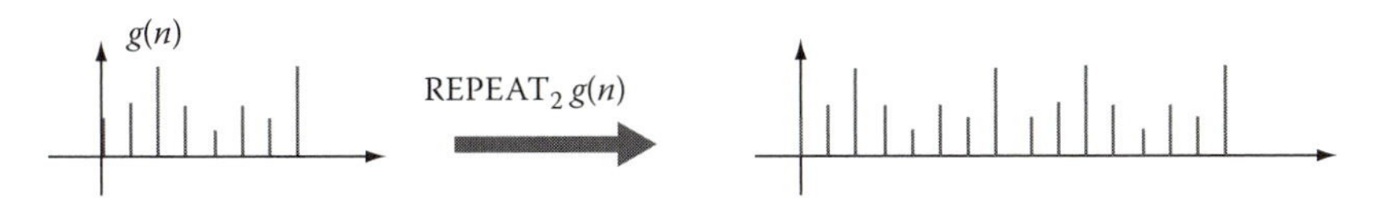

FIGURE 2.9 Repeat of a signal.

Next, we define "circular convolution" for discrete signals $x_1(n)$ and $x_2(n)$ as follows:

$$g_1(n)\times g_2(n)=\sum_{m=0}^{N-1}g_1(m)g_2(n-m)=\sum_{m=0}^{N-1}g_1(n-m)g_2(m) \tag{2.25}$$

In the preceding equation, $x_1(n-m)$ and $x_2(n-m)$ represent the m-point circularly shifted versions of $x_1(n)$ and $x_2(n)$ (as defined earlier). When it comes to Fourier theory, the circular convolution is loosely equivalent to linear convolution for continuous signals. In order to see this more clearly, we describe an important property of DFT as follows:

$$\text{DFT}\{g_1(n)\times g_2(n)\}=\text{DFT}\{g_1(n)\}\times\text{DFT}\{g_2(n)\}=G_1(k)\times G_2(k) \tag{2.26}$$

As can be seen, in the continuous case, DFT can reduce the complex operation of circular convolution by computing the product of the DFTs of the present signals. However, one of the most important properties of the circular convolution can be identified through the next property of DFT:

$$\text{DFT}\{\text{STRETCH}_l\{g(n)\}\}=\text{REPEAT}_l\{\text{DFT}\{g(n)\}\}=\text{REPEAT}_l\{G(k)\} \tag{2.27}$$

or equivalently,

$$\text{STRETCH}_l\{g(n)\}\overset{DFT}{\leftrightarrow}\text{REPEAT}_l\{G(k)\} \tag{2.28}$$

The aforementioned property corresponds to the scaling property of continuous FT, except that in DFT things are more interesting and rather simpler. In other words, this property states that stretching a signal in time would result in the repetition of the signal in frequency domain. This property is used in biomedical signal processing as we will see later.

Before describing the 2-D DFT, let us briefly explore DFT using MATLAB®.

Example 2.5

Consider a time signal shown in Figure 2.10. We will use MATLAB to calculate the DFT of the signal.

The command for DFT calculation in MATLAB is "`fft`". In order to get the magnitude of DFT of a signal, one can use the command "`abs`" to calculate the

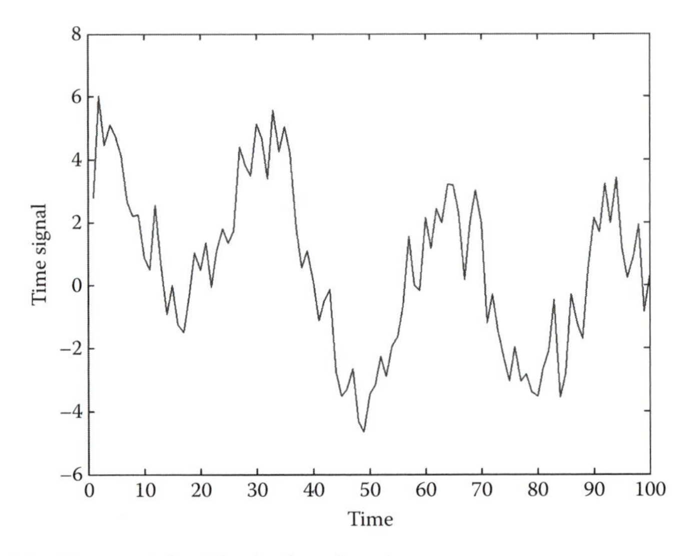

FIGURE 2.10 Signal x defined in the time domain.

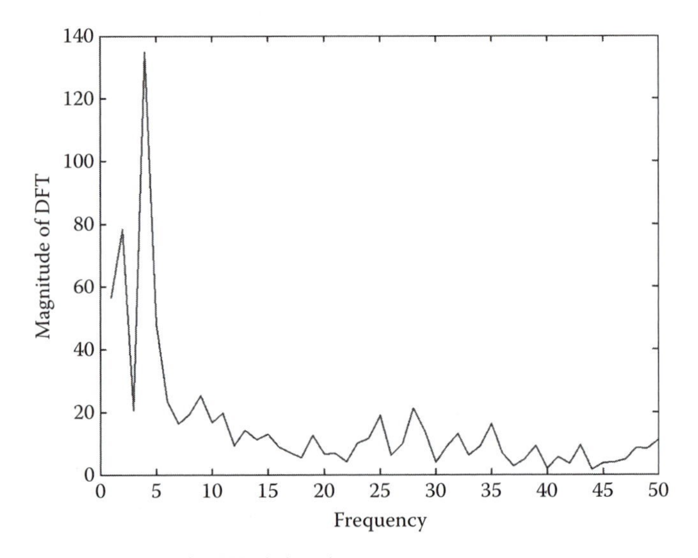

FIGURE 2.11 Magnitude of DFT of signal x.

magnitude of complex variables. The following code generates the graph shown in Figure 2.11, which represents the magnitude of the DFT of the signal x:

```
y = fft(x);
y_magnitude = abs(y);
n = length(y_magnitude);
plot(y_magnitude(1:n/2-1));
xlabel('Frequency');
ylabel('Magnitude of DFT');
```

Since the DFT of a real signal is symmetric across the middle time point (see Problem 2.8), it is often more desirable to see only half of the signal as the remaining half is repetitious. The last two lines are used to label the axes.

2.5 TWO-DIMENSIONAL DISCRETE FOURIER TRANSFORM

Just like in continuous signals, 2-D FT is a rather straightforward extension of the 1-D transform. Mathematically, the 2-D DFT is defined as follows:

$$G(u,v) = \sum_{x=0}^{N-1}\sum_{y=0}^{N-1} g(x,y)e^{-j\frac{2\pi(ux+vy)}{N}} \tag{2.29}$$

where u and v are frequency axes in which $G(u, v)$ is described. The inverse transformation, i.e., 2-D IDFT is then defined as follows:

$$g(x,y) = \sum_{x=0}^{N-1}\sum_{y=0}^{N-1} G(u,v)e^{j\frac{2\pi(ux+vy)}{N}} \tag{2.30}$$

Some of the major conceptual properties of 2-D DFT are essentially the extension of the same conceptual properties in the 1-D DFT. For instance, the high-frequency components of the 2-D DFT represent fast variations in the gray level of the neighboring points in the signal. Such fast variations (i.e., high frequencies) occur at the edges (borders) of the objects or in the texture of an object. Edges by definition are places where the intensity of pixels changes rapidly across a boundary. This rapid change is what we refer to as high frequency. Similarly, texture is defined as the rapid and semirandom changes of intensity in a region. This also identifies high frequencies, i.e., frequencies far from the origin in the 2-D frequency space. Edge detection and texture analysis play important roles in the analysis of biomedical images. For example, the intensity of the points (pixels) in a tumor is often different from their surrounding normal tissues. This difference in intensity identifies an edge between the tumor and its surrounding normal tissues. Tumor detection and segmentation is often performed based on Fourier and similar types of analysis as will be discussed later.

As in 1-D DFT, we will apply MATLAB to calculate 2-D DFT. The following example explores using MATLAB for 2-D DFT images.

Example 2.6

Consider the image $g(x, y)$ shown in Figure 2.12. This is a tomographic image of pulmonary veins in atrial fibrillation. As shown in the following code, the main command in MATLAB for calculating the 2-D DFT of images is "`fft2`". The magnitude of the 2-D DFT of the image g is shown in Figure 2.13. The command "`image`" in MATLAB is used to display an image and is often accompanied by the command "`colormap`", which defines the type and range of gray level or colors to be used for presenting images. Another command, "`imshow`", can also

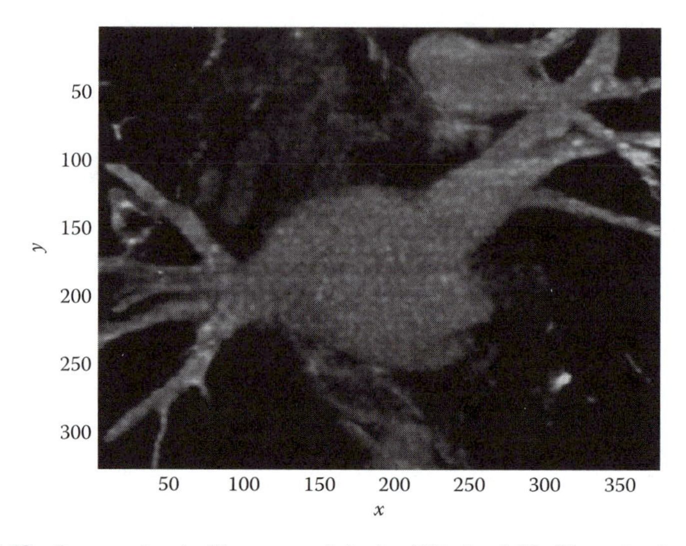

FIGURE 2.12 Image $g(x, y)$. (Courtesy of Andre D'Avila, MD, Heart Institute (InCor), University of Sao Paulo, Medical School, Sao Paulo, Brazil.)

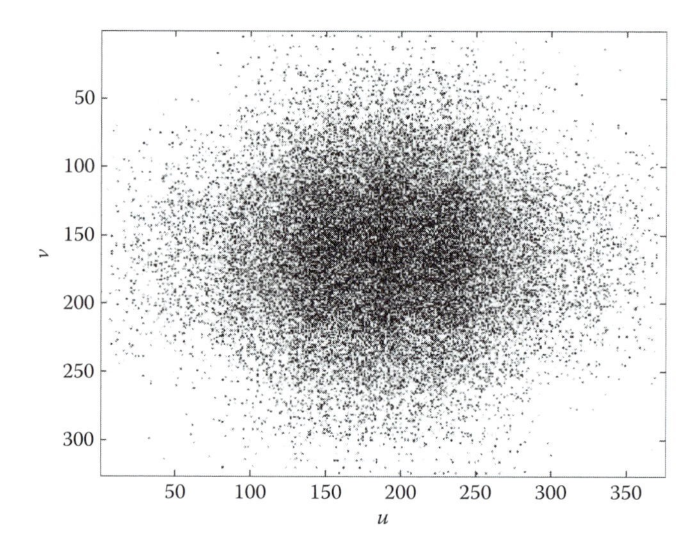

FIGURE 2.13 Magnitude of 2-D DFT of image $g(x, y)$.

be used to display the image. Unlike "`image`", the command "`imshow`" presents the image without numbering the coordinates.

```
colormap(gray(256));
image(g):
y = fft2(g);
xlabel('x');ylabel('y');
figure;
y_magnitude = abs(y);
```

```
image(y_magnitude);
colormap(gray(256));
xlabel('u');
ylabel('v');
```

The center in the DFT image shows the zero frequency, and, as a result, low-frequency components of the signals are the dots close to the origin, while the points far away from the center (origin) represent the high-frequency components of the image.

The properties of 2-D DFT are very similar to continuous signals and 1-D DFT. Some of these properties that play important roles in image processing and are further explored in Problems section.

2.6 FILTER DESIGN

In this section, we discuss using frequency domain or DFT to design practical filters. In preprocessing a signal, it is often the case that some details of the signals must be altered. For example, high frequencies in a signal are often considered to have been corrupted by high-frequency noise (which is the case for many applications). In such cases, one needs to somehow be able to filter the high frequency in the signal. The schematic diagram of Figure 2.14 shows how a filter $H(f)$ can be used to filter a signal (or image) $P(f)$ to generate a processed signal (or image) $Q(f)$.

Often the users of a system have a reasonably reliable idea on the range of frequency for noise. For instance, for high-frequency noise, we may know that majority of the noise energy is at a given frequency and above. In such cases, the ideal scenario is to design a low-pass filter to eliminate the noise. The shape of the ideal low-pass filter is shown in Figure 2.15.

Knowing that $Q(f) = H(f)$, any frequency higher than the cutoff frequency D_0 in the original signal $P(f)$ is eliminated in the filtered signal $Q(f)$. This is ideal filtering of high frequencies using an ideal low-pass filter. Similarly, one can imagine an ideal high-pass filter (Figure 2.16) as well as an ideal band-pass filter (Figure 2.17).

In each case, the desired frequencies are preserved and the unwanted frequencies are eliminated.

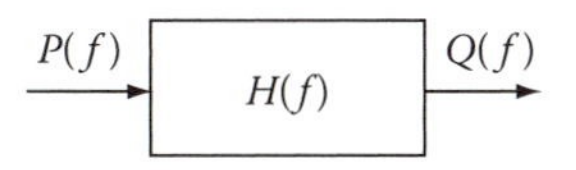

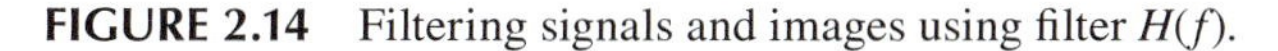

FIGURE 2.14 Filtering signals and images using filter $H(f)$.

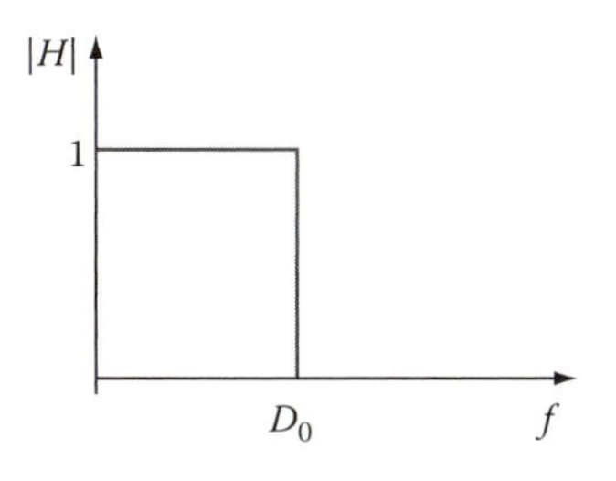

FIGURE 2.15 Ideal low-pass filter.

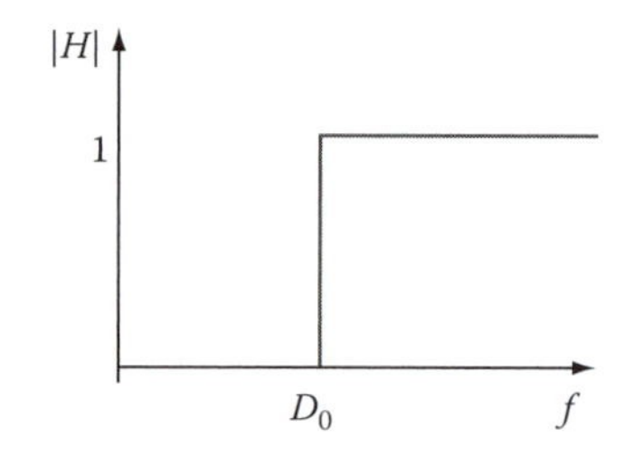

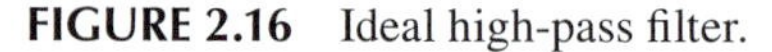
FIGURE 2.16 Ideal high-pass filter.

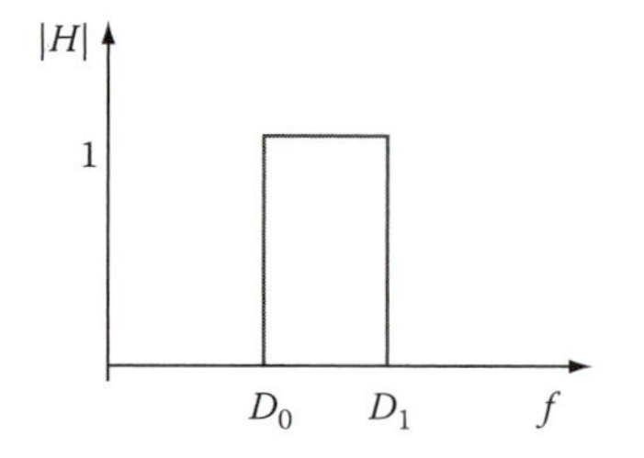

FIGURE 2.17 Ideal band-pass filter.

In practical applications, due to some practical limitations in constructing the ideal filters as well as unwanted effects of abrupt rises or falls in ideal filters, some approximations of these ideal filters are used. These approximations, while similar to the ideal filters in general shape, are smooth and have no sharp jumps in them.

One example of such filter realizations is the family of Butterworth filters. The low-pass Butterworth filter, as shown in Figure 2.18a, has a smooth transition from the amplitude 1 at frequency 0 to amplitude 0 at high frequencies. The high-pass Butterworth filter is shown in Figure 2.18b. As seen, one can roughly approximate the ideal filter with these smooth curves. In these approximations, there is no clear choice for the cutoff frequency; it is often customary to consider the frequency at which the magnitude of the filter falls to $1/\sqrt{2}$ of the peak value (i.e., 1) as the approximate cutoff frequency.

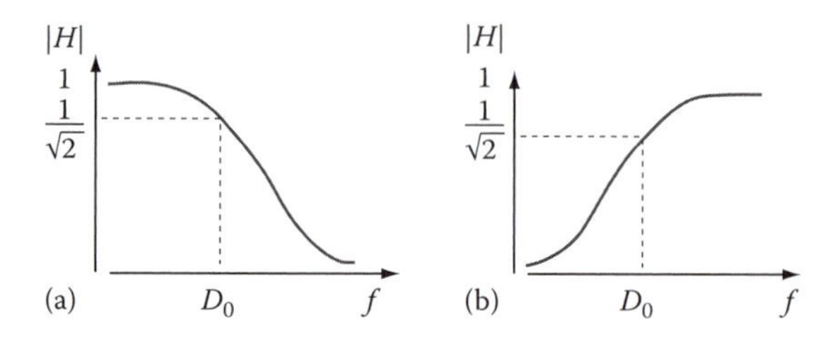

FIGURE 2.18 (a) Low-pass Butterworth filter and (b) high-pass Butterworth filter.

Due to their completely smooth curve, Butterworth filters are also referred to as maximally flat. The mathematical formulation of a Butterworth filter can be written as follows:

$$H(f)=\frac{B(f)}{A(f)}=\frac{b_1(jf)^n+b_2(jf)^{n-1}+\cdots+b_{n+1}}{a_1(jf)^n+a_2(jf)^{n-1}+\cdots+a_{n+1}} \tag{2.31}$$

where j is the imaginary number and the parameters a_i and b_i are the parameters of the filter. The order n identifies both the shape and the complexity of the filter, i.e., the larger n gets, the sharper filter is achieved; however, the sharper filter will be more complex. The field of filter design by itself requires a separate textbook. But describing the details of the filter design process may not provide a meaningful insight to the reader who cares mainly about filter design applications. Here, instead of describing the details of the long and tedious process of filter design, we will simply investigate the filtering process using MATLAB.

In MATLAB, in order to design a Butterworth filter with the order of n, one can use the following command:

```
[b,a] = butter (n,Wn,'s')
```

In this command, n is the order of the low-pass Butterworth filter, `Wn` is the cutoff frequency of the filter, and `s` determines whether the filter is high pass or low pass. The option "`high`" corresponds to high-pass filter and "`low`" gives a low-pass filter.

Example 2.7

In this example, we use MATLAB to design a low-pass Butterworth filter. We are to design a low-pass Butterworth filter of order 10 with the cutoff frequency of 300 Hz. For these specifications, we code the following line in MATLAB and it will provide us the resulting polynomials: `a` and `b`.

```
[b,a] = butter (10,300/500,'low');
```

Next, in order to better visualize the designed filter, we use the command "`freqz`" to draw the frequency response of the aforementioned low-pass Butterworth filter, i.e.,

```
freqz(b,a,128,1000);
```

where 128 is the number of points in which the frequency response is evaluated and 1000 is the sampling frequency. Figure 2.19 shows the frequency response of this low-pass Butterworth filter.

Every concept on filtering of the 1-D signals can be extended to the 2-D case. Just like 1-D signals, images often contain frequencies that need to be filtered out. Two-dimensional low-pass filters, high-pass filters, and band-pass filters are designed to process the images and extract the desired frequency information. Just as in 1-D case, the ideal filters are not very practical, and, as a result, approximations such as Butterworth filters are used for practical applications.

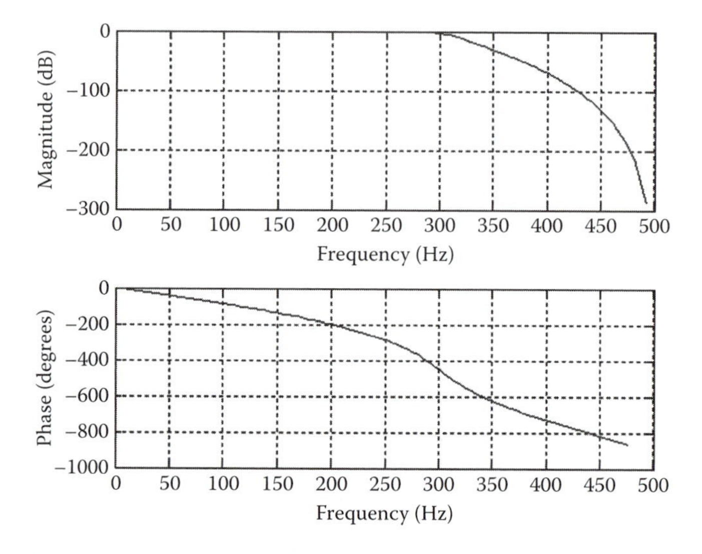

FIGURE 2.19 Frequency response of Butterworth filter designed in Example 2.3.

2.7 SUMMARY

FT is among the most commonly used transformations in signal processing. In this chapter, we have identified the definition, properties, and applications of the FT (both continuous and discrete). We also discussed the 1-D and 2-D formulations of the FT. In addition, we also introduced the ideal and practical filters designed in the frequency domain to process signals and images.

PROBLEMS

2.1 Prove the linearity of FT, i.e., show that for any two signals $g_1(t)$ and $g_2(t)$ and any two scalars α and β,

$$\mathrm{FT}\{\alpha g_1(t)+\beta g_2(t)\}=\alpha \mathrm{FT}\{g_1(t)\}+\chi \mathrm{FT}\{g_2(t)\}=\alpha G_1(f)+\beta G_2(f) \quad (2.32)$$

2.2 Prove the scaling property of the FT, i.e., show that for any signal $g(t)$ and any scalar $\alpha \neq 0$,

$$\mathrm{FT}\{g_1(t)\}=G_1(f)=\frac{1}{\alpha}G\left(\frac{f}{|\alpha|}\right) \quad (2.33)$$

2.3 Prove the time-shift property of the FT, i.e., show that for any signal $g(t)$ and any scalars t_0,

$$\mathrm{FT}\{g(t-t_0)\}=e^{j2\pi f t_0}G(f) \quad (2.34)$$

2.4 Prove the convolution property for FT, i.e., show that

$$\mathrm{FT}\{g_1(t) * g_2(t)\} = G_1(u) \cdot G_2(u) \tag{2.35}$$

2.5 For 2-D DFT, prove that

$$\mathrm{STRETCH}_l\{g(n)\} \overset{\mathrm{DFT}}{\leftrightarrow} \mathrm{REPEAT}_l\{G(k)\} \tag{2.36}$$

2.6 Prove that the DFT of a real signal $g(n)$ is symmetric, i.e., $F(u) = F(-u)$.

2.7 Prove the scaling property of the 2-D DFT, i.e., show that for any 2-D signal $g(x, y)$ and any scalars $\alpha > 0$, $\beta > 0$,

$$\mathrm{FT}\{g_1(x, y)\} = G_1(u, v) = \frac{1}{\alpha\beta} G\left(\frac{u}{\alpha}, \frac{v}{\beta}\right) \tag{2.37}$$

2.8 From the CD, load the file "p_2_9.mat." This gives you a synthetic 1-D signal $x(n)$.

a. Use the command "`fft`" to calculate the DFT of the signal x.
b. Plot the magnitude of the DFT.
c. What are the dominant frequencies in the signal?

2.9 Use command "`imread`" in MATLAB to read the image stores in "p_2_10.jpg," i.e., type "`imread('p _ 2 _ 8','jpg')`". This gives you an image x, which shows an intersection of the heart.*

a. Use the command "`fft2`" to calculate the DFT of the image x.
b. Use the command "`image`" to show the magnitude of the DFT of the image. You may need to adjust the color map of the display using the command "`colormap`".

2.10 Using MATLAB, design a high-pass Butterworth filter of order 9 with cutoff frequency 200 Hz. Plot the frequency response of the filter.

---

* Courtesy of Andre D'Avila, MD, Heart Institute (InCor), University of Sao Paulo, Medical School, Sao Paulo, Brazil.

3 Image Filtering, Enhancement, and Restoration

3.1 INTRODUCTION AND OVERVIEW

The equipments with which we capture images are often influenced by measurement noise; therefore, the resulting images may not provide the quality needed for desired analysis. In addition, even for images with acceptable quality, it is often the case that certain regions, features, or components of the image need to be emphasized and highlighted. As an example, when processing medical images, it is often the case that highlighting certain parts of the image such as tumor-like regions would help physicians make a better diagnosis. In this chapter, the main computational techniques commonly used in image processing to restore and enhance images are discussed.

Image restoration and enhancement techniques can be regarded as computational algorithms that receive an image as their input and generate an enhanced or restored version of this image as their output. This is shown in Figure 3.1.

Image restoration techniques are often described either in space domain or in frequency (Fourier) domain. While almost any space-domain technique has an equivalent frequency-domain method and vice versa, some techniques are easier to understand and/or implement in one domain than another. Some frequency-domain filtering techniques were described in the previous chapter, and in this chapter the focus is given to space-domain techniques. It is not surprising to see that some of the space-domain techniques described in this chapter carry the same name as the ones described in the previous chapter (such as low-pass filtering and high-pass filtering). As we will discuss later, these filters are the space-domain equivalents of the filters described in the previous chapter.

Space-domain image enhancement techniques can be further classified into two general categories: point processing and mask processing techniques. The point processing techniques are the ones in which each pixel of the original (input) image at coordinates (x, y) is processed to create the corresponding pixel at coordinates (x, y) in the enhanced image. This means that the only pixel in the original image that has a role in determining the value of the corresponding pixel in the enhanced image is the pixel located at the exact same coordinate in the original image. In contrast, in mark processing techniques, not only the pixel at (x, y) coordinates of the original image but also some neighboring pixels of this point are involved in generating the pixel at (x, y) coordinates in the enhanced image. The schematic diagrams of the point processing and mask processing techniques are compared with each other in Figure 3.2. These two categories of space-domain image enhancement techniques are further described in this chapter.

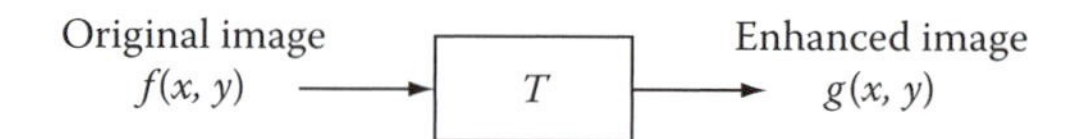

FIGURE 3.1 Schematic diagram of image restoration techniques as computational machines.

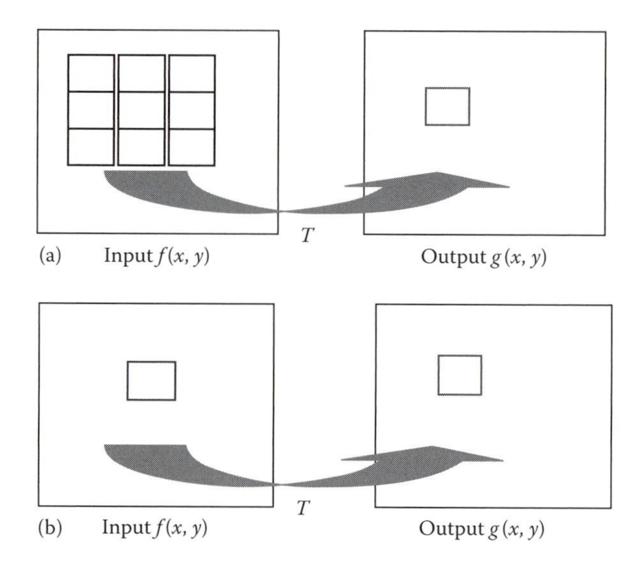

FIGURE 3.2 Schematic diagram of (a) mask processing and (b) point processing techniques.

3.2 POINT PROCESSING

Point processing involves a mathematical transformation that modifies the values of the pixels in the original image to create the values of the corresponding pixels in the enhanced image. The mathematical expression for such a transformation can be described as follows:

$$g(x,y) = T\left[f(x,y)\right] \tag{3.1}$$

where

$f(x, y)$ is the original (input) image
$g(x, y)$ is the enhanced (output) image
T describes the transformation between the two images

The exact choice of the transformation is identified by the exact objectives of the point processing task. Point processing is often performed on an image to improve the quality of an image using the manipulation of the gray-level range of the image. Different methods of point processing and their specific objectives are described in the following.

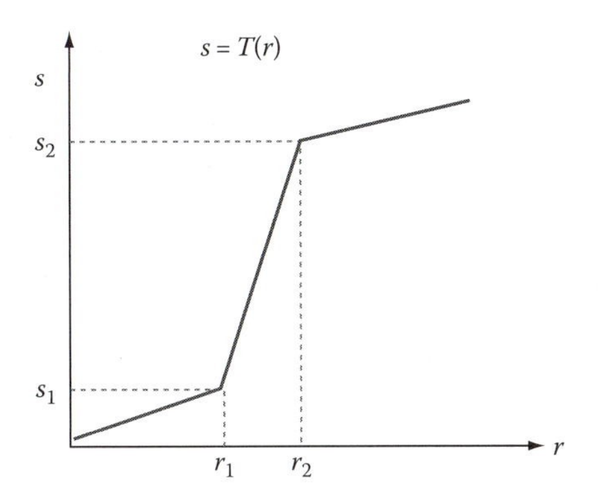

FIGURE 3.3 Contrast enhancement using point processing.

3.2.1 Contrast Enhancement

If the object of interest (to be analyzed) occupies only a specific range of the gray scale, then one may want to manipulate the image such that the object occupies a larger range of the gray level and therefore increase the visibility of the object. In medical images, for example, often one needs to analyze a tumor surrounded by organs that are darker or brighter than the tumor is. If other organs and objects are not the main focus of the analysis, then in order to visualize the tumor better, one can perform contrast enhancement to "stretch" the gray level of the tumor.

Contrast enhancement is a method to create better visibility of a particular range of gray level that corresponds to the object to be studied. This stretch of gray-level range is illustrated in Figure 3.3.

As can be seen in Figure 3.3, the exact shape of the transformation applied for contrast stretching is controlled by values of (r_1, s_1) and (r_2, s_2). It is apparent that the choice of $r_1 = s_1$ and $r_2 = s_2$ would reduce the transformation to a linear operation that has no effect on the gray level of the original image. In practice, we often select these values such that the interval $[s_1, s_2]$ covers the gray-level range of the object of interest and the interval $[r_1, r_2]$ provides the desired range of gray level for a better visibility of the object in the target image. This implies that for a better object visibility "$r_2 - r_1$" must be much larger than "$s_2 - s_1$"; in other words, with this condition, the differences among the gray levels in the region of interest are amplified and enhanced in the target image.

Next, we show how to implement point processing in MATLAB®.

Example 3.1

In this example, we enhance and stretch the gray level of the original image in the interval of [150, 200] to the desired interval of [105, 200]. MATLAB code of this example is shown in the following text. First, we read the original image with "`imread`" command. This image shows that ultrasonic image of the heart and its compartments. We have intentionally chosen a noisy ultrasonic image to better represent the quality of images to be processed in many medical applications.

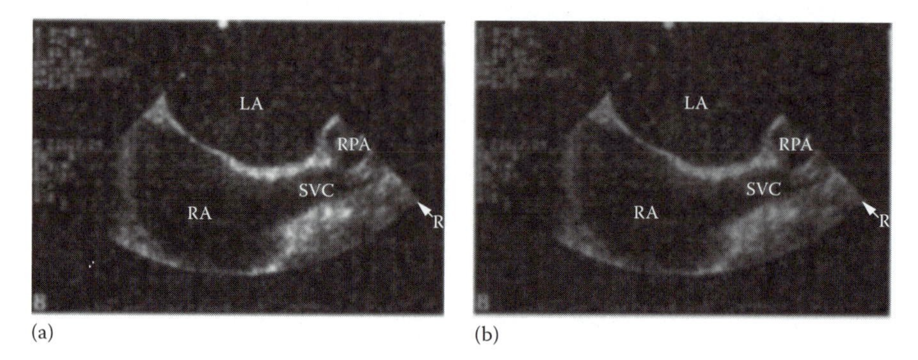

FIGURE 3.4 (a) Original image and (b) image after point processing. (Courtesy of Andre D'Avila, MD, Heart Institute (InCor), University of Sao Paulo, Medical School, Sao Paulo, Brazil.)

As can be seen from the code, in order to do numerical operations on an image, it is often easier to convert the image from unsigned integer format to double format using "double" command. The rest of the code is composed of "for" loops for stretching the interval of [150, 200]. Figure 3.4 shows an ultrasound image of the heart and the image after point processing.

```
I=imread('heart.tif');
S = size(I);
I = double(I);
J = zeros(S(1),S(2));
for i=1:S(1)
    for j=1:S(2)
          if I(i,j) <= 150
                    J(i,j) = I(i,j);
          elseif (150 < I(i,j)) & (I(i,j) < 200)
                    J(i,j)=1.9*(I(i,j)-150)+ 105;
          elseif (I(i,j) >= 200)
                    J(i,j) = .8*(I(i,j)-200) + 200;
          end
    end
end
imshow (I,[0,255]);
imshow (J,[0,255]);
```

Other types of transformation can be used to enhance the quality of an image for particular applications. Figure 3.5a shows a transformation function that creates a binary image from the original image. This transformation is useful for applications where we need to set a threshold value to separate an object from the background. Such applications include the typical scenarios in which a tumor must be separated from the background tissues. However, often we not only need to emphasize and highlight the tumor but also prefer to see the tissues around the tumor to get a better picture of the spatial relation among the tumor and the surrounding tissues or organs. To address this need, a similar transformation shown in Figure 3.5b can be used. This transformation increases

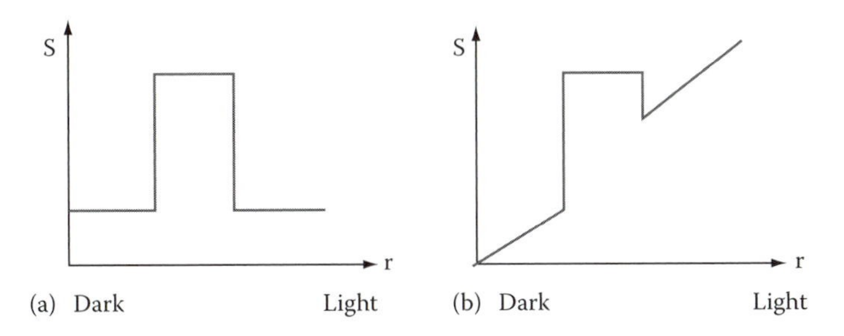

FIGURE 3.5 (a) Transform function that highlights the interested range and sets the other gray levels to a constant low value. (b) Transform function that highlights the interested range and preserves the value of other gray levels.

and highlights the gray level of the region of interest (e.g., tumor), and, to a certain degree, it simultaneously preserves the other gray levels containing the surrounding tissues and organs.

3.2.2 Bit-Level Slicing

In digital computers, the gray level of each pixel in an image is saved as one or more bytes. A byte is a vector of 1 or 0 bits. In digital images, according to the arrangements of these 1's and 0's, a gray level is coded as binary number. For example, in order to encode 256 gray levels, i.e., gray levels of 0, 1, 2,…, 255, one would need 1 B with 8 bit. In such a system, the byte [00000000] would encode for the gray level of 0 and [11111111] represent 255. Similarly, any number between 0 and 255 is encoded by its binary code as 1 B. The bit in the far left side is referred to as "most significant bit," or MSB, because a change in that bit would change the value encoded by the byte significantly. For instance, for an 8-bit byte as described earlier, a change in MSB would alter the value of the encoded gray level by 126 levels, which is a large change. Similarly, the bit in the far right side is referred to as "least significant bit," or LSB, simply because a change in this bit does not change the encoded gray value much. In the 8-bit byte previously discussed, a change in LSB would change the value of the gray level only by 1 level.

Bit-level slicing is a method of representing an image with one or more bit(s) of the byte used for each pixel. For instance, one can choose to only use MSB to represent a pixel, which reduces the original gray level to a binary image. In other applications, one can choose a high value and a low value for the gray levels in the range of interest, maintain the bits in that range to present the image, and discard the rest of the bits. This obviously results to the loss of resolution but at the same time reduces the size of the storage needed to save the image as each pixel is now represented by smaller number of bits.

Generally speaking, bit-level slicing is used to achieve the following three main goals: (1) represent the image with fewer bits and compress the image to an image with lower size while still satisfying a minimum level of quality, (2) convert the gray-level image to a binary image, and (3) enhance the image by focusing on those gray levels that are more important for the task in hand.

Example 3.2

In this example, we explore the implementation of bit-level slicing in MATLAB. In this example, we show that by preserving the four MSBs and discarding the remaining bits of the original image (shown in Figure 3.6a), while maintaining the quality of the original image, one can reduce the size of space needed to store the image. The MATLAB code of this implementation has been shown as follows:

```
I=imread('2.jpg');
I=rgb2gray(I);
imshow(I,[0 255]);
S=size(I);
I=double(I);
I=dec2base(I,2);
newS=size(I);
J= zeros(S(1),S(2));
    for I = 1:newS(1)
            k=char(I(i,:));
            k(5)='0';
            k(6)='0';
            k(7)='0';
            k(8)='0';
            k=base2dec(k,2);
            a=fix(i/S(1))+1;
            b=mod(i,S(1));
                   if b==0
                           b=S(1);
                           a=a-1;
                   end
            J(b,a)=k;
    end
figure,
imshow(J,[0 255]);
```

As can be seen in the code, first, we read each pixel of the original gray-level image in 8 bit. Then, we use a "`for`" loop in which for each pixel, only the four MSBs are preserved and the rest of the bits are set to 0. Figure 3.6 shows both the original image (a) and the image after bit-level slicing (b). Evidently, the image after bit-level slicing has a quality very similar to that of the original image. However, if we discard one or some of the MSBs, for example, the second MSB, the quality of the image will decrease very much. Figure 3.6c shows the image after discarding bits 2, 5, 6, 7, and 8. The low quality of the resulting image indicates how the image quality degrades when some of the MSBs are discarded.

3.2.3 Histogram Equalization

Histogram equalization is among the most popular techniques for image enhancement that is based on the manipulation of images using their histograms. Before describing the technique, the need for such a transformation is explained. Consider cell

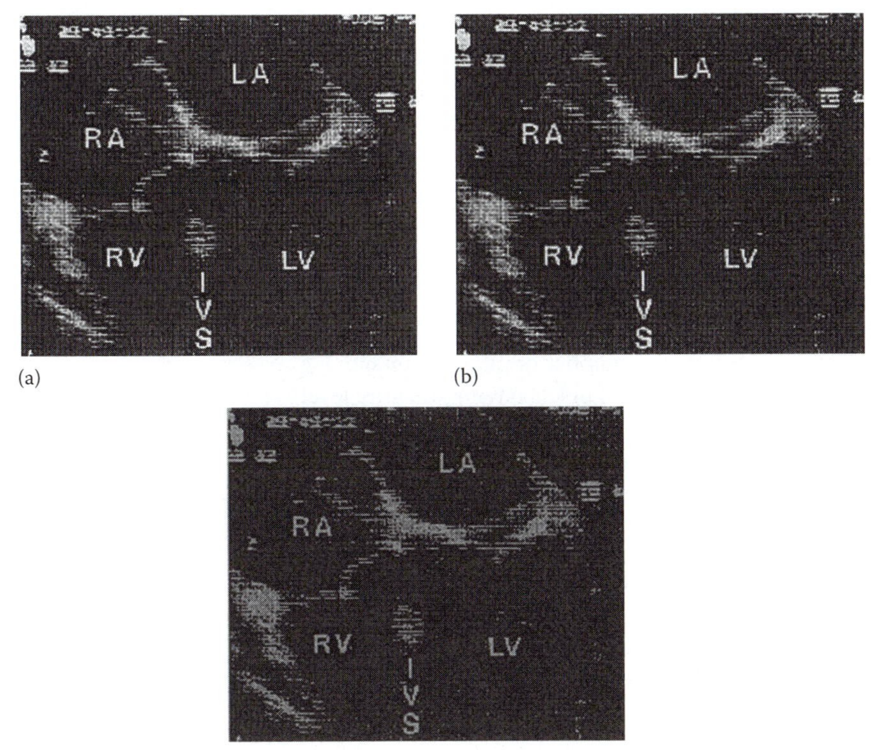

FIGURE 3.6 (a) Original image, (b) resulting image after discarding four of the LSBs, and (c) resulting image setting bits 2, 5, 6, 7, and 8 to zero. (Courtesy of Andre D'Avila, MD, Heart Institute (InCor), University of Sao Paulo, Medical School, Sao Paulo, Brazil.)

images captured from the same cell and its background but at different illumination levels, for example, two cell images captured by the same microscope, one in regular room illumination and one in the presence of extra light sources. Obviously, one of the images will be darker than the other; i.e., the average gray levels as well as the distribution of gray levels would be different in the images. Such differences can cause serious problems if the images are to be analyzed and compared with each other. For instance, the cell in one image can occupy a different gray-level range that in another image; hence, a technique designed to detect the cell in one of the images may not work on another image.

In cell image processing, since the room illumination as well as the lighting settings of microscopes can be very different from one setup to another, designing an image processing method for applications such as nuclei segmentation would not work on all images simply because of the differences in gray-level distribution of the objects caused by different illumination settings. This problem calls for a preprocessing method to "equalize" the gray-level distributions of the image before other processing steps.

Next, we briefly review the concept of image histogram as discussed in Chapter 1. Considering the gray-level values of r, we can define $p_r(r)$ as the probability density function of r. Since we are dealing with digital images, we assume only discrete values for r. The probability density function of r can be estimated according to the pixel values of the image as follows:

$$p_r(r_k) = \frac{n_k}{n}, \quad k = 0,\ 1,\ 2, \ldots,\ L-1 \tag{3.2}$$

where

n represents the total number of pixels in image

n_k is the total number of pixels having the gray level r_k

A graph of $p_r(r_k)$, often referred to as histogram, says a lot about the nature of the image. For dark images, the gray levels close to 0 are very strong, i.e., a considerable portion of the histogram energy is centered on the left-hand side of the histogram. Similarly, for bright images, the balance is visibly shifted toward higher gray levels (i.e., bright gray levels). Then, the task of histogram equalization is both to create a balance between all gray levels and hopefully create an image whose histogram is close to the uniform distribution.

Now, assume that r has been normalized and to the interval of [0, 1]. Then, histogram equalization is a transformation as follows:

$$s = T(r), \quad 0 \le r \le 1 \tag{3.3}$$

where $T(r)$ is the transformation function that creates the value s in the enhanced image from a gray value r in the original image. Further assume that $T(r)$ is monotonically increasing and has values between 0 and 1 for all values of r. The first condition, i.e., monotonically increasing, preserves the order of gray levels in output image, and the second condition ensures that the resulting gray-level values for the output image are also between 0 and 1. Figure 3.7 shows a typical transform function that satisfies these properties. The transformation T is often designed to create images with a more uniform histogram from images whose histograms are not balanced.

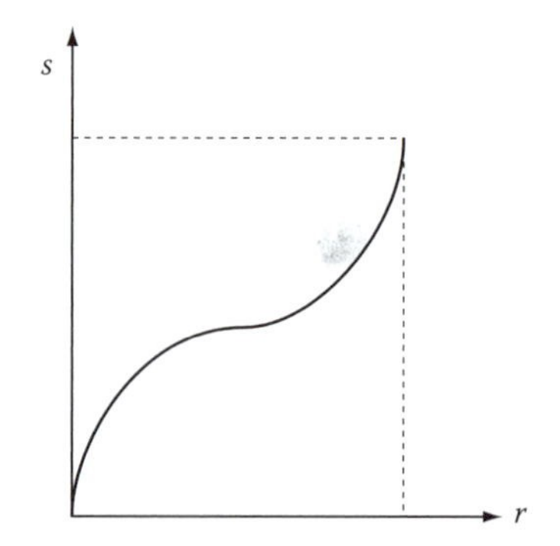

FIGURE 3.7 Typical gray-level transform function.

While in discrete images, theoretically speaking, one can never get a pure uniform probability density function for the transformed image, there are a number of functions (satisfying the conditions described earlier) that provide histograms for the transformed image that are much more uniformly spread compared to the original image. Here, instead of describing the details of these transformations, we focus on using MATLAB for histogram equalization.

Example 3.3

In this example, we explore using MATLAB for histogram equalization. In MATLAB, the command "histeq" performs histogram equalization. Command "imhist" displays histogram of the image. We use command "imhist" to show the histograms of the image before and after equalization. The MATLAB code for this process is as follows:

```
I=imread('7.jpg');
I=rgb2gray(I);
J=histeq(I)
Imshow(I),
figure
Imshow(J)
figure,
Imhist(I,64)
figure,
Imhist(J,64)
```

Figure 3.8 shows the image and its histogram before and after histogram equalization. As can be seen, the quality of the image has improved in the processed image.

3.3 MASK PROCESSING: LINEAR FILTERING IN SPACE DOMAIN

It is often the case that instead of linear processing of images using filters described in frequency domain, space-domain linear filters are used in typical image processing applications. This is mainly to the fact that frequency-domain description of two-dimensional (2-D) filters is often more complex than the one-dimensional (1-D) filters. In principle, space-domain linear filters approximate the impulse response of various kinds of typical frequency-domain filters with a 2-D mask. In spatial filtering, as described before, a weight mask is used to express the effect of the filter on each pixel of the image in an insightful fashion. A typical mask has been shown in Figure 3.9. In this section, we introduce some of the most popular mask filters that are applied in space domain.

The pixel value for the pixel (x, y) in the processed image, $g(x, y)$, is computed as a sum of products of the filter coefficients and the original image f, i.e.,

$$g(x,y)=\sum_{s=-a}^{a}\sum_{t=-b}^{b}\omega(s,t)f(x+s,y+t) \tag{3.4}$$

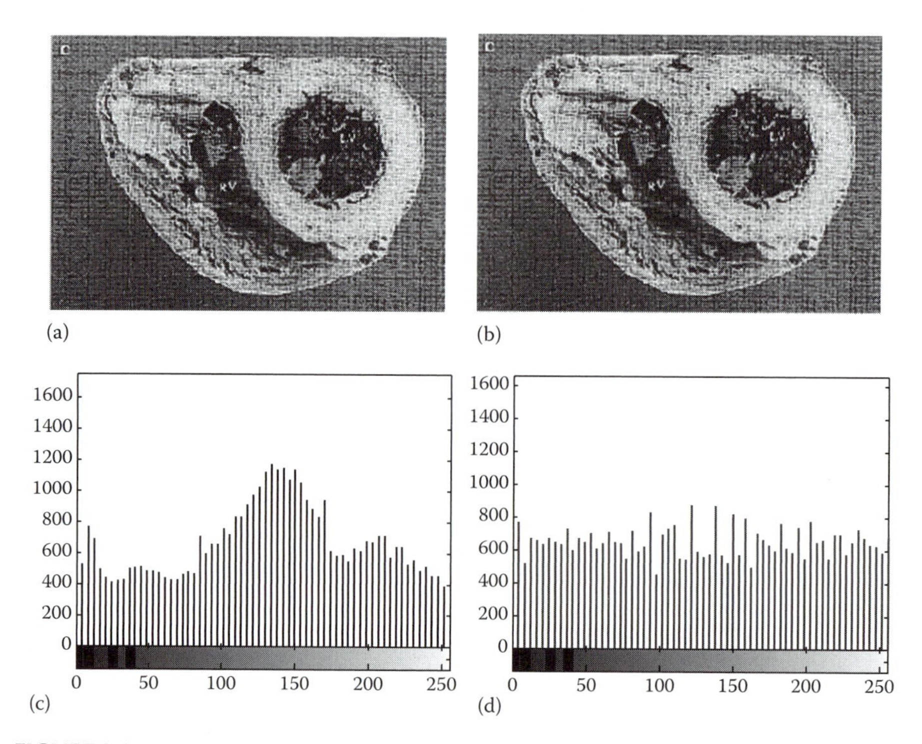

FIGURE 3.8 (a) Original image. (b) Transformed image after histogram equalization. (c) Gray-level histogram of the original image. (d) Histogram of the image after histogram equalization. (Courtesy of Andre D'Avila, MD, Heart Institute (InCor), University of Sao Paulo, Medical School, Sao Paulo, Brazil.)

$\omega(-1, -1)$	$\omega(-1, 0)$	$\omega(-1, 1)$
$\omega(0, -1)$	$\omega(0, 0)$	$\omega(0, 1)$
$\omega(1, -1)$	$\omega(1, 0)$	$\omega(1, 1)$

FIGURE 3.9 Typical 3×3 mask.

Masks can be thought of as the truncated space-domain response of the typical linear filters to the impulse function. For instance, we will introduce masks for low-pass filters that are simply approximation of the space-domain representation of the ideal low-pass filters typically designed in the frequency domain. As one can expect, there are four popular types of space-domain linear filters commonly used in image processing: low-pass filters, high-pass filters, high-boost filters, and band-pass filters.

3.3.1 Low-Pass Filters

Low-pass filters attenuate or eliminate high-frequency components of an image such as edges, texture, and other sharp details. Low-pass filters that are often used for applications such as smoothing, blurring, and noise reduction provide a smooth

	1	1	1
(1/9)*	1	1	1
	1	1	1

(a)

	1	2	1
(1/16)*	2	4	2
	1	2	1

(b)

FIGURE 3.10 (a and b) Two typical masks used for low-pass filtering.

version of the original image. A low-pass filter is sometimes used as a preprocessing step to remove unimportant details from an image before object extraction. Such filters are also used to bridge small gaps in lines and curves as an interpolating technique. Low-pass filters, however, suffer from certain disadvantages. For instance, low-pass filters attenuate edges and some sharp details that are often important in many applications.

Two typical masks used for low-pass filtering have been shown in Figure 3.10.

Focusing on the mask shown in Figure 3.10a, it is evident that the filter using this mask will calculate the average of pixel values around a pixel to generate the corresponding pixel in the filtered image. In other words, the task of this filter is averaging of pixel points to form a smoother image. This filter has nine equal coefficients and is called a box filter. The mask shown in Figure 3.10a is a 3×3 mask, but one can define a larger mask for averaging. The larger the mask becomes, the more attenuation in high-frequency components is achieved.

In the filter shown in Figure 3.10b, the coefficients are not equal. In this filter, we assign a higher value to the central coefficient of the mask to emphasize and accentuate the importance of the central pixel. The values assigned to other coefficients are often inversely proportional to their distance from the central coefficient. Therefore, the coefficients in diagonal squares will have the least values. Such a mask will partially avoid the unwanted blurring effect.

Example 3.4

In this example, we explore the implementation of a low-pass filter H in MATLAB. In the following code, choosing H as defined in the code will set the mask as the low-pass filter defined in Figure 3.10a. Then, the command "imfilter" is used to apply the filter H on image I. Figure 3.11a shows the original image, and Figure 3.11b shows the image after applying the low-pass filter.

```
I=imread('image.jpg');
I=rgb2gray(I);
H=(1/9)*[1 1 1; 1 1 1; 1 1 1];
smooth_image = imfilter(I,H);
imshow(I);
figure,
imshow(smooth_image);
```

As can be seen, Figure 3.11b is more blurred than the original image. Increasing the dimension of the mask to higher values will result in more blurring effect.

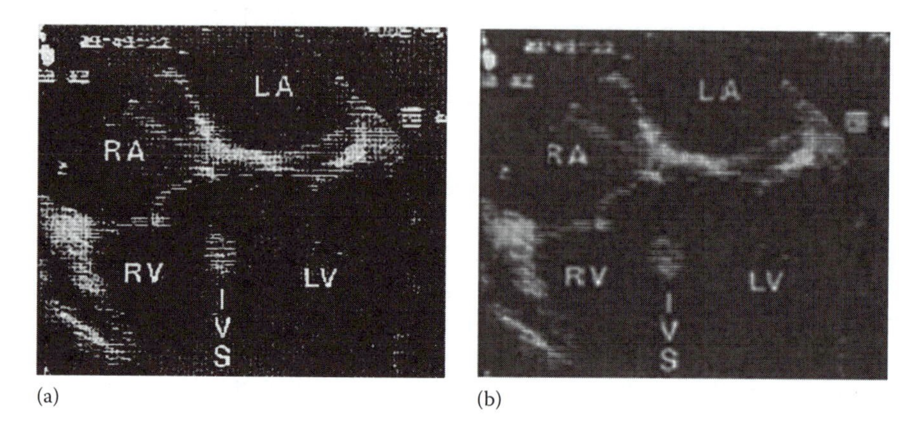

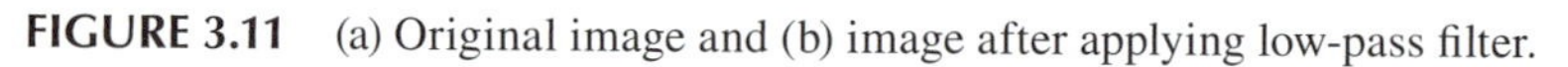
FIGURE 3.11 (a) Original image and (b) image after applying low-pass filter.

3.3.2 Median Filters

Median filters are statistical nonlinear filters that are often described in the space domain. Median filters are known to reduce the noise without eliminating the edges and other high-frequency contents. Median filters (also referred to as order statistics filters) perform the following operations to find each pixel value in the processed image:

Step 1: All pixels in the neighborhood of the pixel in the original image (identified by the mask) are inserted in a list.
Step 2: This list is sorted in ascending (or descending) order.
Step 3: The median of the sorted list (i.e., the pixel in the middle of the list) is chosen as the pixel value for the processed image.

As defined earlier, median filter create pixel values of the filtered image based on the sorting of the gray level of pixels in the mask around the central pixels in the original image.

Example 3.5

The performance of a 3 × 3 median filter on a subimage is illustrated in Figure 3.12.

As can be seen from Figure 3.12, the median filter selects the median of the gray-level values in the 3 × 3 neighborhood of the central pixel and assigns this value as the output. In this example, the median filter is to select the median of following set: {8 10 10 12 12 23 45 64}. According to the sorted list, the response of the filter is 12.

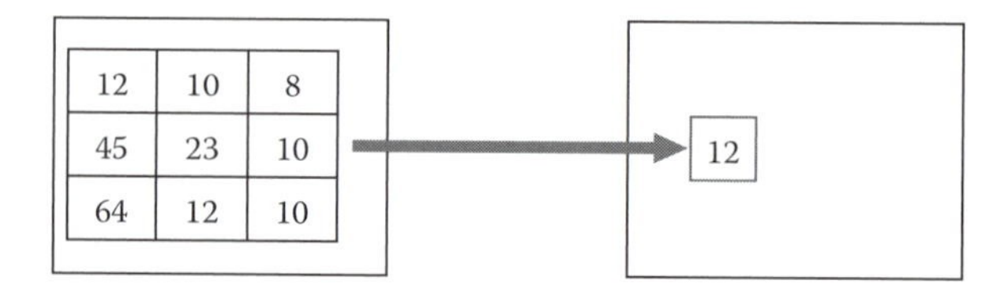

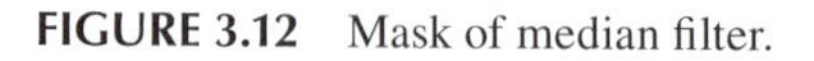
FIGURE 3.12 Mask of median filter.

Intuitively, when median filters are applied to an image, pixels whose values are very different from their neighboring pixels will be eliminated. By eliminating the effect of such odd pixels, values are assigned to the pixels that are more representative of the values of the typical neighboring pixels in the original image.

The main advantage of median filter is reducing the random noise without eliminating the useful high-frequency components such as edges. This means that while median filter provides smoothing effects similar to linear low-pass filter, it avoids blurring effects that are associated with linear smoothing filters.

Example 3.6

In this example, we discuss the simulation of median filter in MATLAB. In order to explore the performance of median filters, we select a non-noisy image and intentionally add some noise to it. Then, we apply median filter to remove the added noise. In order to do so, we use "imnoise" command to add some noise to the image. The command "medfilt2", which is the 2-D median filter, is then used to filter the noise. Finally, both the noisy image and the filtered image are graphed.

```
I=imread('no_noisy_image.jpg');
I=rgb2gray(I);
J=imnoise(I,'salt&pepper',.2);
k=medfilt2(J);
imshow(J);
figure,
imshow(k);
```

Figure 3.13 shows the two images. Figure 3.13a shows an image, which was contaminated by salt and pepper noise, while Figure 3.13b shows the median-filtered image.

As can be seen in Figure 3.13, median filter has reduced the noise in the image without destroying the edges. This is the main advantage of the median filters over the linear low-pass filters. This difference is further illustrated in the following example.

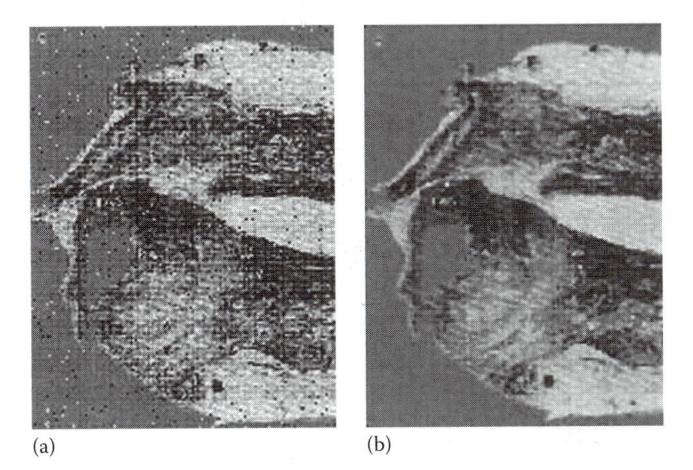

FIGURE 3.13 (a) Noisy image and (b) median-filtered image. (Courtesy of Andre D'Avila, MD, Heart Institute (InCor), University of Sao Paulo, Medical School, Sao Paulo, Brazil.)

Example 3.7

In this example, we focus on the original image shown in Figure 3.14a, and its noisy version shown in Figure 3.14b. Figure 3.14c shows the effect of median filter on the noisy image, while Figure 3.14d illustrates the results of low-pass filtering of the noisy image.

Evidently, the low-pass filter has reduced the noise level in the image; however, at the same time, the filter has blurred the image. On the other hand, while median filter has also reduced the noise, it has preserved the edges of the image almost entirely. Again, this difference is due to the fact that the median filter forces the pixels with distinct intensities to be more like their neighbors and therefore eliminates isolated intensity spikes. Such a smoothing criterion will not result in significant amount of filtering across edges.

Median filters, however, have certain disadvantages. When the number of noisy pixels is greater than half of the total pixels, median filters give a poor performance. This is because, in such cases, median value will be much more influenced by dominating noisy values than the non-noisy pixels. In addition, when the additive noise is Gaussian in nature, median filters may fail to provide a desirable filtering performance.

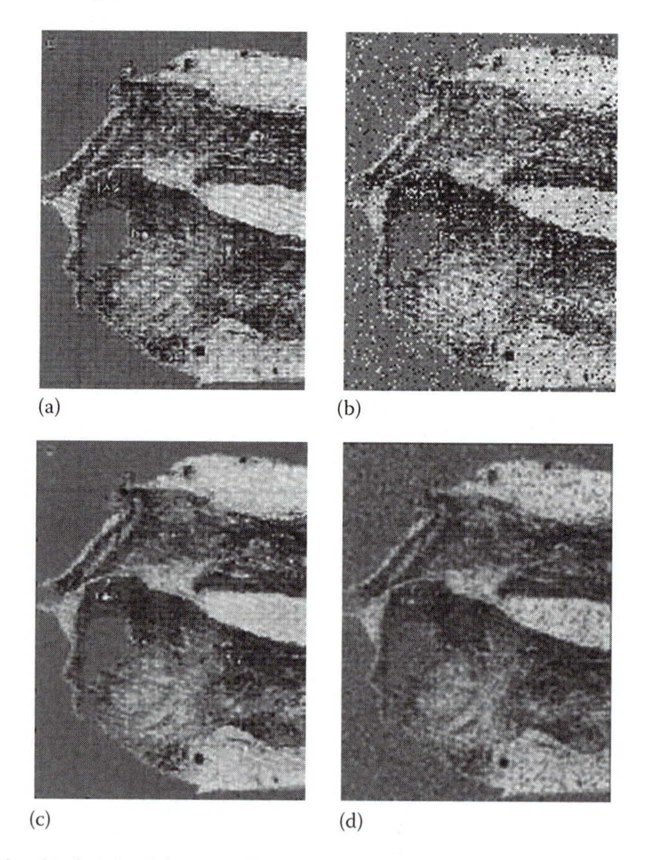

FIGURE 3.14 (a) Original image, (b) noisy image, (c) image after low-pass filter, and (d) image after median filter. (Courtesy of Andre D'Avila, MD, Heart Institute (InCor), University of Sao Paulo, Medical School, Sao Paulo, Brazil.)

3.3.3 Sharpening Spatial Filters

Sharpening filters are used to extract and highlight fine details from an image and also to enhance some blurred details. A typical usage of such filters is deblurring of an image to provide sharper and more visible edge information. There are many applications for sharpening filters including medical imaging, electronic printing, industrial inspection, and autonomous guidance in military systems.

There are three important types of sharpening filters: high-pass filters, high-boost filters, and derivative filters.

3.3.3.1 High-Pass Filters

As in linear low-pass filters, the masks used for high-pass filtering are nothing but the truncated approximations of the space-domain representation of the typical ideal high-pass filters. As such, in high-pass filters the shape of impulse response should have (+) coefficients near its center and (–) coefficients in the outer periphery.

Example 3.8

Figure 3.15 shows an example of a high-pass filter. As can be seen, the central value of the box is positive and the peripheral values are negative.

As in linear low-pass filters, while this set of numbers might form the most popular high-pass mask, there is nothing special about these specific numbers, and similar high-pass masks with different set of numbers can be defined as long as the general rule of "positive in center and negative in peripherals" is observed.

Next, we discuss the implementation of this filter mask in MATLAB.

Example 3.9

As shown in the following code, we first define matrix `H` as the mask defined in Figure 3.15:

```
I=imread('med_image.jpg');
I=rgb2gray(I);
H=(1/9)*[1 1 1; 1 -8 1; 1 1 1];
sharpened = imfilter(I,H);
imshow(I);
figure,
imshow(sharpened);
```

	−1	−1	−1
(1/9)*	−1	8	−1
	−1	−1	−1

FIGURE 3.15 Typical mask of linear high-pass spatial filter.

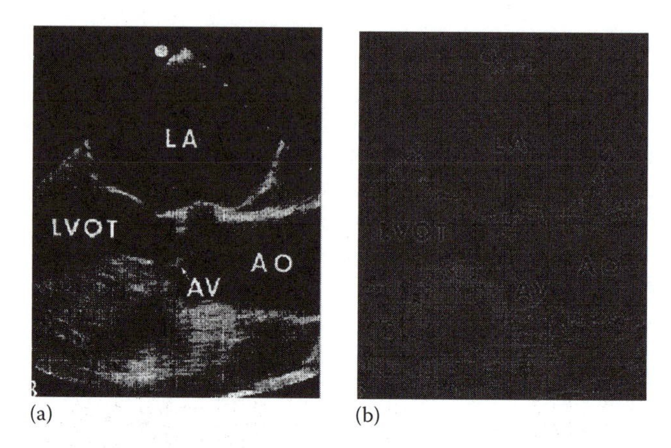

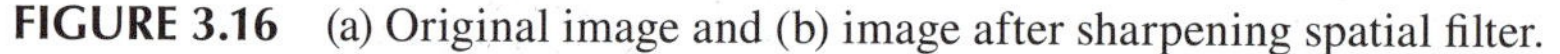
FIGURE 3.16 (a) Original image and (b) image after sharpening spatial filter.

Then, we apply the mask to the medical image `I` shown in Figure 3.16a. Figure 3.16b shows the effect of the high-pass filter on the image.

Figure 3.16b shows how high-pass filters remove all the information of the image except for the edges and other high-frequency components such as texture. If the purpose of using high-pass filter is to improve the overall quality of an image through sharpening, high-pass filters by themselves may not be the solution. Specifically, if we are using high-pass filters only to extract edges, they might be the right tools, but they are not the best filters to simply improve the quality of a blurred image. This is again due to the fact that high-pass filters eliminate all important low-pass components that are necessary for an improved image. Another problem with high-pass filters is the possibility of generating negative numbers as the pixel values of the filtered image. This is due to the negative numbers used in the applied mask.

The solution to the previously mentioned problems with high-pass filters is a similar filter called "high boost."

3.3.3.2 High-Boost Filters

Some extensions of high-pass filters, while highlighting the high frequencies, preserve some low-frequency components and avoid negative pixel values. The most commonly used extensions of high-pass filters are high-boost filters that are also referred to as high-frequency emphasis filters.

Before creating a mask for high-boost filters, note that a $k \times k$ mask with only one nonzero value in the center and zero everywhere else does not change the frequency contents of the image. More specifically, if the nonzero value is 1, then the mask would not change any pixel in the original image. Such a mask is often referred to as "all-pass filter" or "all-pass mask."

A high-boost filter can be simply defined as a weighted combination of the original image and the high-pass-filtered version of the image. In this combination, the high-pass components are highlighted more than the low-pass ones, i.e.,

$$\text{High-boost filtered image} = (A-1)\,\text{original image} + \text{high-pass filtered image} \tag{3.5}$$

	0	0	0		−1	−1	−1		−1	−1	−1
(A − 1)	0	1	0	+1/9	−1	8	−1	=1/9	−1	W	−1
	0	0	0		−1	−1	−1		−1	−1	−1

FIGURE 3.17 High-boost mask.

Or simply, in terms of filters

$$\text{High-boost filter} = (A - 1)\ \text{all-pass filter} + \text{high-pass filter} \tag{3.6}$$

As can be seen, setting $A = 1$ would result in the standard high-pass filter. But in a typical high-boost filter by setting $A > 1$, a weighted version of the original image is added back to the high-pass components. Such choices of A maintain the low-frequency components lost in the pure high-pass filtering and therefore produce improved images that not only emphasize the high frequencies (i.e., sharpen the image) but also show almost all low-frequency components that are often lost in the standard high-pass filters.

Figure 3.17 shows a high-boost filter. This mask is simply the weighted summation of the all-pass mask and the high-pass mask. The coefficient A determines the share or weight of the original image on the filtered image. As it can be seen, the second mask is nothing but a simple high-pass filter mask.

From the diagram of Figure 3.17, it should be apparent that $W = 9A - 1$ and any choice of A will create a different high-boost filter with a different influence of the original image on the final image.

The following example shows how MATLAB can be used to form a high-boost filter. It also shows the impact of the parameter A on the filter performance.

Example 3.10

In this example, we explore the implementation of a high-boost filter in MATLAB. In this implementation, we add a weighted version of the identity matrix K to the matrix H. Figure 3.18 shows the effect of the high-boost filters on the original image for different values of A.

```
I=imread('test.jpg');
I=rgb2gray(I);
A=1.2;
H=(1/9)*[1 1 1;1 -8 1; 1 1 1];
K=[0 0 0;0 1 0;0 0 0];
HB=((A-1).*K) + H;
sharpened = imfilter(I,HB);
imshow(I);
figure,
imshow(sharpened);
```

The best value of A for a particular image is often found by trial and error, but, in many images, values around $A = 1.15$ provide desirable performances.

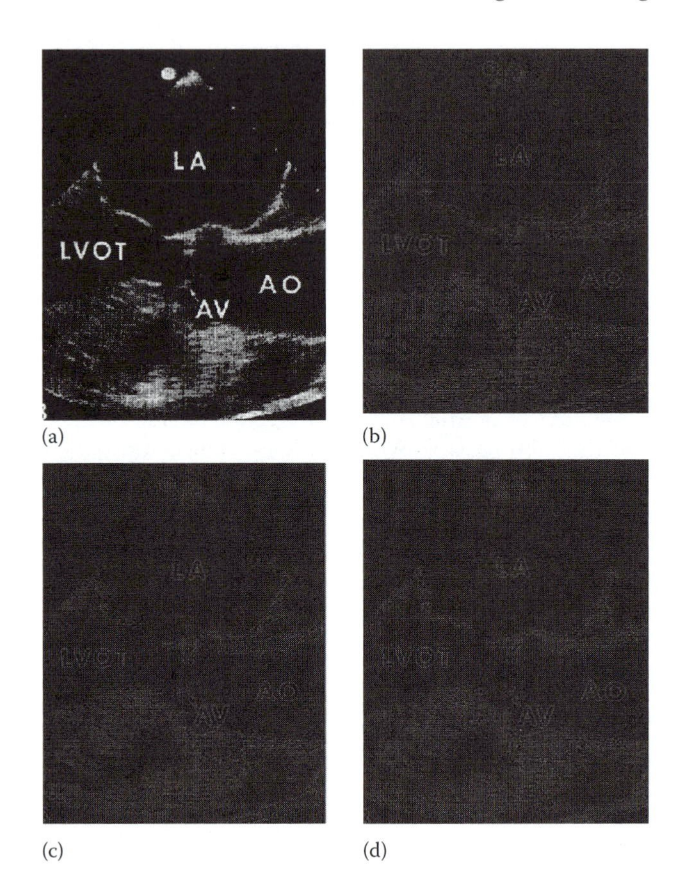

FIGURE 3.18 (a) Original image, (b) filtered image with $A = 1.1$, (c) filtered image with $A = 1.15$, and (d) filtered image with $A = 1.2$.

3.3.3.3 Derivative Filters

As we saw in the previous sections, image blurring can be caused by averaging. Since averaging is simply the discrete version of spatial integration, one can expect that spatial differentiation would result in image sharpening. This observation about spatial differentiation is the main idea behind a family of sharpening filters called "derivative filters." In order to find suitable masks for spatial differentiation, we need to study the concept of differentiation in digital 2-D spaces more closely.

Since an image is a 2-D signal, instead of simple 1-D differentiation, the directional differentiations must be calculated in both horizontal and vertical directions. This leads to spatial gradient defined as follows:

$$\nabla f = \begin{bmatrix} \frac{\partial f}{\partial x} \\ \frac{\partial f}{\partial y} \end{bmatrix} \tag{3.7}$$

The partial differentiations such as $\partial f/\partial x$ can be approximated in discrete image simply by calculating the difference in the gray level of two neighboring pixels, i.e.,

$$\begin{aligned}\frac{\partial f(x,y)}{\partial x} &\cong \frac{f(x,y)-f(x-1,y)}{x-(x-1)} \\ &= \frac{f(x,y)-f(x-1,y)}{1} \\ &= f(x,y)-f(x-1,y)\end{aligned} \tag{3.8}$$

Note that since the smallest value to approximate ∂x is one pixel, we ended up replacing this value with 1. Also note that the final value in Equation 3.7 is an integer (positive or negative). This is due to the fact that subtraction of two integers (i.e., $f(x, y) - f(x - 1, y)$) would always give an integer value. Back to the continuous gradient, the magnitude of the gradient vector is given by

$$|\nabla f| = \left[\left(\frac{\partial f}{\partial x}\right)^2 + \left(\frac{\partial f}{\partial y}\right)^2\right]^{1/2} \tag{3.9}$$

Now, note that storing integers in digital computers is significantly more efficient than storing real numbers that require floating points. In addition, performing calculations with integers are faster and more efficient than doing calculations with real numbers. These two observations strongly encourage the use of integers for image processing in which large images must be stored and processed. Since the result of Equation 3.8 is almost always a real number, we need to approximate this operation such that the resulting number stays an integer.

The approximation of Equation 3.8 typically used in image processing is as follows:

$$|\nabla f| \cong \left|\frac{\partial f}{\partial x}\right| + \left|\frac{\partial f}{\partial y}\right| \tag{3.10}$$

This approximation does not only give us a positive integer, but it also reduces the time complexity of calculating the magnitude of the gradient vector.

In digital image processing, we often work with digital images and therefore need to define approximation of Equation 3.9 in digital case. Specifically, in calculating Equation 3.9, the values $\partial f/\partial x$ and $\partial f/\partial y$ are substituted with their discrete approximations, as introduced earlier. Implementing these approximations will define the masks for spatial differentiation. In order to form these masks, we start with analyzing a small subimage as shown in Figure 3.19. In this figure, z_is are the gray levels of the corresponding pixels.

z_1	z_2	z_3
z_4	z_5	z_6
z_7	z_8	z_9

FIGURE 3.19 3 × 3 part of original image.

−1	0
0	1

−1	0
0	1

FIGURE 3.20 Robert Cross gradient operators.

Figure 3.19 shows a 3 × 3 region of an image. As mentioned earlier, the first directional derivatives of this image can be approximated as follows:

$$\frac{\partial f}{\partial x} = G_x = z_9 - z_5 \tag{3.11}$$

and

$$\frac{\partial f}{\partial y} = G_y = z_8 - z_6 \tag{3.12}$$

Therefore, the magnitude of the gradient vector ∇f can be approximated as follows:

$$\left|\nabla f\right| \cong \left|z_9 - z_5\right| + \left|z_8 - z_5\right| \tag{3.13}$$

Figure 3.20 shows masks that can be used as the implementation of Equation 3.13. These masks are often called Robert Cross gradient operators.

Masks such as the one introduced earlier are applied for image sharpening through spatial differentiation. However, just like the scenario we discussed for high-pass filters, simple derivative filters are too unforgiving to the low-pass components of images, and, therefore, often these filters are combined with some low-pass components of the original image to provide a better performance.

3.4 FREQUENCY-DOMAIN FILTERING

Two-dimensional discrete Fourier transform (2-D DFT) of a digital image, as discussed in the previous chapters, expresses the spatial relationship among the pixel gray levels in the frequency domain and describes the frequency variations in images. Specifically, low-frequency components correspond to slow variations in gray levels of the image, while high frequencies quantify fast variations in gray levels such as edges and texture.

The linear filters previously discussed in spatial domain (e.g., low-pass, high-pass, and high-boost filters) can also be defined in frequency domain using 2-D DFT. To apply the frequency-domain filters on a digital image, first the DFT of the original image, $P(u, v)$, is computed and then DFT of the original image is multiplied by the impulse response function of the frequency-domain filter, $H(u, v)$. This gives the DFT of the filtered image, $Q(u, v)$. In other words,

$$Q(u,v) = H(u,v) \cdot P(u,v) \tag{3.14}$$

The calculation of the IDFT of $Q(u, v)$ gives the filtered image in the space domain. As in the space-domain linear filtering, there are two major types of frequency-domain filters: smoothing (low-pass) filters and sharpening (high-pass) filters. Other filters such as band-pass filters and high-boost filters can be formed using a linear combination of low-pass and high-pass filters.

As mentioned earlier, unlike the 1-D signals where frequency filtering is more insightful and computationally efficient, in filtering of images, spatial filtering using masks is often more straightforward and institutively insightful. However, we describe these frequency filters in the following using a simple description of their mathematical details.

3.4.1 Smoothing Filters in Frequency Domain

The main objective in smoothing an image is to decrease the noisy fast variations in the gray levels of the image. Since the fast variations in gray level of digital images correspond to high frequencies in DFT of the image, a filter that attenuates the high-frequency values of the DFT of the original image is simply a low-pass filter.

Next, we discuss the ideal 2-D low-pass filter in the frequency domain and its approximation using 2-D Butterworth filters.

3.4.1.1 Ideal Low-Pass Filter

In an ideal low-pass filter, all frequencies inside a circle in the frequency domain with radius D_0 (centered at the origin) are allowed to pass through, and all the frequencies outside this circle are eliminated. An ideal low-pass filter $H(u, v)$ can be defined as follows:

$$H(u,v) = \begin{cases} 1 & D(u,v) \le D_0 \\ 0 & D(u,v) > D_0 \end{cases} \tag{3.15}$$

where

$$D(u,v) = (u^2 + v^2)^{1/2} \tag{3.16}$$

Figure 3.21 shows the three-dimensional (3-D) representation of this filter. As mentioned before, due to some undesirable effects of abrupt jumps in the ideal filters together with some limitations in implementation of the ideal filters, it is desirable to approximate the ideal low-pass filters using filters such as Butterworth filters.

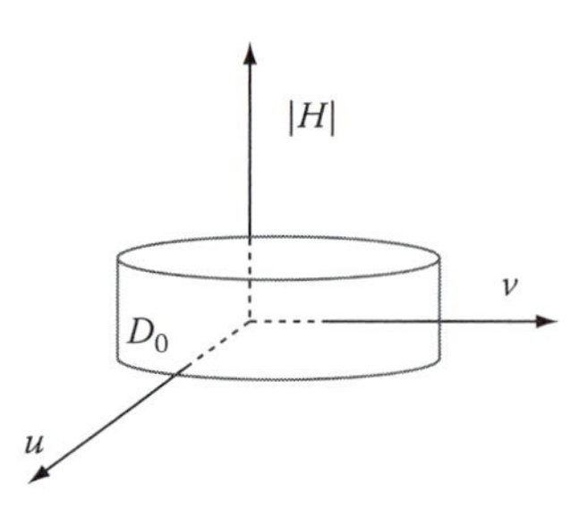

FIGURE 3.21 Three-dimensional representation of low-pass filter.

3.4.1.2 Butterworth Low-Pass Filters

Butterworth filters were introduced for 1-D signals in the previous chapters. The definition of the 2-D low-pass Butterworth filter is the straightforward extension of the 1-D case, i.e.,

$$H(u,v) = \frac{1}{1+\left[D(u,v)/D_0\right]^2} \tag{3.17}$$

where $D(u, v)$ is the distance from the origin in the frequency domain, as previously defined.

3.4.2 Sharpening Filters in Frequency Domain

The most fundamental sharpening filters defined in frequency domain are high-pass filters and high-boost filter. As defined earlier, high-boost filters can be easily formed as a linear combination of the high-pass filters and the all-pass filters; consequently, we only focus on the mathematical definition of high-pass filter. The all-pass filters in frequency domain are simply defined as filters in which $H(u, v) = 1$.

As a result, in order to implement sharpening filters in the frequency domain, it is sufficient to know how to implement high-pass filters, i.e., high-boost filters can be easily formed based on high-pass filters.

3.4.2.1 Ideal High-Pass Filters

High-pass filters in the frequency domain are also defined using $D(u, v)$, the distance from the origin in the frequency domain, as follows:

$$H(u,v) = \begin{cases} 0 & D(u,v) \le D_0 \\ 1 & D(u,v) > D_0 \end{cases} \tag{3.18}$$

This definition simply states that the high-pass filter only allows the high frequency of the image to pass through the filter and that all of the other frequencies are blocked by the filter.

As in the low-pass filters, it is often preferred to use a smooth approximation of the high-pass filter such as high-pass Butterworth filter.

3.4.2.2 Butterworth High-Pass Filters

High-pass Butterworth filters are the straightforward extensions of the 1-D case, i.e.,

$$H(u,v) = \frac{1}{1+\left[D_0/D(u,v)\right]^2} \tag{3.19}$$

where $D(u, v)$ is the distance from the origin in the frequency domain.

3.5 SUMMARY

In this chapter, we discussed different methods of image filtering, restoration, and enhancement. We started with the discussion that image enhancement and filtering can be performed in either space or frequency domains. Space-domain techniques are divided into two categories. The first category includes point processing and histogram equalization, and the methods in the second group are implemented as mask filtering techniques. In the description of the frequency-domain processing methods, we explained different types of filters such as low-pass and high-pass filters. We also discussed the approximations of these filters using Butterworth functions.

PROBLEMS

3.1 We are to improve the quality of an image using a point processing transformation. The transformation function will have the general form:

$$s = a + be^{cr} \tag{3.20}$$

where
a, b, and c are constants
r and s are normalized gray levels in the original and processed images, respectively

The desired transformation will map $r = 0$ to $s = 0$, $r = 1$ to $s = 1$, and $r = 0.85$ to $s = 0.5$.

a. Calculate the values of a, b, and c that provide all desired specifications.
b. Apply the resulting transformation to the mouse vertebra image given in "p_3_1.jpg".* Note that the gray level of the original image is not normalized and that the gray levels in the image need to be normalized first. Show both images, and interpret the effects of the designed transformation on the image.

3.2 Read the MR image in "p_3_2.jpg".† This image shows the MRI of the brain. In almost all of the hospitals across the world, the MRI technology is used

* Courtesy of Dr. Helen Gruber, Carolina Medical Center, Charlotte, NC.
† From Goldberger, A.L. et al. (2000).

to capture a large number of brain images that need to be saved in physical medium such as a hard disk or a CD. Therefore, it is essential to compress these images to avoid the excessive cost of digital storage. Even though the image in this problem is already compressed (using JPEG technology), we would like to explore compressing this image using bit slicing.

a. Eliminate the three LSBs of the image and compare the quality of the resulting image with the original one.
b. Eliminate the four LSBs of the image and compare the quality of the resulting image with the original one.
c. Continue eliminating the bits as long as the quality of the resulting image is visually satisfactory. How many bits can be eliminated before the quality is unsatisfactory? What compression percentage is achieved?

3.3 Read the mouse vertebra image "p_3_3.jpg".* Using MATLAB, perform histogram equalization and compare the quality of the resulting equalized image with the original one.

3.4 Load the MRI image in "p_3_4.mat." This image is essentially the MRI image of Problem 3.2 that is corrupted by additive noise. As can be seen, the quality of the image is rather poor due to the noise. Conduct the following processing steps using MATLAB to improve the image quality:

a. Use the low-pass masks shown in Figure 3.10 to filter the image.
b. Compare the visual performance of the two masks.
c. Design a similar mask (by changing the numbers in the aforementioned masks) to outperform the masks used in part "a."
d. Use a 3×3 median filter to filter the image and compare the resulting image with those of the previous parts.

3.5 Load the image in "p_3_5.mat." In this image, we would like to improve the quality of the image by sharpening of the edges. Conduct the following processing steps using MATLAB:

a. Apply a high-boost filter on the image using A = 1, 1.05, 1.10, 1.15, and 1.20.
b. Compare the results of the part "b" and identify the value of A that gives the best performance.
c. Use a derivative filter to emphasize the edges and compare the results with those of part "a."
d. How would you modify the derivative filters for image improvement applications?

REFERENCE

Goldberger, A.L., Amaral, L.A.N., Glass, L., Hausdorff, J.M., Ivanov, P.Ch., Mark, R.G., Mietus, J.E., Moody, G.B., Peng, C.K., and Stanley, H.E. (2000, June 13). PhysioBank, PhysioToolkit, and PhysioNet: Components of a new research resource for complex physiologic signals. *Circulation* 101(23):e215–e220. [Circulation Electronic Pages; http://circ.ahajournals.org/cgi/content/full/101/23/e215].

* Courtesy of Dr. Helen Gruber, Carolina Medical Center, Charlotte, NC.

4 Edge Detection and Segmentation of Images

4.1 INTRODUCTION AND OVERVIEW

In medical image processing, as well as many other applications of image processing, it is necessary to identify the boundary between the objects in the image and separate the objects from each other. For example, when analyzing a cell image (captured by a microscope), it is vital to design image processing algorithms to segment the image and distinguish the objects in the cell from each other, for example, identify the contour of a nucleus. In many practical applications, segmentation and edge detection techniques allow separation of objects residing in an image and identify the boundary among them.

In principle, there are two approaches for edge detection and segmentation. In the first approach, differences and dissimilarities of pixels in two neighboring regions (objects) are exploited to segment the two regions, while, in the second approach, the similarities of the pixels within each region are used to separate the region from the neighboring regions. As can be seen, while the two approaches are based on rather related ideas, they apply different criteria. We discuss several examples of each of these two approaches in this chapter.

4.2 EDGE DETECTION

In this section, some of the main edge detection techniques, commonly used in biomedical image processing, are reviewed and compared with each other.

4.2.1 Sobel Edge Detection

The Sobel technique is one of the most popular edge detection techniques that is also computationally simple. In this technique, a 3 × 3 simple mask is used to magnify the differences among the points on the opposite sides of a boundary and eliminate the smooth gray-level changes in the pixels located on the same side of the boundary. The Sobel mask to magnify horizontal edges is as follows:

$$S_H = \begin{bmatrix} -1 & -2 & -1 \\ 0 & 0 & 0 \\ 1 & 2 & 1 \end{bmatrix} \tag{4.1}$$

Before describing the Sobel mask for detecting vertical lines, an example of the application of the horizontal Sobel mask mentioned earlier is provided that further illustrates the concept of the Sobel edge detection.

Example 4.1

In order to better understand how Sobel masks highlight edges, let us consider the image block shown in Figure 4.1a. The image has three gray levels: 0, 1, and 2, where level 0 represents a completely dark pixel, level 2 encodes a completely bright pixel, and level 1 illustrates points with medium gray-level intensity.

As it can be seen in Figure 4.1, there are two regions in the image and a border (edge) in between. Now, let us consider three pixels: pixel (4, 4) located on the edge and pixels (2, 4) and (6, 4) that are not located on the edge. For the pixels at coordinates (4, 4), (2, 4), and (6, 4), the gray level of the corresponding points in the edge-detected image using the Sobel mask will be 2, 0, and 0, respectively. Note that while the calculated value for the first point is 6, this value must be then floored to 2 since we have only three allowed gray levels. As the aforementioned numbers indicate, the resulting edge-enhanced image has a very small value for the points away from the edge (i.e., it sets the nonedge pixels to 0), while it has large gray levels for the pixels on the edge. In other words, the resulting edge-detected image shown in Figure 4.1b clearly highlights the edge between the two regions and replaces the points inside the regions on either side of the edge with 0.

As previously mentioned, the Sobel mask introduced in Equation 4.1 is capable of detecting horizontal edges. The Sobel mask that best extracts the vertical edges is as follows:

$$S_V = \begin{bmatrix} -1 & 0 & 1 \\ -2 & 0 & 2 \\ -1 & 0 & 1 \end{bmatrix} \tag{4.2}$$

In practical images such as medical images, very few edges are either vertical or horizontal. This implies that in real applications, a combination of the

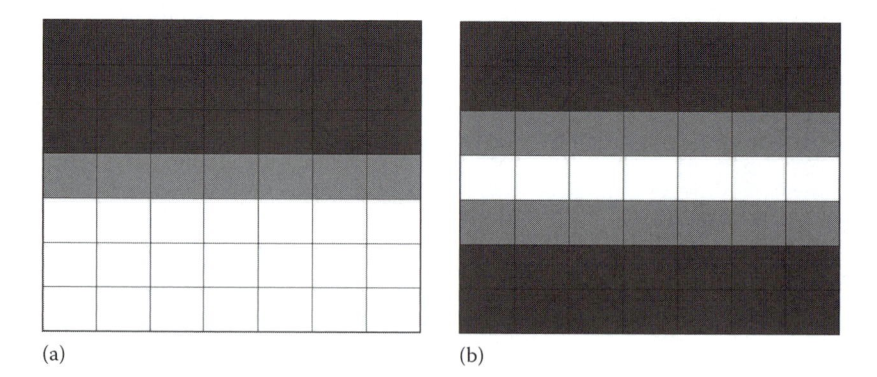

FIGURE 4.1 (a) Original image and (b) edge-enhanced image.

horizontal edge-detecting and vertical edge-detecting masks must be used to capture the edges. However, in small scale, any edge can be approximated by a number of short horizontal and vertical edge components that can be detected by the masks described earlier. As a result, in Sobel edge detection, the image is often divided into smaller blocks, and then, in each block, a combination of vertical and horizontal Sobel edge detection is performed. Then, the detected edges in smaller blocks are combined with each other to form the edges in the complete image.

In MATLAB®, Sobel edge detection is provided as one of the options in the command "edge". The application of this command is described in the following example:

Example 4.2

The following code reads an image called "image.jpg" and performs edge detection on the image using "edge" command. In "edge" command, one needs to determine which edge detection method is to be used. For example, here we use the option "sobel" to implement the Sobel method.

```
I = imread('image.jpg');
I = rgb2gray(I);
Imshow(I);
J = edge(I,'sobel');
Figure,
Imshow(J);
```

The image processed in this example is a photographic image of an intersection of the heart. As it can be seen in Figure 4.2, the edge-detected image (Figure 4.2b) extracts some of the edges in the original image.

While Sobel masks are used in some practical applications, they are known to be outperformed by two other edge detection methods such as Laplacian of Gaussian and Canny edge detection methods.

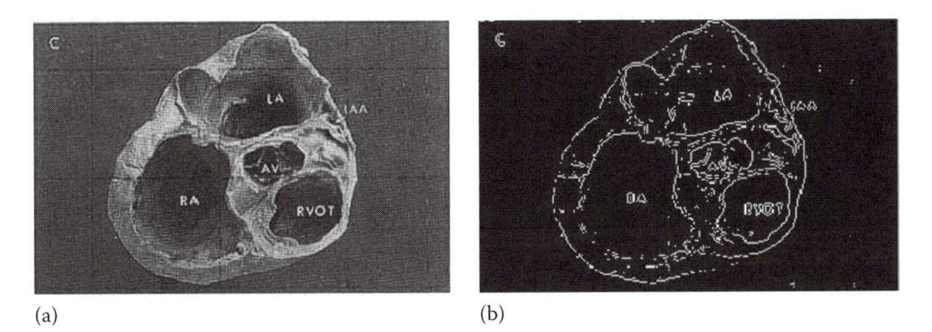

(a) (b)

FIGURE 4.2 (a) Original image and (b) edge-detected image. (Courtesy of Andre D'Avila, MD, Heart Institute (InCor), University of Sao Paulo, Medical School, Sao Paulo, Brazil.)

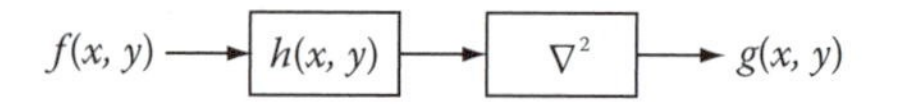

FIGURE 4.3 Schematic diagram of edge detection using Laplacian of Gaussian.

4.2.2 Laplacian of Gaussian Edge Detection

This edge detection technique, as the name may suggest, is a straightforward combination of a Laplacian operator and a Gaussian smoothing filter. The method is described in the block diagram of Figure 4.3.

In Figure 4.3, the Laplacian operator $\nabla^2(.)$ is defined as follows:

$$\nabla^2 f = \left(\frac{\partial f}{\partial x}\right)^2 + \left(\frac{\partial f}{\partial y}\right)^2 \tag{4.3}$$

In addition, the Gaussian low-pass filter, $h(x, y)$, is defined as follows:

$$h(x,y) = \exp\left(-\frac{x^2+y^2}{2\sigma^2}\right) \tag{4.4}$$

The use of a Laplacian operator for edge detection is inspired by the fact that for weak edges, the first derivatives (estimated in masks such as Sobel) may not be large enough to distinguish the edge points, and, therefore, a weak edge can go undetected by such methods. Taking the second derivate of the points or Laplacian amplifies the changes in the first derivative and therefore increases the chances of detecting a weak edge. However, the second derivative or Laplacian if used alone also magnifies the noise in the image, which increases the chances of detecting false edges. This is why a Gaussian smoothing filter, $h(x, y)$, is used to filter out the high-frequency noise before applying Laplacian operator.

Example 4.3

The following code reads "`image.jpg`" and performs edge detection on the image using "`edge`" command based on both Sobel and Laplacian of Gaussian methods. The option keyword in "`edge`" command that identifies Laplacian of Gaussian method is "`log`".

```
I = imread('image.jpg');
I = rgb2gray(I);
Imshow(I);
J = edge(I,'sobel');
Figure,
Imshow(J);
JL = edge(I,'log');
Figure,
Imshow(JL);
```

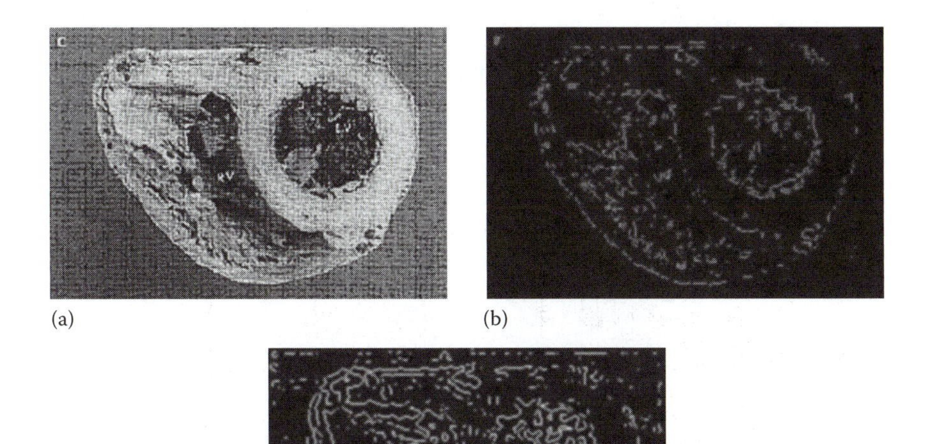

(a) (b)

(c)

FIGURE 4.4 (a) Original image, (b) edge-detected image using Sobel, and (c) edge-detected image using Laplacian of Gaussian. (Courtesy of Andre D'Avila, MD, Heart Institute (InCor), University of Sao Paulo, Medical School, Sao Paulo, Brazil.)

In Figure 4.4, the effect of Laplacian of Gaussian edge detection technique on the heart image is shown and compared with Sobel technique.

As can be seen, the Sobel method is clearly outperformed by the Laplacian of Gaussian method, as the edges discovered by Laplacian of Gaussian method are closer to the complete set of true edges in the image.

4.2.3 Canny Edge Detection

Canny edge detection is among the most popular edge detection techniques and has a number of specialized versions. All Canny edge detection systems, however, have the following four fundamental steps:

Step 1: The image is smoothed using a Gaussian filter (as defined earlier).

Step 2: The gradient magnitude and orientation are computed using finite-difference approximations for the partial derivatives (as discussed in the following).

Step 3: Non-maxima suppression is applied to the gradient magnitude to search for pixels that can identify the existence of an edge.

Step 4: A double thresholding algorithm is used to detect significant edges and link these edges.

The details of the aforementioned steps are given as follows. Assume that $I(i, j)$ denotes the image and $G(i, j, \sigma)$ is a Gaussian smoothing filter where σ is the spread of the Gaussian controlling the degree of smoothing. The output of the smoothing filter, $S(i, j)$, is related to the original image and the smoothing filter as follows:

$$S(i, j) = G(i, j) * I(i, j) \tag{4.5}$$

In the next step, in order to calculate the magnitude and orientation (direction) of the gradient vector, the gradient of the smoothed image is used to produce the horizontal and vertical partial (directional) derivatives $P(i, j)$ and $Q(i, j)$, respectively. These directional derivatives are calculated as follows:

$$P(i, j) \approx \frac{S(i, j+1) - S(i, j) + S(i+1, j+1) - S(i+1, j)}{2} \tag{4.6}$$

and

$$Q(i, j) \approx \frac{S(i, j) - S(i+1, j) + S(i, j+1) - S(i+1, j+1)}{2} \tag{4.7}$$

As it can be seen, $P(i, j)$ is calculated as the average of the horizontal derivate at pixels (i, j) and $(i + 1, j)$. The value of $Q(i, j)$ is calculated similarly using the average of the vertical derivative at pixels (i, j) and $(i, j + 1)$. The magnitude $M(i, j)$ and orientation $\theta(i, j)$ of the gradient vector are then given as follows:

$$M(i, j) = \sqrt{P(i, j)^2 + Q(i, j)^2} \tag{4.8}$$

and

$$\theta(i, j) = \tan^{-1}\left[\frac{Q(i, j)}{P(i, j)}\right] \tag{4.9}$$

In the third step, a thresholding operation is applied to identify the ridges of the edge pixels. In Canny method, an edge point is defined as a point whose gradient's magnitude identifies a local maximum in the direction of the gradient. The process of searching for such pixels, which is often called "non-maxima suppression," thresholds the gradient magnitude to find potential edge pixels. This step will result to an image $N(i, j)$, which is 0 except at the local maxima points.

After applying non-maxima suppression, there are often many false edge fragments in the image often caused by either noisy pixels or by edge-like fragments in the image that do not represent a true edge. To discard these false edge fragments, one can apply thresholds to $N(i, j)$ and set all of the values below the threshold value to 0. After thresholding, an array including the edges of the image, $I(i, j)$, is obtained. As the description of the thresholding step implies, the selection of the right threshold values is a sensitive choice. While small threshold values can allow many false

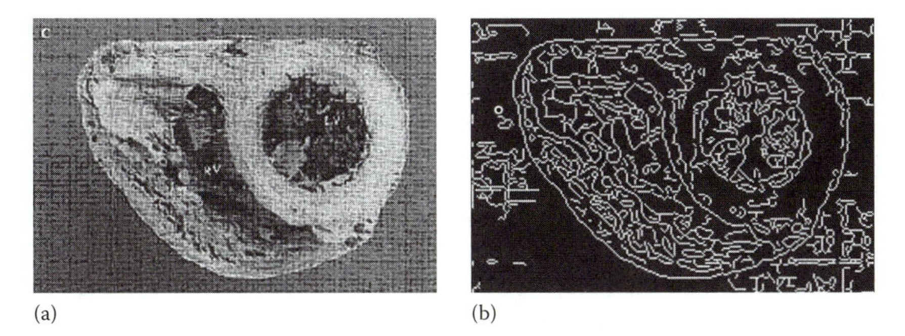

(a) (b)

FIGURE 4.5 (a) Original image and (b) Canny edge-detected image. (Courtesy of Andre D'Avila, MD, Heart Institute (InCor), University of Sao Paulo, Medical School, Sao Paulo, Brazil.)

edges, excessively large thresholds can miss the true edges. At this step, the surviving edge pixels are connected to each other to form complete edges.

As mentioned earlier, there are many varieties of Canny edge detection methods. In this chapter, we focus on using MATLAB for Canny edge detection.

Example 4.4

In this example, the heart image used in the previous example is edge detected using Canny edge detection method. The option "canny" in "edge" command identifies Canny method. The MATLAB codes are as follows:

```
I = imread('image.jpg');
I = rgb2gray(I);
Imshow(I);
J = edge(I,'canny');
Figure,
Imshow(J);
```

The results shown in Figure 4.5 indicate the strength and capabilities of Canny edge detectors. As can be seen, the performance of this edge detection method is almost comparable with that of Laplacian of Gaussian. This is the reason that in the majority of medical image processing applications either Laplacian of Gaussian or Canny method is used for the standard edge detection step.

4.3 IMAGE SEGMENTATION

In almost all biomedical image processing applications, it is necessary to separate different regions and objects in an image. In fact, image segmentation is considered as the most sensitive step in many medial image processing applications. For instance, in processing of cytological samples, we need to segment an image into regions corresponding to nuclei, cytoplasm, and background pixels. The main techniques for image segmentation are introduced in the following sections.

As described earlier, the image segmentation techniques can be classified into two general categories. In the first category of techniques, segmentation is conducted based on the discontinuity of the points across two regions, while, in the second group of segmentation methods, the algorithms exploit the similarities among the points in the same region for segmentation. We first focus on the first category.

The main methods in the first category include detecting gray-level discontinuities such as points, lines, and edges. Another popular method in the first category is thresholding. In thresholding, a part of the image is selected based on its gray-level difference from the other parts of the image. Here, we first introduce some methods for detection of points and lines in an image. Then, we will describe image segmentation methods that detect regions and objects in an image using thresholding ideas.

4.3.1 Point Detection

In point detection methods, the intention is to detect the isolated points in an image. The main factor that can help us detect these isolated points or pixels is the difference between their gray levels and gray levels of their neighboring pixels. This observation suggests using masks that magnify these differences to distinguish these points from the surrounding pixels. The mask shown in Figure 4.6 is simply designed to amplify the gray-level differences of the center pixel from its neighbors.

If the value obtained by applying this mask to a pixel is shown as F, then based on this value one can decide whether the pixel is an isolated one or not. In practical applications, it is often the case that the value F is compared with a prespecified threshold T. Formally speaking, for any point in the image, the point detection method checks the following condition:

$$F \geq T \tag{4.10}$$

If the condition holds, then the point is marked as an isolated point that stands out and needs to be investigated. While in biomedical image processing applications many singular points in images are caused by "salt and pepper" type of noise, some isolated pixels (or small cluster of pixels) can represent small abnormalities (e.g., small tumors in early stages of growth). This emphasizes the importance of point detection methods.

−1	−1	−1
−1	8	−1
−1	−1	−1

FIGURE 4.6 Mask for point detection. (Courtesy of David Malin Images, Anglo-Australian Observatory [AAO], Epping, New South Wales, Australia. http://www.davidmalin.com).

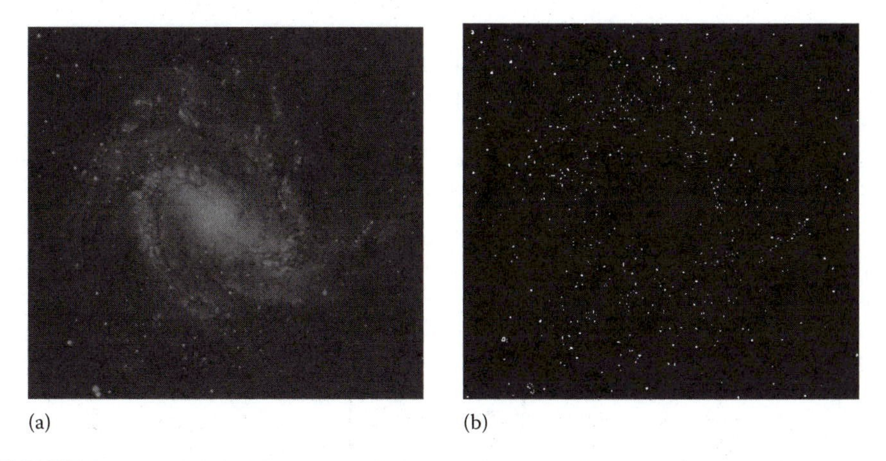

(a) (b)

FIGURE 4.7 (a) Original image and (b) image after point detection.

Example 4.5

In this example, we show how to use MATLAB to detect singular points in a typical image in astronomy. We first apply the mask shown in Figure 4.6 and then compare the response of the pixels in the image with a threshold value. In this example, the threshold value is set to 90% of the maximum observed gray-level value in the image. Figure 4.7 shows the original image and the image after point detection.

```
I = imread('synthetic.jpg');
I = rgb2gray(I);
Maxpix = max(max(I));
H = [-1 -1 -1;-1 8 -1;-1 -1 -1];
Sharpened = imfilter(I,H);
Maxpix = double(Maxpix);
Sharpened = (sharpened > .9*Maxpix);
Imshow(I);
Figure,
Imshow(sharpened);
```

The main singular points in the original image are highlighted and shown in the processed image.

4.3.2 Line Detection

Line detection methods are designed using a variety of line detection masks that are useful in magnifying and detecting horizontal lines, vertical line, or lines with any prespecified angles (e.g., 45°).

Figure 4.8 shows four masks that can be used for detecting horizontal lines, vertical lines, rising lines with the angle of 45°, and falling lines with the angle of –45°. For example, the first mask in Figure 4.8 that detects horizontal lines sweeps through the image enhancing and magnifies the horizontal lines.

−1	−1	−1
2	2	2
−1	−1	−1

−1	2	−1
−1	2	−1
−1	2	−1

−1	−1	2
−1	2	−1
2	−1	−1

2	−1	−1
−1	2	−1
−1	−1	2

FIGURE 4.8 Line detection masks. From left to right: horizontal lines, vertical lines, rising lines with 45° angle, and falling lines with −45° angle.

In practical application, for each single point in the image, the masks for all four directions are applied. Then, through a thresholding on the response for each point, the algorithm decides whether the point belongs to a line in a specific direction or not. Often, only the line with maximum mask response will be chosen as the line the point belongs to.

Example 4.6

In this example, we illustrate the effects of the line detection masks introduced in Figure 4.8 on a satellite image. In MATLAB, code for this example is shown as follows. In the first few lines of the code, we define the first three masks of Figure 4.8 and then we apply these masks to the original image.

```
I = imread('18.jpg');
I = rgb2gray(I);
Hh = [-1 -1 -1;2 2 2;-1 -1 -1];
Hv = [-1 2 -1;-1 2 -1;-1 2 -1];
H45 = [-1 -1 2;-1 2 -1;2 -1 -1];
Hlinedetected = imfilter(I,Hh);
Vlinedetected = imfilter(I,Hv);
Line45detected = imfilter(I,H45);
Imshow(I);
Figure,
Imshow(Hlinedetected);
Figure,
Imshow(Vlinedetected);
Figure,
Imshow(Line45detected);
```

Figure 4.9 shows an image of the vascular system and images after line detection. It can be seen that in the image of Figure 4.9b, most of the horizontal lines representing the horizontally oriented blood vessels have been detected. Similarly, most of the vertical lines have been detected in the image of Figure 4.9c. The image in Figure 4.9d extracts the diagonal lines from the original image. There is nothing special about the 3 × 3 size of the defined masks, and the masks can be extended to larger masks such as 5 × 5 and 7 × 7 line detection masks.

4.3.3 Region and Object Segmentation

Previously, we discussed the detection of points and lines in an image. Next, we focus on processing techniques to distinguish and detect regions representing different objects. These methods are particularly important for biomedical image

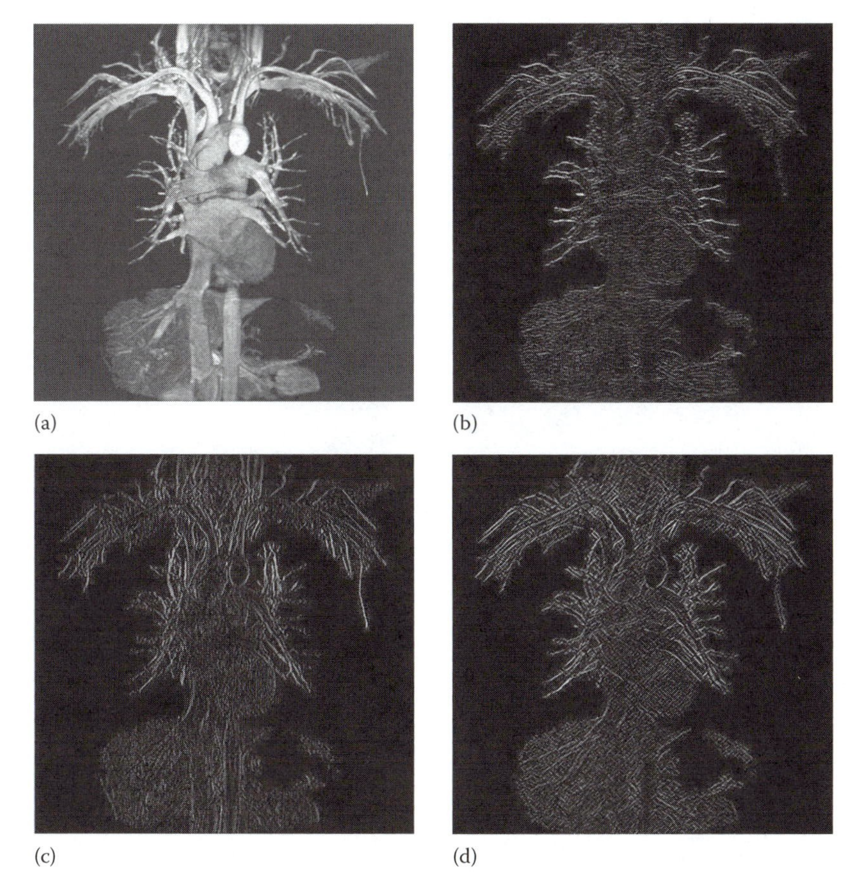

FIGURE 4.9 (a) Original image, (b) image after horizontal line detection, (c) image after vertical line detection, and (d) image after 45° line detection. (Courtesy of Andre D'Avila, MD, Heart Institute (InCor), University of Sao Paulo, Medical School, Sao Paulo, Brazil.)

processing because in a typical medical image analysis, one needs to detect regions representing objects, such as tumors, from the background. Next, we describe two general methods for region and object detection.

4.3.3.1 Region Segmentation Using Luminance Thresholding

In many biomedical images, the pixels in the objects of interest have gray levels that are either greater or smaller than the gray levels of the background pixels. In these images, one can simply extract the objects of interest from the background using the differences in the gray level. When the object is bright and the background is dark (or vice versa), separating the interested object from the image can be performed with a simple thresholding of histogram as described in the following.

Figure 4.10 shows a synthetic cell image that contains cells that are much darker than the bright background. Also, Figure 4.10 shows the histogram of this, which shows two almost entirely separate peaks and intervals in the histogram.

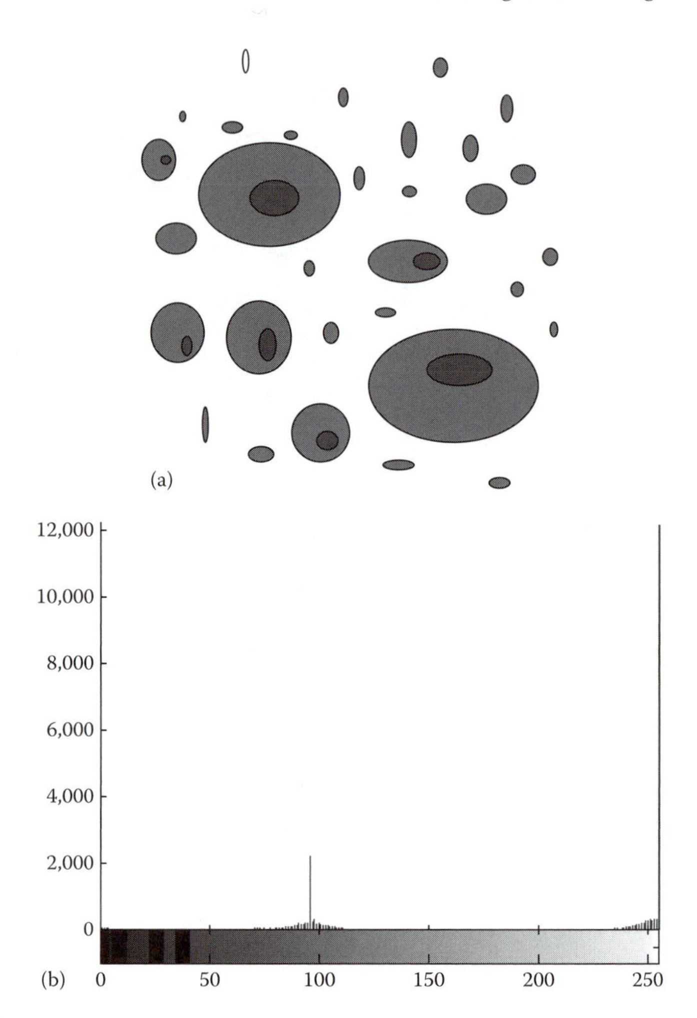

FIGURE 4.10 (a) Original image and (b) image histogram.

Specifically, the histogram contains a very strong bright region in the far right-hand side of the graph that represents the background, moderately bright region representing the cytoplasm, and a small dark interval close to the origin that represents the nuclei. This separation indicates that the three parts of the histogram can be rather easily separated from each other by thresholding.

While in the synthetic images, such as the one shown in Figure 4.10, the separation process is rather easy; in real biomedical images, the gray-level separation process is often much more complicated. This fuzziness occurs because in such images both the background and the interested object often occupy gray-level ranges that overlap with each other. In such cases, a simple thresholding may not work at all. In addition, in images with poor illumination, it might be difficult to segment histogram of the image into two parts, and again, a simple thresholding process may not provide desirable results.

A typical solution for these problems is dividing the original image into some subimages in such a way that the histogram of each subimage can be easily separated into two parts with a simple thresholding process. This means that for each subimage one must select a suitable threshold to segment the histogram of that subimage into two parts. Then, the segmented subimages are put together to form the overall segmented image. The bottleneck of this method is designing a reasonable process to divide the original image into subimages. Selecting threshold values for the resulting subimages is another issue to be dealt with.

4.3.3.2 Region Growing

The methods introduced so far belonged to the first category of segmentation algorithms. These methods are based on finding differences and boundaries between parts of an image. In other words, the methods discussed earlier use discontinuities among gray levels of entities in an image (e.g., point, line, edge, and region) to segment different parts of the image. In this section, we focus on the second category of segmentation techniques that attempt to find segmented regions of the image using the similarities of the points inside image regions.

In region growing methods, segmentation often starts by selecting a seed pixel for each region in the image. Seed pixels are often chosen close to the center of the region or object. For example, if we are to segment a tumor from the background, it is always advisable to select the seed point for the tumor in the middle of the tumor and the seed point for the background somewhere deep in the background region. Then, the region growing algorithm expands each region based on a criterion, which is defined to determine similarity between pixels of each region. This means that starting from the seed points and using the criterion, algorithm decides whether the neighboring pixels are similar enough to the other points in the region, and if so, these neighboring pixels are assigned to the same region that the seed point belongs to. This process is performed on every pixel in each region until all the points in the image are covered.

The most important factors in region growing are selecting a suitable similarity criterion and starting from a suitable set of seed points. Selecting similarity criteria mainly depends on the type of the application in hand. For example, for the monochrome (gray level) images, similarity criterion is often based on the gray-level features and spatial properties such as moments or textures.

Example 4.7

In this example, a subimage shown in Figure 4.11a is segmented through growing of the seed points for the two regions shown in Figure 4.11a. The range of gray level in this image is from 0 to 8. As can be seen, the gray level of each pixel is also shown in Figure 4.3a, and the seed points are marked by red-underlined gray levels. In this example, the similarity criterion is defined as follows: two neighboring pixels (i.e., horizontal, vertically, or diagonally neighboring pixels) belong to the same region if the absolute difference of their gray levels is less than $T = 3$. With this criterion and starting the identified seeds in Figure 4.11a, the segmented image of Figure 4.11b is obtained.

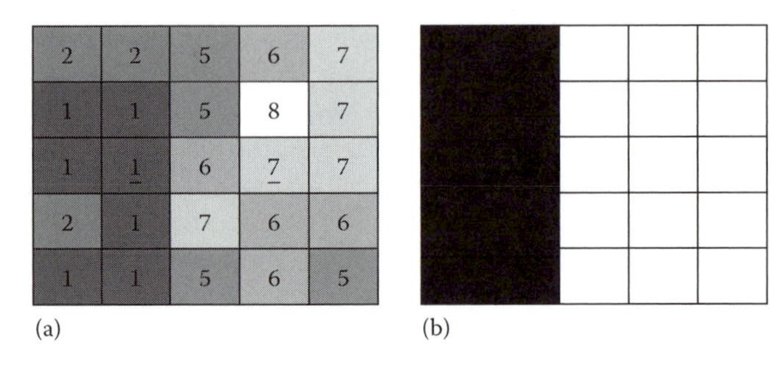

FIGURE 4.11 (a) Subimage with only the seed points and (b) segmented subimage using region growing method.

In Figure 4.11b, one region is represented by a completely dark gray level (i.e., 0) and another by a completely bright gray level (i.e., 8). As it can be seen, the resulting segmented image is truly representing two regions in the subimage.

For region growing segmentation of color images, color features are often used as the similarity criteria. Another choice in region growing is how to stop the growing of regions. As mentioned earlier, the region growing algorithm is often stopped when there are no other pixels satisfying the similarity criteria of segmentation.

4.3.3.3 Quad-Trees

A more sophisticated region segmentation algorithm that does not rely on a set of seed pixels for segmentation is called a quad-tree. In a typical quad-tree algorithm, unlike the region growing, the algorithm does not start segmentation from the initial seeds; rather, this method divides the image into a set of disjointed regions and then uses splitting and merging of pixels or regions to obtain the segmented regions that satisfy a prespecified criterion. This criterion is essentially the same as the similarity criterion that identifies the range of gray-level variations for a region, as shown in the previous example. In quad-tree methods, if the gray levels of the pixels in two regions are not in the same range, they are assumed to belong to different objects, and, therefore, the region is split into a number of subregions.

To see this more clearly, let us presume that the entire image is initially marked as one region only, R. First, the algorithm divides the entire region R into some subregions R_i. Since in quad-trees a region is often split into four quadrants, the method is named as quad-trees. Then, the algorithm makes it sure that each quadrant region R_i is truly different from the other subregions (based on the defined criterion). If the pixel values in some of these subregions are not different enough from each other, these corresponding subregions are merged with each other again; otherwise, they are left as different regions. The algorithm continues dividing the image into smaller parts until, based on the defined condition, no more splitting of regions is possible. If the algorithm only splits regions, in the end it will produce some adjacent regions that are almost identical and must be merged with each other. Therefore, it is often the case that after splitting is complete, the algorithm merges the adjacent regions that have identical or similar properties to obtain more continuous regions.

Quad-tree algorithms are often too computationally time consuming and less accurate than the previously discussed method such as seed growing algorithm. This is primarily due to the fact that they do not require seed points. However, in biomedical image processing, it is often the case that physicians have reliable estimates of the seed points that can be used for simple seed growing methods. This fact rather eliminates the need for quad-trees in many biomedical applications. In addition, since in medical diagnostics physicians prefer to supervise and control the segmentation and classification steps (as opposed to completely relying on machine decision), supervised region growing with seeds has proved to be more applicable than fully automated quad-trees for medical applications.

4.4 SUMMARY

In this chapter, we discussed the computational techniques used for edge detection and segmentation of images. While many edge detection and segmentation methods are based on differences among pixels and regions, there are a number of methods that utilize the similarities for segmentations. In this chapter, we covered the main segmentation methods in each of the two groups. We also gave MATLAB examples and simulations for the introduced methods.

PROBLEMS

4.1 Load the image in the file "p_4_1.mat" and show the image. This image is a fluoroscopic image of the heart and a catheter that is inserted in the blood vessels. In such images, it is desirable to extract the edges and lines representing important objects such as blood vessels and catheter.

a. Apply horizontal Sobel mask to extract horizontal edges in the image. Show the resulting image.
b. Apply vertical Sobel mask to extract vertical edges in the image. Show the resulting image.
c. Apply Laplacian of Gaussian method to extract all edges in the image. Show the resulting image.
d. Apply Canny edge detection method to extract all edges in the image. Show the resulting image.
e. Compare the results of the previous sections and comments on the differences. Which method can highlight the catheter more effectively?

4.2 Load the image in the file "p_4_2.mat" and show the image. This image is also a fluoroscopic image of the heart and a catheter inserted in the blood vessels. As mentioned earlier, in fluoroscopic images, the objective is to highlight the lines formed by important objects such as blood vessels and catheter.

a. Apply horizontal line detection mask to highlight the horizontal linear objects and show the resulting image.
b. Apply vertical line detection mask to highlight the vertical linear objects and show the resulting image.
c. Apply the mask for detection of rising lines with the angle of 45° line to highlight these linear objects and show the resulting image.

d. Apply the mask for detection of falling lines with the angle of −45° line to highlight these linear objects and show the resulting image.
e. Explain what object(s) in the image each of the masks was able to extract or highlight the best. Which mask was the most useful mask for this image?

4.3 In description of the Laplacian of Gaussian edge detection method, we use two subsystems, i.e., Laplacian and Gaussian smoothing in series. Combine the two subsystems to describe the entire edge detection method with one mathematical expression. (*Hint*: Apply the Laplacian operator on the Gaussian smoothing function.)

4.4 Load the image in the file "p_4_4.mat" and show the image. This image represents the 2-D representation of the 3-D reconstruction of multislice tomographic image of a large part of the cardiovascular system. Repeat all steps of Problem 4.2 for this image.

4.5 Load the image in the file "p_4_5.mat" and show the image. This is a photographic image of the heart in which different objects such as arteries and veins of the heart are shown. Note the areas marked as SVC, AAO, PV, RB, RBA, LB, PA, DAO, and LPA. For each of these regions, find the coordinates of a seed point inside the region that well represents the region. Then, design a suitable similarity criterion based on the gray-level ranges of the regions mentioned. Using the seeds and the similarity criterion, perform seed growing to segment the image. Discuss the results.

5 Wavelet Transform

5.1 INTRODUCTION AND OVERVIEW

This chapter is dedicated to the concepts and applications of the wavelet transform (WT). The WT has become an essential tool for all types of signal and image processing applications as this transformation provides capabilities that may not be achieved by other transformations. We start this chapter with justifying the need for such a transform and then take an intuitive approach toward the definition of the WT.

5.2 FROM FT TO STFT

Despite the numerous capabilities of the Fourier transform (FT), there exists a serious concert over the use of the FT for certain applications. This concern can be better described using the following examples.

Example 5.1

Consider the two time signals shown in Figure 5.1. Each of the signals is formed of three sinusoidal components with the same duration. The only difference between the two signals is the order at which these sinusoidal components appear in the signal. It is evident that order or relative location of these three components is indeed an important characteristic that allows differentiating the two signals from each other.

Next, we calculate the magnitude of the discrete Fourier transform (DFT) for these two signals, as in Figure 5.2. As can be seen in Figure 5.2, the magnitude of the DFT for the two signals is exactly the same. In other words, if we limit ourselves only to the magnitude of the DFT, all the information regarding the order of the three sinusoidal components is lost.

Before leaving this example, we have to emphasize that the order information is not truly lost; rather, the order information is contained in the phase of the DFT of the signals. In other words, if someone observes and interprets the phase of the two signals, he or she must be able to discover the order of the three sinusoidal components, even though this may not be an easy task at all. However, as mentioned in the previous chapters, interpreting and dealing with the phase of the DFT of a signal is often considered as a relatively difficult task and one would rather focus on the magnitude of DFT only.

In the next example, the shortcomings of relying only on the magnitude of the FT are further emphasized.

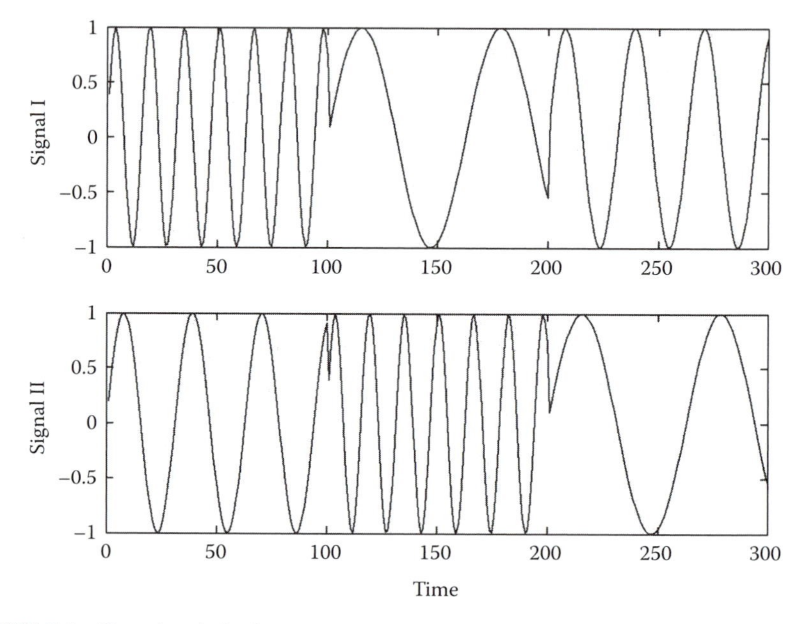

FIGURE 5.1 Two signals in time.

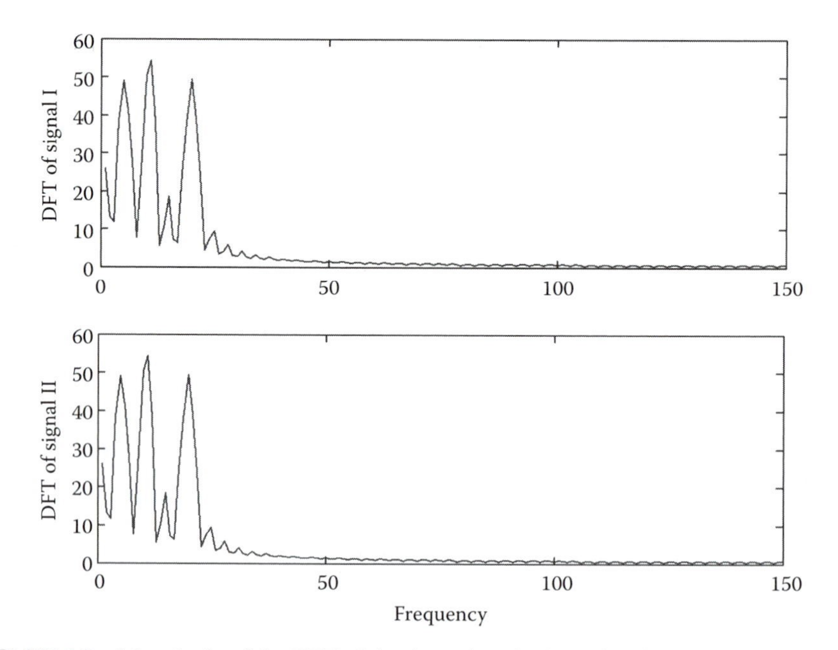

FIGURE 5.2 Magnitude of the DFT of the three signals shown in Figure 5.1.

Example 5.2

Consider the signals shown in Figure 5.3a and b. As can be seen, the signal in Figure 5.3a is a rectangular pulse that starts very close to the origin while the second pulse shown in Figure 5.3b begins at a much later time.

While these two pulses are very different from each other (i.e., they start and end at different times), as can be seen in Figure 5.3c and d, the magnitude of their DFT is exactly the same. Even though one could distinguish these two signals from the phase of their DFT, as we discussed before, in typical signal and image processing applications, we often like to work with the magnitude of the DFT, and if we do so, we lose the pulse localization information.

The problem observed in the earlier examples can be restated as follows: Focusing only on the magnitude of FT, the localization of the information is lost. In other words, from the magnitude of FT, one cannot identify when and in what order "events" are occurring. In Example 5.1, if we define our events as the exact times a particular sinusoidal variation starts and ends, then the event localization information is lost in the magnitude of FT.

Next, we attempt to define a new version of the FT in which the time localization is preserved. This attempt leads us to the definition of a particular form of the FT called the short-time Fourier transform or STFT. For a signal $x(t)$, the STFT is defined as

$$X_{\mathrm{STFT}}(a,f) = \int_{-\infty}^{+\infty} x(t)g^*(t-a)e^{-j2\pi ft}dt \tag{5.1}$$

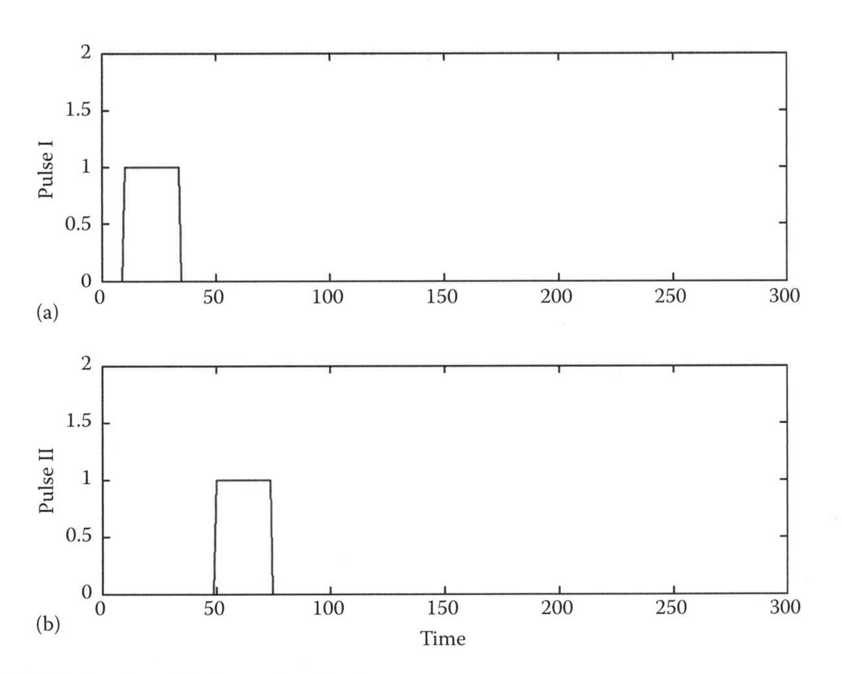

FIGURE 5.3 (a and b) Two pulses in time.

(continued)

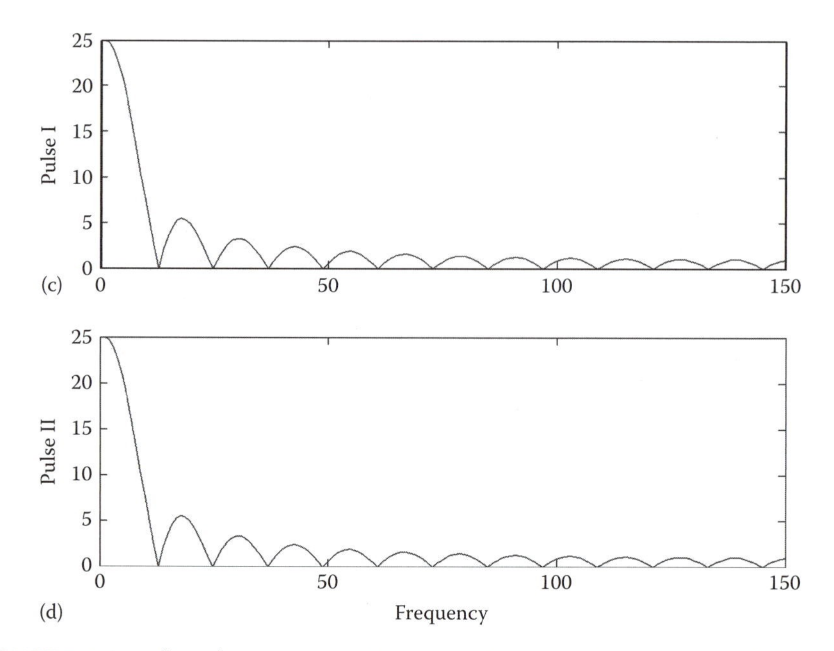

FIGURE 5.3 (continued) (c and d) The magnitude of the FT of the two pulses in time shown in (a) and (b).

In the previous definition, $g(t - a)$ is a shifted version of a time window (gate) $g(t)$ that extracts a portion of the signal $x(t)$. In other words, the gate $g(t - a)$, having a limited time span, selects and extracts only a portion of the signal $x(t)$ to be analyzed by the FT. This time window is often a real-time function, and, therefore,

$$g^*(t - a) = g(t - a) \tag{5.2}$$

Simply put, in STFT, a time window selects a portion of $x(t)$ and then the regular FT is calculated for this selected part of the signal. By changing the amount of shift parameter a, one obtains not only the FT of every part of the signal, but also the time localization of each part as these portions are extracted at known time intervals identified by the shift factor a. In other words, the STFT analyzes both time and frequency information of every selected portion of the signal. However, as evident from the earlier definition, the STFT has two parameters, f and a. This means that there is more computation (compared to FT) involved in the process. The following examples explain how the STFT partially addresses the issues we had with the FT.

Example 5.3

Consider the signal shown in Figure 5.4. The signal contains two time-limited events, namely, a triangular pulse centered around $t = 1$ and a sinusoidal variation starting at $t = 8$.

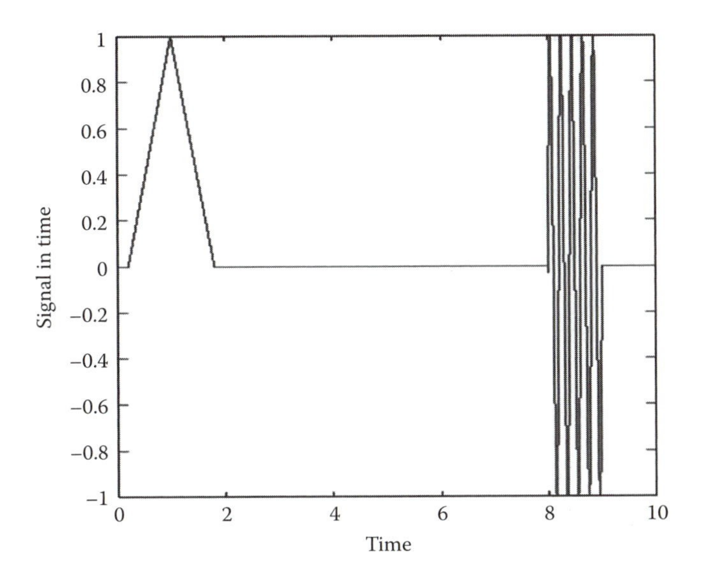

FIGURE 5.4 A given time signal with two time events.

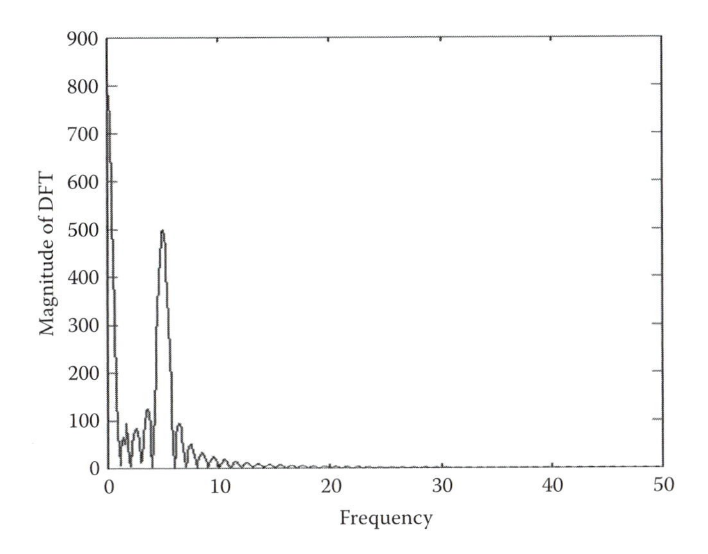

FIGURE 5.5 FT of the signal in Figure 5.4.

As one can expect, the FT of the signal would "mask" the order and localization of the two time events, as shown in Figure 5.5.

Now, we calculate the STFT for this signal for some values of a. The time gate used for this analysis, i.e., $g(t)$, is shown in Figure 5.6. This rectangular window is among the most popular windows used for the STFT.

The magnitude of the STFT of the signal for $a = 1$ is shown in Figure 5.7a. As can be seen, the shifted gate captures the first time event, the triangular pulse, and calculates the frequency contents of this event.

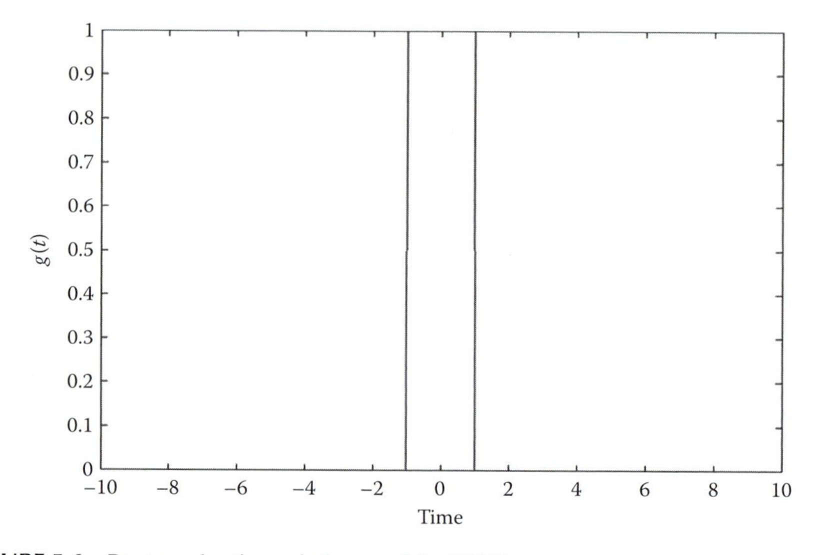

FIGURE 5.6 Rectangular time window used for STFT.

For the shift values $3 \le a \le 7$, the STFT will be zero as the shifted window captures a zero part of the signal that contains no time events. For $a = 8$ (Figure 5.7b), the STFT captures the second event in the signal, i.e., the sinusoidal variations.

Again, for $10 \le a \le +\infty$, no event is captured by the STFT, and, therefore, no particular information is in this part of the signal.

As can be seen in the previous example, the STFT seems to address the disadvantage of the FT being blind to the time localization. In reality, several different types of time windows are used for the STFT. These popular windows include triangular windows as well as trapezoidal windows. Such windows, even though distort the amplitude of the extracted portion of the signal, assign more

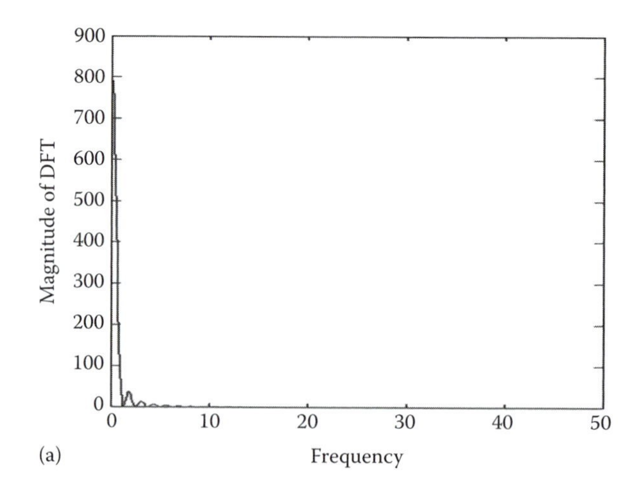

FIGURE 5.7 (a) Magnitude of STFT for $a = 1$.

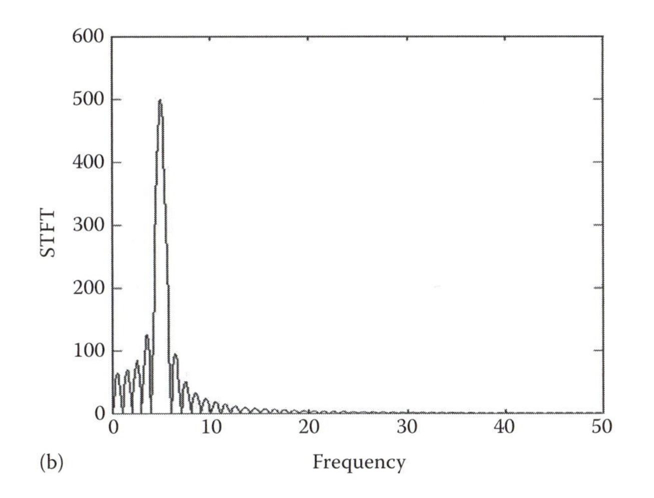

FIGURE 5.7 (continued) (b) The magnitude of STFT for $a = 8$.

weight to the central part of the captured events and therefore reduce the negative effect of the overlap between the neighboring events. Such windows are becoming more popular in analysis of the biomedical signals in which events often overlap and one may need to attempt to separate the events from each other using triangular windows.

Despite the favorable properties of the STFT, this transform is not the best solution to address the time and frequency localization of the signal events. The first simple factor that identifies the shortcomings of the STFT is the choice of the window length. A too short window may not capture the entire duration of an event, while a too long window may capture two or more events in the same shift. For instance, consider the signal in Example 5.3 and a window with duration 0.1. Such a time window would never capture any of the events mentioned earlier even in its entirety. At the same time, a time window with duration 10 could never capture only one of the events without including at least a part of another event. In practice, we would like to capture all events with any duration without supervising the transformation (i.e., without manually adjusting the length of the window). This disadvantage of the STFT calls for another transform in which all window sizes are tested.

Another disadvantage of the STFT deals with the nature of the basis functions used in the FT, i.e., complex exponentials. The term $e^{-j2\pi ft}$ describes sinusoidal variations in real and complex spaces. Such sinusoidal functions exist in all times and are not limited in time span or duration. However, by definition, events are variations that are typically limited in time, i.e., they start at a certain point in time and end at another. The fact that the sinusoidal basis functions that are time unlimited are used to analyze the time-limited variations (i.e., events) explains why the STFT may not be the best solution for even detection. At this point in our search for an ideal transformation for even detection, it makes perfect sense to use time-limited basis functions to decompose and analyze the time-limited events.

These two disadvantages of the STFT lead us to the definition of the WT that is extremely useful for biomedical applications.

5.3 ONE-DIMENSIONAL CONTINUOUS WAVELET TRANSFORM

Before introducing WT, we need to take a closer look at the basic definition of "frequency" as the fundamental concept of the FT. We need to focus on the definition of frequency at this point because we are to use time-limited basis functions for the new transform as opposed to the periodic time-unlimited functions used in the FT. This means that since we will not be using periodic sinusoidal basis functions for the new transform, we need to think of a concept that replaces frequency. Time-limited basis functions are obviously not periodic, and therefore, we need to invent a new concept that can represent a concept similar to frequency.

In order to find a replacement for frequency, we need to see what interesting features are captured by frequency. Consider a sinusoidal basis function with frequency 0.1 Hz. Having a basis function with this frequency, another basis function in the Fourier decomposition of the signal would be the second harmonic of this basis function, i.e., a sinusoidal basis function with frequency 0.2 Hz. The harmonic relation among the basis signals is the fundamental concept of signal transformation and decomposition. Therefore, the relation among harmonics is something that we need to somehow represent by our new concept that will replace frequency.

In order to find this new concept, we make the following important observation about harmonics: warping the time axis "t" allows us to obtain the harmonics from the original signal, for example, replacing the time axis "t" in the original signal with "$2t$" time axis results in the second harmonic. This is essentially "scaling" the signal in time to generate other basis functions. We claim here that the main characteristic of harmonic frequencies can be drawn from a more general concept that we call "scale." Scale, as a replacement of frequency, can reflect the same interesting properties in terms of the harmonic relation among the basis functions. The interesting part is that unlike frequency that is defined only for periodic signals, scale is equally applicable to nonperiodic signals. This proves that we have found a new concept, i.e., scale, to replace frequency. Using scale as a variable, the new transform, which will be based on time-limited basis function, can be meaningfully applied to both time-unlimited and time-limited signals.

With the introduction provided earlier, we are ready to define the continuous wavelet transform (CWT) of a time signal $x(t)$ as follows:

$$W_{\Psi,X}(a,b) = \frac{1}{\sqrt{|a|}} \int_{-\infty}^{+\infty} x(t)\Psi^*\left(\frac{t-b}{a}\right)dt, \quad a \neq 0 \tag{5.3}$$

In this equation, which is also referred to as the CWT analysis equation, $\Psi(t)$ is a function with limited duration in time, b is the shifting parameter, and a is the scaling parameter (replacing frequency parameter f). As can be seen, the basis functions of the CWT are the shifted and scaled version of the $\Psi(t)$, i.e., $\Psi^*((t-a)/b)$. Due to the central role of the function $\Psi(t)$ in generating the basis functions of the

CWT, this function is often referred to as the mother wavelet. In addition, now it becomes clearer why this transformation is called "wavelet transform." A closer look at the definition of the mother wavelet tells that this function must be limited in duration and therefore looks like a decaying small wave. All other basis functions are the shifted and scaled version of the mother wavelet. In contrast with the STFT, instead of using sinusoidal functions in order to generate the basis functions, a mother wavelet is continuously shifted and scaled to create all basis functions in CWT.

Now that we have discussed the analysis equation or the CWT, it is the best time to describe the synthesis equation that allows forming the time signal based on its WT. The inverse continuous wavelet transform or ICWT is defined as

$$x(t) = \frac{C_{\Psi}^{-1}}{a^2} \int_{-\infty}^{+\infty} \int_{-\infty}^{+\infty} W_{\Psi,X}(a,b)\Psi\left(\frac{t-b}{a}\right) da\, db, \qquad a \neq 0 \tag{5.4}$$

In this equation, C_{Ψ}^{-1} is a constant whose value depends on the exact choice of the mother wavelet $\Psi(t)$. As can be seen, while the CWT equation is a single integral, the ICWT is a double integral based on two dummy variables a and b.

Every choice of the mother wavelet gives a particular CWT, and as a result, we are dealing with infinite number of transformations under the same name CWT (as opposed to only one transform for the continuous Fourier transform [CFT]). Any choice of the mother wavelet gives certain unique properties that make the resulting transformation a suitable choice for a particular task. A mother wavelet called Mexican hat is shown in Figure 5.8. The reason this mother wavelet is called Mexican hat (or sombrero) is evident from its waveform. The waveform represented by this signal is the general shape of the most popular mother wavelets.

Daubechies (dbX) wavelets are among the most popular mother wavelets that are commonly used in signal and image processing. The index "X" in dbX identifies the exact formulation of the function. These mother wavelets are simply the functions

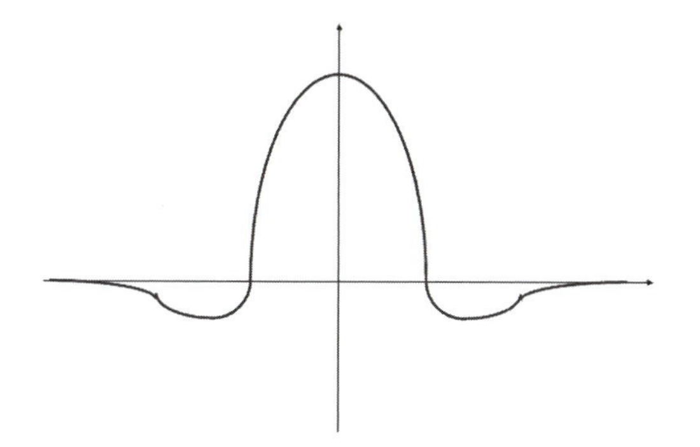

FIGURE 5.8 Mexican hat mother wavelet.

belonging to parameterized family of functions that have different levels of complexity. For example, while all dbX functions look more or less similar, db2 is a simpler mother wavelet than db3 or db4. As a rule of thumb, more complex mother wavelet may be needed to analyze more complex signals. For instance, in order to process medical signals such as ECG, one would limit X to 10 or 15, while, in processing of complex signals such as speech signals, much more complex mother wavelets such as db30 or even higher provide better performances.

Other popular mother wavelets are Mexican hat or sombrero (as shown previously), Coiflets, Symlets, Morlet, and Meyer. The details about the exact mathematical definition of these functions are outside the scope of this book, and the interested readers are referred to the introduced references for further studies. In this book, we will focus on the applications of the wavelets for biomedical signal processing.

The most logical question at this point is how to choose a mother wavelet for a particular application. This question, to the most part, is an open problem, and it does not appear to have a definite answer. However, two intuitive rules of thumb are widely followed when choosing a mother wavelet: (1) complex mother wavelets are needed for complex signals (as discussed earlier) and (2) the mother wavelet that resembles the general shape of the signal to be analyzed would be a more suitable choice.

As in the CFT, there are some major issues with the CWT that encourages the invention and use of a discrete version of the CWT. While some of the concerns are the same as the concerns applicable to the CFT (such as the dominance of the digital processing and storage systems), the CWT suffers from a more computationally serious problem. A closer look at the CWT reveals that this transformation requires the calculations based on all continuous shifts and all continuous scales. This obviously makes the computational complexity of the CWT and the ICWT unsuitable for many practically important applications. This leads us to the discrete version of this transform.

5.4 ONE-DIMENSIONAL DISCRETE WAVELET TRANSFORM

Discrete wavelet transform (DWT) accepts continuous signals and applies only discrete shifts and scales to form the transform. This means that if the original signal is sampled with a suitable set of scaling and shifting, the entire continuous signal can be reconstructed from the DWT. In order to see how this is done, we start with providing the equations for the DWT. Define

$$a_{jk} = a_0^j, \quad b_{jk} = ka_0^j T \tag{5.5}$$

where

T is the sampling time
a_0 is a positive nonzero constant

Also define

$$\Psi_{jk}(t) = \frac{1}{\sqrt{a_{jk}}}\Psi\left(\frac{t-b_{jk}}{a_{jk}}\right) = a_0^{-j/2}\,\Psi\left(a_0^{-j}t - kT\right) \tag{5.6}$$

where $\Psi(t)$ is the continuous mother wavelet, $0 \le j \le N-1$, and $0 \le k \le M-1$. Then, the coefficients of the DWT are calculated as

$$W_{jk} = \int_{-\infty}^{+\infty} x(t)\Psi_{jk}^{*}(t)dt \tag{5.7}$$

The aforementioned analysis equation calculates a finite set of discrete coefficients directly from a continuous signal. This makes the DWT somewhat different from the DFT that accepts only discrete signals as its input. The beauty of the DWT becomes clearer from the synthesis equation in the following:

$$x(t) = c\sum_{j=0}^{N-1}\sum_{k=0}^{M-1} W_{jk}\Psi_{jk}(t) \tag{5.8}$$

In this equation, c is a constant that depends on the exact choice of the mother wavelet. The interesting thing about this equation is the fact that we can reconstruct the continuous signal directly from a set of discrete coefficients. This capability makes the DWT and the IDWT particularly interesting and useful for the applications where a continuous signal must be decomposed to and reconstructed from a finite set of discrete values. A closer look identifies the DWT as the equivalent of the Fourier series as opposed to the DFT.

A relevant question at this point is how to choose the number of basis functions for a given signal. Specifically, how many shifted and scaled versions of the mother wavelet are needed to decompose a signal. We start this discussion by describing the difference between a frame and a basis. A frame is a set of basis functions that can be used to decompose a signal. This set can be minimal or nonminimal, i.e., if the number of basis functions in the frame is minimal and any other frame would need the same number or more basis functions, the frame is called a basis. From the definitions given earlier, in order to minimize the number of basis functions and therefore the required computations in calculating the DWT and the IDWT, one would like to use a basis for the operation as opposed to a nonminimal frame. To see the differences between a frame and a basis more clearly, consider the energy of a signal $x(t)$:

$$E_x = \int_{-\infty}^{+\infty} |x(t)|^2 dt \tag{5.9}$$

Now consider a frame formed based on the functions $\Psi_{jk}(t)$ defined earlier. For such a frame, it can be proved that there exist some bounded positive values A and B such that

$$A.E_x \le \sum_{j=0}^{N-1}\sum_{k=0}^{M-1} |W_{jk}|^2 \le B.E_x \tag{5.10}$$

This relation intuitively means that the energy of the wavelet coefficients for a frame is bounded on both upper and lower sides by the true energy of the signal. In the case of a basis (i.e., a minimal frame), the values A and B in the aforementioned inequality become the same, i.e., $A = B$. This means that for a basis we have

$$E_x = \sum_{j=0}^{N-1} \sum_{k=0}^{M-1} \left| W_{jk} \right|^2 \quad (5.11)$$

This indicates the energy of the coefficients is exactly the same as the energy of the signal. This is something we saw in DFT before and reminds us that the complex exponential basis used in the DFT indeed forms a basis. The next important question to ask here is: "What are the properties of the functions that allow the function sets to form a basis?" The most popular basis sets are the orthogonal ones, i.e., the function sets whose members are orthogonal to each other. There is an extensive literature on how orthogonal basis function sets for DWT are formed.

Despite the usefulness of DWT computed from continuous signals, this transformation is not very popular. This is due to the fact that the original time signals are often discrete and not continuous. As a result, the next definition of the WT that is computed over discrete signals is more popular.

5.4.1 Discrete Wavelet Transform on Discrete Signals

As indicated in our discussion of DFT, in almost all practical applications, signals are formed of discrete measurements, and therefore in practice we normally deal with sampled signals. This means that we need to focus on calculating DWT from discrete signals. At this point, we assume that the discrete signal, if sampled from a continuous signal, has been sampled according to the Nyquist rate (or faster). This guarantees that all information of the continuous signal is preserved in the discrete signal. For such a discrete signal, DWT can be calculated in different ways based on the exact type of mother wavelets used for transformation. As mentioned in the previous section, the best types of mother wavelets are the ones that form an orthogonal set.

The question here is how to form such basis sets systematically. The method described next, called Mallat pyramidal algorithm or quadrature mirror filter (QMF), allows systematic creation of an unlimited number of orthogonal basis sets for DWT. The interesting feature of this method is the fact that the method relies only on the choice of a digital low-pass filter $h(n)$, and once this filter is chosen, the entire algorithm is rather mechanical and straightforward. In reality, the restrictions on $h(n)$ are so relaxed that many such filters can be easily found, and, therefore, many mother wavelets can be formed based on different choices of the low-pass filter $h(n)$. This method can be best described using the schematic diagram of Figure 5.9.

Based on the QMF algorithm, the DWT for a one-dimensional (1-D) signal is systematically calculated as follows. Assuming a digital filter $h(n)$, we form another filter $g(n)$ as follows:

$$g(n) = h(2N - 1 - n) \quad (5.12)$$

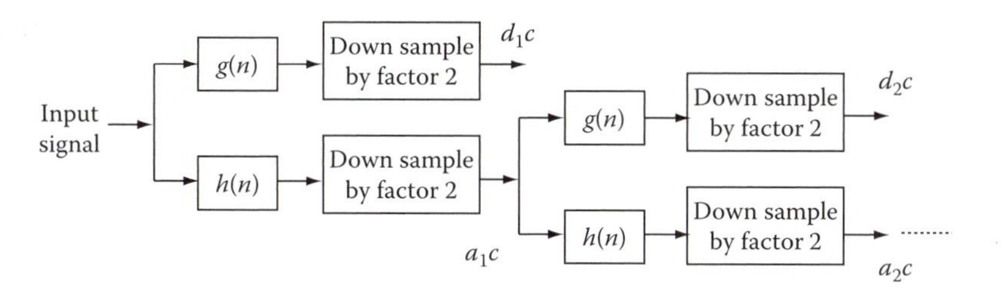

FIGURE 5.9 Schematic diagram of QMF algorithm for DWT.

As can be seen, once $h(n)$ is chosen, $g(n)$ is automatically defined. This means that even though in the block diagram of Figure 5.9 there are two filters, only one of them is selected and the other one is calculated from another. From Equation 5.12, we can observe that when $h(n)$ is a low-pass filter, $g(n)$ would turn out to be a high-pass filter automatically.

As can be seen in the schematic diagram of Figure 5.9, the first step in transformation is filtering the signal once with the low-pass filter $h(n)$ and once with the high-pass filter $g(n)$. Then the filtered versions of the signal are downsampled by a factor of 2. This means that every other samples of the signal are preserved and the remaining samples are discarded. At the first glance, one might feel that the downsampling operation would result in the loss of information, but, in reality, since now we are dealing with two copies of the signal (one high-pass and one low-pass version), no information is truly lost. We can also ask another relevant question about downsampling: "How would downsampling fit into the general ideas of the DWT?" Without getting into the mathematical details of the process, one can see that downsampling somehow creates the description of the signal at a different scale and resolution. This matches the basic idea of the DWT in expressing and decomposing a signal into different levels.

As evident from Figure 5.9, the signal transformation and decomposition can be repeated for as many levels as desired. If one wishes to terminate the operation at the first level, two coefficients are found, d_1c (the high-pass coefficient on the first level) and a_1c (the low-pass coefficient on the first level). However, in reality, we often prefer to decompose the high-pass version of the signal even further, and, as a result, another level of decomposition is performed using the same subsystem used for the first level of decomposition. This would result in two new coefficients: d_2c (the low-pass coefficient on the second level) and a_2c (the high-pass coefficient on the second level). This decomposition process can be repeated for several levels, and, in each level of decomposition, more scales of the signal are separated and quantitatively expressed using the wavelet coefficients.

Before describing the IDWT, let us answer a simple but fundamental question: "What is the mother wavelet of the QMF algorithm?" It seems that we were so emerged in the description of the algorithm using the low-pass filter $h(n)$ that we did not notice the apparent absence of the mother wavelet involved in the process. The QMF is indeed based on a mother wavelet that is represented by the low-pass filter $h(n)$. In reality, each choice of this filter results to one specific discrete mother wavelet $\Psi(n)$ according to the following iterative relations:

$$\Psi(n) = \sum_{i=0}^{N-1} g(i)\Phi(2n-i) \tag{5.13}$$

where

$$\Phi(n) = \sum_{i=0}^{N-1} h(i)\Phi(2n-i) \tag{5.14}$$

The function $\Phi(n)$ is often referred to as the "scaling function" and, in the previous equation, helps the calculation of the mother wavelet. From the preceding equations, one can see that the mother wavelet of the operation is uniquely identified and represented by the filter $h(n)$ or, in other words, the role of the mother wavelet is somehow replaced by $h(n)$. The complexity of the iterative process of Equations 5.13 and 5.14, on the one hand, and the simple structure of the schematic diagram of Figure 5.9, on the other hand, clearly state why in QMF algorithm one would prefer to focus on the concept of $h(n)$ as opposed to the direct use of the mother wavelet. It can be shown that all popular discrete wavelets such as dbX can be formed using QMF algorithm.

Another question, which is to the most part an open problem, is as follows: "How many decomposition levels are needed for a suitable transform?" An intuitive criterion to choose the level of the decomposition would be continuing decomposition until the highest known frequencies in the signal of interest are extracted and identified. Loosely speaking, if one needs to have more detailed decomposition of the signal in higher frequencies, he or she would need to calculate higher levels of decomposition. This simply would allow more specific description of high-frequency components of a signal.

As expected, the IDWT is formed in a similar multilevel process shown in Figure 5.10.

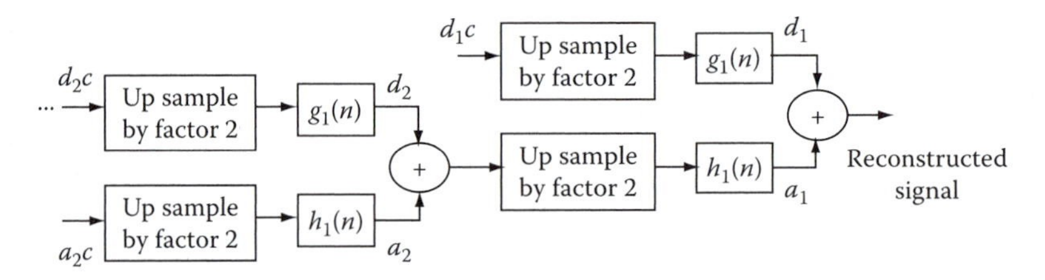

FIGURE 5.10 Schematic diagram of IDWT using QMF algorithm.

In the diagram of IDWT, the filters $h_1(n)$ and $g_1(n)$ are defined based on $h(n)$ and $g(n)$ as follows:

$$h_1(n) = (-1)^{1-n} h(1-n) \tag{5.15}$$

and

$$g_1(n) = h_1(2N-1-n) \tag{5.16}$$

As can be seen, the structure and operations in IDWT are very similar to those of DWT, and therefore, with some minor changes, the same codes written to calculate DWT can be used to calculate IDWT.

An interesting feature of the DWT and IDWT is the possibility of reconstructing the signal only based on a few of the levels (scales) of decomposition. For example, if we want to extract only the main trend of the signal and ignore the medium and fast variations, we can easily decompose the signal to several levels using DWT, but use only the first (or first few) low-pass components to reconstruct the signal using IDWT. This allows bypassing the medium- and high-frequency components. Similarly, if the objective is to extract only the fast variations of signal, in the reconstruction phase, we can easily set the coefficients of the low frequency (high scales) to zero while calculating the IDWT. This would eliminate the low-frequency trends of the signal. Such approaches are very similar to low-pass and high-pass filtering using DFT except that due to the advantages of the DWT mentioned at the beginning of the chapter, DWT is often preferred over DFT.

The following example exhibits some of the DWT capabilities discussed earlier when it is applied for biomedical signal processing.

Example 5.4

In this example, an EEG signal (described in Part II of this book) is decomposed using the QMF method. First we use the "`wavemenu`" command in MATLAB® to activate the interactive wavelet toolbox in MATLAB. Then, on Wavelet Toolbox Main Menu, under One-Dimensional, we select Wavelet 1-D. Now, on the Wavelet 1-D, we load and read the EEG signal. In order to analyze the signal, several options for the mother wavelet as well as decomposition levels are provided by MATLAB. We select db3 wavelet and decompose the signal to the seventh levels. Figure 5.11 shows the original signal, *S* (top graph), and reconstructed versions of the signal at different levels for all seven levels.

As can be seen, the first reconstruction of the signal (i.e., the second signal from the top) has only the low-frequency trend of the signal, while the last signal captures only noise-like fast variations of the signal. If the signal is believed to be corrupted by high-frequency noise, we can simply reconstruct the signal using only the first few components to eliminate the high-frequency noise. For denoising and filtering of the signal using DWT, more efficient techniques are often applied that will be discussed later in this chapter.

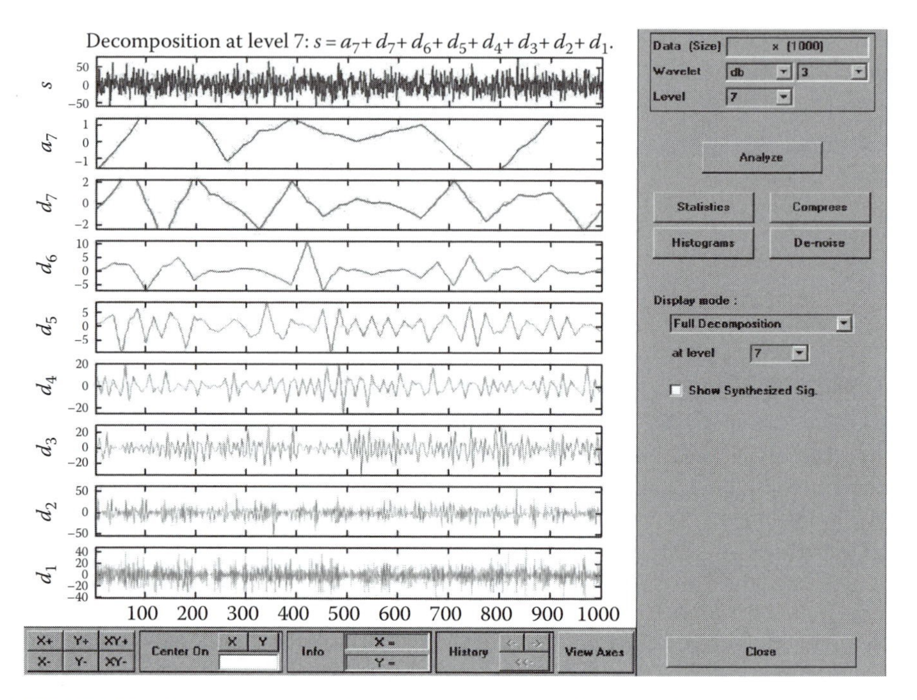

FIGURE 5.11 Decomposition and reconstruction of an EEG signal at different resolutions.

The strength (power) of the reconstructed signals at different levels has important physiological meanings and applications. For instance, in an EEG signal, a very strong low-frequency component (second graph from the top) identifies that the patient might be asleep or about to fall asleep. This will be further discussed in a chapter dedicated to EEG.

5.5 TWO-DIMENSIONAL WAVELET TRANSFORM

The basic idea of the WT can be extended to two-dimensional (2-D) space. This extension can be made both in continuous and discrete environments. However, as the FT, the main 2-D application of the WT in biomedical sciences is processing of biomedical images, and since all 2-D entities processed in biomedical sciences are digital images, the CWT is not a particularly useful transform for biomedical image processing. As a result, in this section, the focus is given only to the 2-D DWT that operates on the digital images.

The approach we take in this section to describe the 2-D DWT is based on the main concepts described for the 1-D DWT, which allows a better understanding and implementation of the 2-D DWT.

5.5.1 Two-Dimensional Discrete Wavelet Transform

The 2-D DWT can be easily described and implemented using the block diagram of Figure 5.12 that applies the principles and operations of the 1-D DWT.

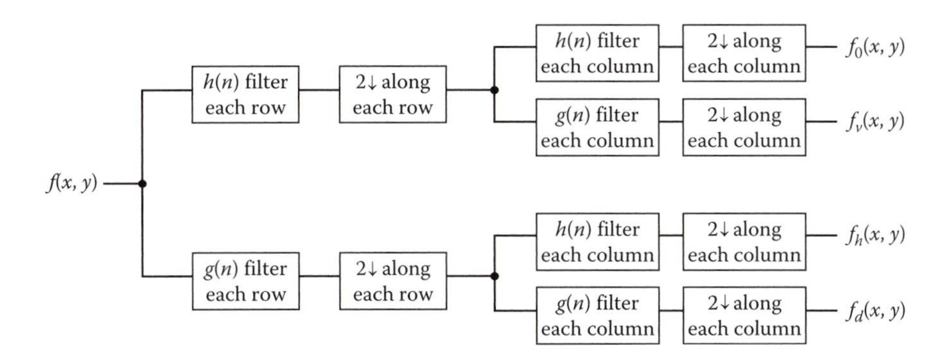

FIGURE 5.12 Schematic diagram of 2-D DWT.

As can be seen from the diagram of Figure 5.12, an $N \times N$ image $f(x, y)$ is regarded once as a series of 1-D row signals and once as a series of 1-D column signals. When assuming the image as N rows of 1-D signals, each with N points, the 1-D DWT of each row is calculated. These N rows of numbers are put together to form a matrix X_h. The same process is repeated on the columns of the image to form X_v. At this point, X_h contains primarily the information regarding the horizontal variations at different levels, and X_v comprises the decomposition and analysis of the vertical variations in the image.

Next, the same operation is reappeared for X_h and X_v. More specifically, in the case of X_h, the DWT of the row is computed and named as X_{hh}, and the DWT of the columns is calculated and named as X_{hv}. The same process is repeated for X_v, generating X_{vv} and X_{vh}. The components X_{vv} and X_{hh} will then have the second-level vertical and horizontal decompositions, respectively, while X_{hv} and X_{vh} will represent the diagonal information of the image.

The 2-D DFT will be further described in the following example.

Example 5.5

In this example, we decompose an image using the 2-D DWT and observe the image reconstructed in every scale. The image to be analyzed is a digital image of coronary arteries captured during an imaging process called angiography. Analyzing the image using the 2-D DWT gives a set of images shown in Figure 5.13. This figure shows the low-frequency component of the original image (top left), the horizontal component (top right), the vertical component (bottom left),and diagonal information (bottom right).

The first observation is that the low-pass component (top left) is almost enough to perceive the entire image. This is a witness to the compression capabilities of DWT. In other words, while the size of the DWT coefficients needed to reconstruct the low-pass components of the image is 25% of the original image, almost all information of the original image is preserved in the low-pass component. In addition, as can be seen in Figure 15.3, the horizontal component captures the horizontal information of the image (e.g., horizontal lines identify the arteries that are mainly in the horizontal direction), the vertical component represents the vertical information (e.g., vertical arteries), and diagonal information (e.g., diagonal lines and texture) is captured by the diagonal component. In other words, the

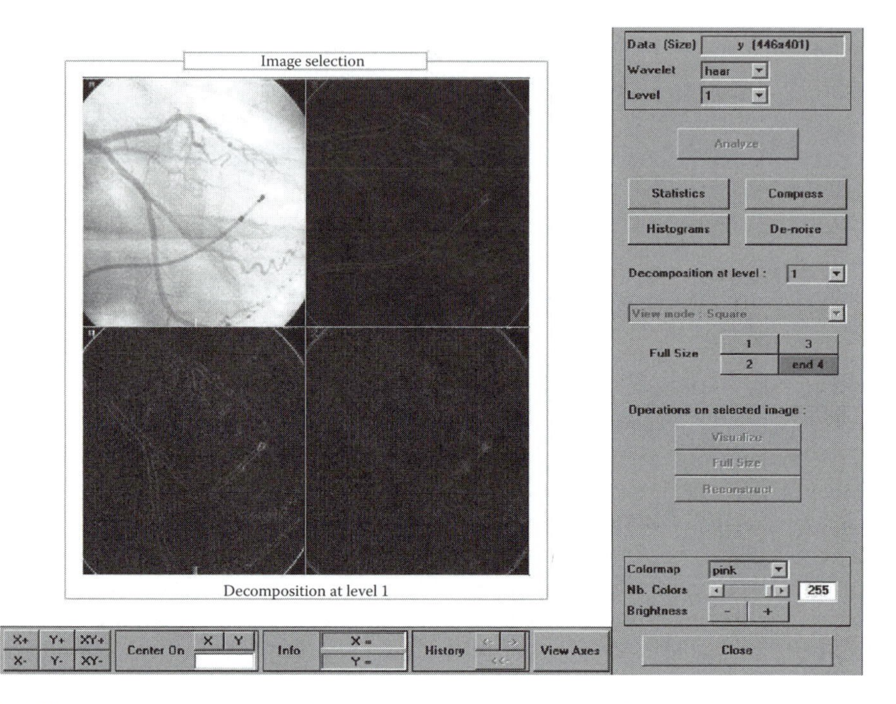

FIGURE 5.13 Decomposition of an image to the first level using DWT. (Courtesy of Andre D'Avila, MD, Heart Institute (InCor), University of Sao Paulo, Medical School, Sao Paulo, Brazil.)

arteries that are mainly horizontal are more visible in the horizontal components and the vertical arteries are more highlighted in the vertical components.

Nothing tells us to stop at the first level of decomposition, and we can easily continue decomposing the signal to another level. Figure 5.14 shows the decomposition of the image into the second level. The second-level components provide a higher resolution in expressing the contents of the image in each direction and therefore can capture more detailed information regarding the image.

5.6 MAIN APPLICATIONS OF DWT

The main applications of DWT in biomedical signal and image processing are filtering, denoising, compression, and extraction of scale-based features. Filtering and denoising are very similar in the sense that they both deal with eliminating some scales (frequencies) from the signal and extracting some targeted components. We start the discussion with denoising and filtering.

5.6.1 Filtering and Denoising

As mentioned earlier, it is often the case that noise exists in high frequencies (i.e., low scales) of signals and images. For instance, electromagnetic drifts that appear in the wires and electrodes are high-frequency noise. Such a noise appears in almost all biomedical signals such as electroencephalogram and electrocardiogram

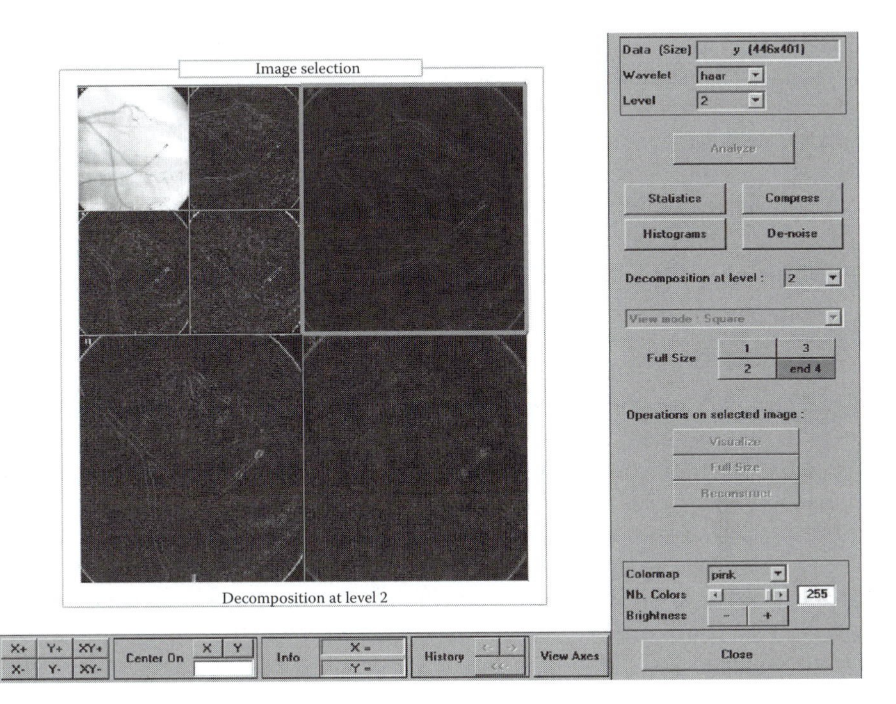

FIGURE 5.14 Decomposing the image into the second level.

(as will be discussed later in this book). It is desirable to filter out such noise and extract the informative part of the recorded signals. In DWT domain the denoising often translates into reducing or eliminating the high-frequency variations in the low scales.

Two main types of DWT-based denoising are used in signal processing: hard thresholding and soft thresholding. In hard thresholding, all coefficients of some particular levels of decomposition that are less than a threshold are set to zero, and the remaining coefficients are used for reconstruction of the signal. In other words, denoting the threshold value as ξ and the original coefficients j at level k as d_{jk}, the coefficients after hard thresholding are calculated according to the following criterion:

$$d_{jk}^{hard} = \begin{cases} d_{jk} & \text{if } |d_{jk}| > \xi \\ 0 & \text{Otherwise} \end{cases} \tag{5.17}$$

In soft thresholding, just as in hard thresholding, all coefficients below the threshold value ξ are eliminated; however, unlike hard thresholding, all other coefficients are also adjusted by the threshold amount, i.e.,

$$d_{jk}^{hard} = \begin{cases} d_{jk} - \xi & \text{if } d_{jk} > \xi \\ 0 & \text{if } |d_{jk}| \le \xi \\ d_{jk} + \xi & \text{if } d_{jk} < -\xi \end{cases} \tag{5.18}$$

As can be seen, soft thresholding can be thought of as an extension of hard thresholding that avoids creating discontinuities. Soft computing is often considered as a relatively more successful algorithm for automated denoising. The main factor that affects the performance of both algorithms is the selection of a suitable threshold value ξ. As discussed later, MATLAB toolbox for WT provides several techniques for this selection; however, often the manual selection of the threshold value seems to be the most appropriate method for a given image or signal. As a result, we leave exploring this selection process to the readers as an exercise in the Problems section.

5.6.2 Compression

In many biomedical applications, long signals and large images are created. The storage of all these signals and images creates a serious issue. The main objective here is to design techniques to reduce the size of a signal or image without compromising the information contained in the signal or image.

The process of compression using the DWT is very similar to denoising: first, the signal or image is decomposed to its DWT coefficients, and then the coefficients that are less than a threshold value are eliminated. Since there are often many coefficients that are too small to make a sensible difference in the signal, when a signal is reconstructed using only the surviving coefficients, a good approximation of the signal is obtained.

The second rule for compression states that since noise often corrupts the high-frequency components, by eliminating too-high-frequency components, the useful information in a signal would not change considerably.

The third rule for compression states that too-low-frequency components may not contain vital information, and their corresponding coefficients can be eliminated or reduced in the compression process. This rule can be better understood if we think of some undesirable trends in signals such as electrocardiogram that contain no relevant information, and, therefore, it makes sense to eliminate them before saving the signal. In a typical electrocardiogram, the low-frequency variations caused by the patient's respiration constitute the trend that is often eliminated by discarding the high-scale (low-frequency) coefficients in the DWT domain.

The compression performance of the DWT will be further illustrated in the following example.

Example 5.6

As previously mentioned, in decomposing of the image given in Figure 5.13, the low-pass component requires only 25% of the storage space to provide an almost identical version of the original image. The second-level decomposition of the image is shown in Figure 5.14. As shown, the low-pass component, while having only 6.25% of the original image, still provides an acceptable approximation of the original image. These observations demonstrate the capabilities of the DWT in compression applications. This is why the newer versions of image compression technologies such as some JPEG standards apply the DWT for compression.

5.7 DISCRETE WAVELET TRANSFORM IN MATLAB®

In MATLAB, a complete toolbox is dedicated to the WT and its applications in signal and image processing. Even though we are not to cover the detailed description of this toolbox, we encourage the reader to explore these capabilities using the visual user interface provided for most of these capabilities. The command "`wavedemo`" provides a demonstration of these capabilities, and "`wavemenu`" activates the user interface of the wavelet toolbox. While `wavedemo` helps the reader understand the different DWT commands and options provided by MATLAB, `wavemenu` provides the means to visually conduct almost all aforementioned applications of the DWT. These applications include denoising, compression, and filtering. MATLAB also provides a set of commands for direct calculation of the DWT coefficients as well as the IDWT. These commands include `dwt`, `idwt`, `dwt2`, and `idwt2`. In using each of these commands, one needs to identify the type of the mother wavelet and the level of decomposition (or reconstruction).

The readers are further guided to systematically explore these capabilities in the Problems section.

5.8 SUMMARY

In this chapter, the concept of continuous and discrete WTs was presented. We started with the need for such a transformation and then described the mathematical formulation as well as the applications of WT such as denoising, filtering, and compression.

PROBLEMS

5.1 A biomedical image that was corrupted by additive noise is given in the file "p_5_1.mat." This image shows a fluoroscopic image of arteries.*

a. Read the image using "`load`" command.
b. Calculate the 2-D DWT of the image using "`dwt2`" command (assume only one level of decomposition). Use Daubechies 2 ("`db2`" in MATLAB) as the mother wavelet.
c. Apply hard and soft thresholding for denoising of the image assuming $\xi = 0.01$, $\xi = 0.05$, and $\xi = 0.1$.
d. Use "`idwt2`" command to reconstruct the filtered image for all three values of ξ for both hard and soft thresholding, compare the results, and identify the setting with the best results.

5.2 An EEG signal is to be denoised using DWT.† The signal is given in "p_5_2.mat."

a. Read the EEG signal using "`load`" command and plot the signal.

---

* Courtesy of Andre D'Avila, MD, Heart Institute (InCor), University of Sao Paulo, Medical School, Sao Paulo, Brazil.

† Courtesy of Dr. Henri Begleiter, Neurodynamics Laboratory, State University of New York Health Center at Brooklyn, Brooklyn, NY.

b. Calculate the DWT of the signal using "dwt" command (use as many levels of decomposition as you need for better results). Use Harr mother wavelet, which is the same as Daubechies 1 ("db1" in MATLAB).
c. Apply soft thresholding for denoising of the signal assuming $\xi = 0.01$, $\xi = 0.05$, and $\xi = 0.1$.
d. Use "idwt" command to reconstruct the filtered signal for all three values of ξ, compare the results, and identify the setting with the best results.

5.3 We are to compress an image given in "p_5_3.mat." This image shows a multislice tomographic image of the pulmonary vein in a patient with fibrillation. In this problem, we will explore the effects of using different mother wavelets for compression of the given image.*

a. Read the image using "load" command and show it using "image".
b. Calculate the 2-D DWT of the image using "dwt2" command (assume two levels of decomposition). Use the following three mother wavelets for this purpose: Daubechies 2, Harr, and Coiflets 1 ("coif1" in MATLAB).
c. Apply hard thresholding for denoising of the image assuming $\xi = 0.01$, $\xi = 0.05$, and $\xi = 0.1$.
d. Use "idwt2" command to reconstruct the compressed image for all three values of ξ for all mother wavelets, compare the results, and identify the setting with the best results.

5.4 In this problem, we explore forming QMF algorithm for a given filter $h(n)$. This problem also allows us to generate a new mother wavelet. Assume that this filter is given as

$$h(n) = \begin{cases} e^{-2n}, & n \geq 0 \\ 0 & \text{otherwise} \end{cases} \tag{5.19}$$

a. In order to form the decomposition process, first find the corresponding $g(n)$.
b. For this set of $h(n)$ and $g(n)$, find the mother wavelet as well as the scaling function.
c. For reconstruction process, we will need to know two functions: $h_1(n)$ and $g_1(n)$. Use $h(n)$ and $g(n)$ to calculate these functions.

* Courtesy of Andre D'Avila, MD, Heart Institute (InCor), University of Sao Paulo, Medical School, Sao Paulo, Brazil.

6 Other Signal and Image Processing Methods

6.1 INTRODUCTION AND OVERVIEW

In this section, some other techniques used in biomedical signal and image processing are discussed. In order to avoid an excessively long chapter, the introduced techniques are described in a brief and concise manner. The first part of this chapter deals with the complexity measures computed mainly for one-dimensional (1-D) signals and their roles in biomedical signal processing. The second part of the chapter focuses on an important transformation in signal and image processing called cosine transform. In addition, a part of this chapter is dedicated to a brief review of coding and information theory, which is heavily used in both signal and image processing. Finally, a brief review of the methods for coregistration of images is presented.

6.2 COMPLEXITY ANALYSIS

A main characteristic of the biomedical and biological systems is their high complexity. For instance, complexity is often considered as the key feature that allows biomedical and biological systems to adapt to the dramatic environmental changes. In processing of a biomedical system, it is often the case that the complexity of the signals created by the system needs to be identified and evaluated using signal processing method. Evaluation of the biomedical complexity has become an important factor in diagnostics of the biomedical systems. A rule of thumb in biomedical sciences states that the normal and healthy biomedical systems are often very complex, and once a disease or abnormality occurs, the complexity of the system drops. An example of this rule is the significant decrease in all complexity measures of electroencephalogram (EEG) in diseased cases such as epilepsy (compared to the normal EEG). The same rule is applicable in other physiological units such as cardiovascular system, where a sharp drop in electrocardiogram (ECG) is associated with diseases such as flutter. These observations will be further described in Part II of the book.

Knowing the importance of the complexity measures in biomedical signals and systems, we start the description of some popular complexity measures with two local measures of complexity: "signal complexity" and "signal mobility."

6.2.1 Signal Complexity and Signal Mobility

These two features can quantitatively measure the level of variations along a signal. They are often used in the analysis of biomedical signals quantifying the first- and second-order variations in signals. Signal mobility addresses the normalized first-order variations of the signal, while signal complexity deals with the second-order variations. Consider a biomedical signal x_i, $i = 1,\ldots, N$. Also, let signal d_j, $j = 1,\ldots, N - 1$, represent the vector of the first-order variations in x, i.e.,

$$d_j = x_{j+1} - x_j \tag{6.1}$$

Moreover, define the signal g_k, $k = 1,\ldots, N - 2$, as the vector of the second-order variations in x, i.e.,

$$g_k = d_{k+1} - d_k \tag{6.2}$$

Then, using the concepts x, d, and g, we define the following fundamental first- and second-order factors:

$$S_0 = \sqrt{\frac{\sum_{i=1}^{N} x_i^2}{N}}, \tag{6.3}$$

$$S_1 = \sqrt{\frac{\sum_{j=2}^{N-1} d_j^2}{N-1}}, \tag{6.4}$$

$$S_2 = \sqrt{\frac{\sum_{k=3}^{N-2} g_k^2}{N-2}}, \tag{6.5}$$

Now, we can define signal complexity and signal mobility as follows:

$$\text{Signal complexity} = \sqrt{\frac{S_2^2}{S_1^2} - \frac{S_1^2}{S_0^2}} \tag{6.6}$$

and

$$\text{Signal mobility} = \frac{S_1}{S_0} \tag{6.7}$$

These two measures are heavily used in biomedical signal processing specially in processing of EEG, ECG, and electromyogram (EMG) signals as described in Part II of this book.

6.2.2 Fractal Dimension

Fractal dimension, which is frequently used in analysis of biomedical signals such as EEG and ECG, is a nonlocal measure that describes the complexity of the fundamental patterns hidden in a signal. Fractal dimension can also be considered as a measure of self-similarity of a signal. Informally speaking, assume we have printed a signal on a piece of paper and have a number of magnifiers with different zoom power. First, we look at the entire signal without a magnifier and observe the signal pattern. Then, we focus only on a portion of the signal and use a magnifier. In biological and biomedical signal, we often notice that the observed pattern with the magnifier has a high degree of similarity to the entire signal. If we continue focusing on smaller and smaller portions of the signal using magnifiers with higher and higher zoom powers, we observe more or less similar patterns. This proves the "self-similarity" of the biomedical signals. Fractal dimension is a measure that quantitatively assesses the self-similarity of a signal. Knowing that almost all biomedical signals are to some degree self-similar, evaluating the fractal dimension allows us to distinguish between the healthy and diseased signals.

In the signal processing literature, several methods are introduced to estimate the fractal dimension. Among all the fractal-based complexity measures, the Higuchi algorithm is known to be one of the most accurate and efficient methods to estimate self-similarity. Here, we briefly describe the estimation of fractal dimension using Higuchi's algorithm.

From a time series X with N points, first a set of k subseries with different resolutions are formed, i.e., a set of k new time series X_k are defined as follows:

$$X_k^m\colon\ x(m), x(m+k), x(m+2k), \ldots, x\left(m + \left\lfloor \frac{N-m}{k} \right\rfloor k\right) \tag{6.8}$$

where m indicates the initial time indices ($m = 1, 2, 3, \ldots, k$). The length of the curve X_k^m, $l(k)$, is then calculated as follows:

$$l(k) = \frac{\left(\sum_{i=1}^{\lfloor N-m/k \rfloor} \left|x(m+ik) - x(m+(i-1)k)\right| (N-1)\right)}{\left(\left\lfloor (N-m)/k \right\rfloor\right) k} \tag{6.9}$$

Then, the average length is calculated as the mean of the k lengths l_k for $m = 1, \ldots, k$. This is repeated for each k ranging from 1 to k_{max}. The slope of the plot $\ln(l(k))$ versus $\ln(1/k)$ is the estimation of the fractal dimension. We use the Higuchi dimension to express the complexity of biomedical signals in the following chapters.

6.2.3 Wavelet Measures

Another group of nonlocal complexity measures used in signal processing includes the wavelet-based measures. Wavelet transform, as introduced in Chapter 5, uses a function called a mother wavelet and fits the scaled and shifted versions of this function to decompose a sequence. This transform can also measure self-similarity at different scales of the sequence. In biomedical signal processing applications, the coefficients of the wavelet transform in each subband as well as the normalized power of coefficients in each subband are used as complexity features. The use for the wavelet-based measures is encouraged by the fact that in detecting specific changes in a diseased signal (compared to normal signals), we need to know not only the exact shape of these changes but also the length of the separation between the changes (i.e., the scale of the change).

The wavelet measures commonly used in the biomedical studies are the wavelet coefficients in high frequencies, which reflect the detailed high-frequency changes across the signal. In order to better understand the use of high-frequency coefficients, assume we are comparing two signals that are apparently similar to each other, for example, a healthy and a diseased signal with high degree of similarities. The overall similarity of the two signals indicates that the wavelet coefficients describing the overall approximation of the two signals are very similar (or the same). This means that the wavelet coefficients in the low frequencies (i.e., large scales) are very similar. But assuming that the two signals are indeed different, the wavelet theory also asserts that the coefficients describing the details of the two signals must be different. This means that a comparison of the high-frequency (low-scale) coefficients should reveal the differences of the two signals.

6.2.4 Entropy

Entropy is another measure of complexity, defined in information theory that is commonly used in biomedical signal and image processing. This measure is defined later in this chapter when describing the fundamentals of coding and information theory.

6.3 COSINE TRANSFORM

In the previous chapters, we emphasized the importance of the techniques to compress a signal or an image. A popular technique for compression that is frequently used in biomedical signal and image processing is cosine transform. Even though in many compression applications, the cosine transform is being replaced by the wavelet transform, we will briefly review this very useful technique. Since only discrete cosine transform (DCT) is commonly used in real applications, we focus on the DCT. For a discrete 1-D signal $g(n)$, where $n = 0,1,\ldots, N-1$, 1-D DCT is described as follows:

$$C(u) = a(u)\sum_{n=0}^{N-1} g(n)\cos\left[\frac{(2n+1)\pi u}{2N}\right], \quad u = 0,1,\ldots,N-1 \tag{6.10}$$

In the preceding equation, "u" represents the variable of the cosine domain and $a(u)$ is defined as follows:

$$a(u) = \begin{cases} \sqrt{\dfrac{1}{N}} & \text{for } u = 0 \\ \sqrt{\dfrac{2}{N}} & \text{for } u = 1,2,\ldots,N-1 \end{cases} \tag{6.11}$$

The inverse discrete cosine transform (IDCT) is defined using the same function $a(u)$:

$$g(n) = \sum_{u=0}^{N-1} a(u)C(u)\cos\left[\frac{(2n+1)\pi u}{2N}\right], \quad n = 0,1,\ldots,N-1 \tag{6.12}$$

As can be seen, the preceding equations have similarities to both DFT and DWT. Before showing some applications of the DCT, we define the two-dimensional (2-D) DCT. The 2-D DCT of an image $g(x, y)$, where $x = 0,1,\ldots, N-1$ and $y = 0,1,\ldots, N-1$, is defined as follows:

$$C(u,v) = a(u)a(v)\sum_{x=0}^{N-1}\sum_{y=0}^{N-1} g(x,y)\cos\left[\frac{(2x+1)\pi u}{2N}\right]\cos\left[\frac{(2y+1)\pi v}{2N}\right],$$

$$u = 0,1,\ldots,N-1, \quad v = 0,1,\ldots,N-1 \tag{6.13}$$

In the preceding equation, $a(u)$ is exactly what we defined earlier for the 1-D DCT and $a(v)$ is the same function with variable v. The 2-D IDCT is defined as follows:

$$g(x,y) = \sum_{u=0}^{N-1}\sum_{v=0}^{N-1} a(u)a(v)C(u,v)\cos\left[\frac{(2x+1)\pi u}{2N}\right]\cos\left[\frac{(2x+1)\pi v}{2N}\right],$$

$$x = 0,1,\ldots,N-1, \quad y = 0,1,\ldots,N-1 \tag{6.14}$$

The formulations of DCT and IDCT are evidently very similar to each other, and this similarity is utilized in implementation of the two formulae. In order to better understand the application of the DCT in image compression, we present the following example:

Example 6.1

In this example, the MR image shown in Figure 6.1a is transformed to the DCT domain. The resulting DCT coefficients are shown in Figure 6.1b. The code for this example is given as follows:

```
X=imread('image1.jpg');
X=double(X);
figure;
colormap(gray(256));
image(X);
Y=dct2(X);
figure;
colormap(gray(256));
image(Y);
```

```
Yc=zeros(256,256);
Yc(1:128, 1:128)=Y(1:128, 1:128);
Xc=idct2(Yc);
figure;
colormap(gray(256));
image(Xc);
```

As can be seen, only a small number of DCT coefficients located in the top left corner of the DCT domain (i.e., the low frequency coefficients with small u and v indices) are significant and the rest of the coefficients are very close to 0. This means that if we keep only the significant coefficients (e.g., the coefficients whose absolute values is larger than a threshold value), the only coefficients that will survive are the ones in the top left corner. As shown in Figure 6.1c, reconstruction of the image using only the coefficients in the top left quadrant of the DCT domain results to a high-quality approximation of the image. In other words, using only a quarter of the original DCT coefficients will allow producing a high-quality reconstruction of the original image. This compression process is the principal idea of some practical systems such as the older versions of the JPEG technology.

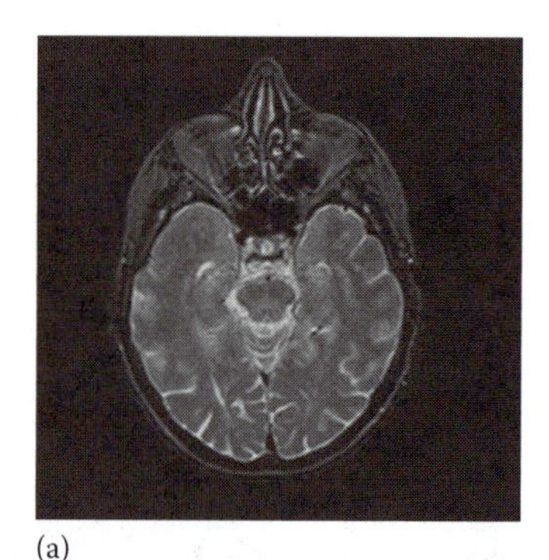

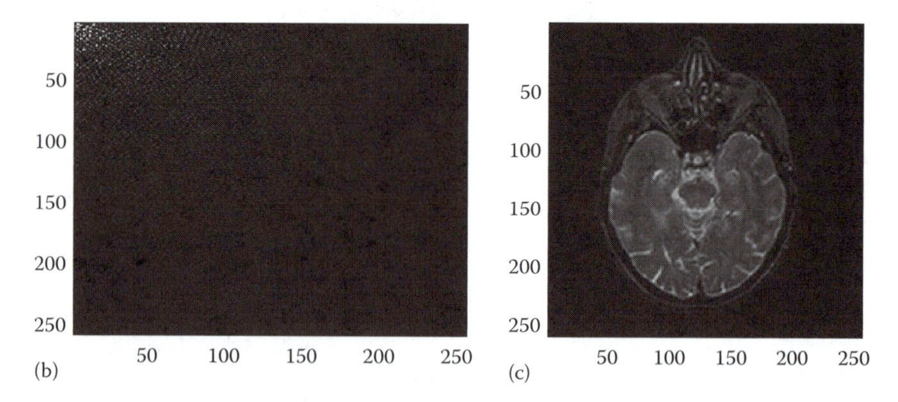

FIGURE 6.1 (a) Original image, (b) DCT of the image, and (c) reconstructed image using only the coefficients in the top left quadrant of the DCT domain. (From Goldberger, A.L. et al., *Circulation*, 101(23), e215, 2000, Circulation Electronic Pages; http://circ.ahajournals.org/cgi/content/full/101/23/e215).

As in DWT, there are several techniques for choosing a suitable threshold value for compression, and this issue is still an open problem. As shown in the aforementioned code, in MATLAB®, the commands "`dct`" and "`dct2`" are used for 1-D DCT and 2-D DCT, respectively. The inverse commands "`idct`" and "`idct2`" are used for decompression of the signals and images, respectively.

In more practical image processing applications, instead of compressing the entire image in one shot, the image is split into a number of subimages (often using a rectangular grid) and then each subimage is compressed using DCT separately. In reconstruction, first, each small subimage is decompressed and then the subimages are put together to form the final reconstructed image. This will be further explored in one of the problems in the Problems section.

6.4 INTRODUCTION TO STOCHASTIC PROCESSES

Most of the techniques described so far are applicable to "deterministic" signals and systems. If every time a signal is recorded or registered the exact same values are obtained, the signal is called to be deterministic. As evident from the definition, there are very few quantities in nature that give the exact same signals in all measurements. In other words, most of the signals, including biomedical signals, are "stochastic." A stochastic signal, even though statically similar in all recordings, contains some stochastic variations in each of the recordings. A stochastic process, $x(w, t)$, is represented by two variables where t is time and the variable w identifies a particular outcome of the stochastic process. The variable w emphasizes the fact that each measurement of the variable x at a specific time can result in a different value.

An interesting stochastic process is the "white noise." White noise defines a stochastic process in which the value of the signal has absolutely no relation or dependency on the value of the signal at any other times. An example of such a process is a sequence of numbers obtained in consecutive tosses of a fair coin. In such a process, the outcome of each toss does not depend on the past or future outcomes. As biomedical example, consider a faulty recording of an ECG machine where the electrodes are not properly attached to the patient's chest. Observing absolutely no pattern in the recording signal, i.e., getting only white noise, often tells the technicians that the electrodes are disconnected. What is really measured during such situations is the background noise, often caused by the thermal and radiation sources of noise. It is interesting to know that often, even when electrodes are properly connected, we still capture some of this white noise that has to be filtered. The study of the white noise and the techniques to detect or remove it from a signal is a dynamic field of research.

6.4.1 Statistical Measures for Stochastic Processes

When dealing with a stochastic process and in order to make the notation shorter and simpler, often the variable w is dropped from the notation and $x(t)$ is used to represent $x(w, t)$. Hereafter, when dealing with a stochastic process, while keeping in mind the random nature of the processes, the shorter notation is used.

The difference between a deterministic signal and a stochastic process is the fact that once we have one recording of a deterministic signal, we know everything about it; however, every measurement of a stochastic signal is merely one outcome of a random sequence and therefore may not be used to represent all aspects of the stochastic process. The question then becomes how a stochastic process can be described. The answer is simply using a probability function to express the likelihood of having a value for a signal at any time t. The probability density function (PDF) of a process $x(w, t)$ is represented as $p_X(w, t)$ or simply $p_X(t)$. As in probability theory, once the PDF is available, it is always desirable to know the average of a stochastic process at a particular time t. In practical applications where we have many recording of a stochastic signal, we can average all the available recordings at time t and consider this value as the estimation of $m(t)$, i.e., mean of the signal at time t. Mathematically, the actual value of the mean function at all times can be computed as follows:

$$m(t) = E(x(t)) = \int_{-\infty}^{+\infty} x(t) p_X(t) dx(t) \tag{6.15}$$

The function $E(.)$ is called the expectation function, or ensemble averaging function. For a discrete stochastic process $x(w_i, n)$ that is defined at time points n, the mean function is defined as follows:

$$m(n) = E(x(w_i, n)) = \sum_{i=-\infty}^{+\infty} x(w_i, n) p_X(w_i, n) \tag{6.16}$$

where $p_X(w_i, n)$ is the probability of having outcome w_i at time n.

Often only one function, i.e., mean, is not sufficient to represent an entire stochastic process. Variance is another popular function that is very effective in expressing the average variations and scattering of the data around the mean. This function is defined as follows:

$$\sigma(t) = E\left((x(t) - x)^2\right) = \int_{-\infty}^{+\infty} (x(t) - m(t))^2 p_X(t) dx(t) \tag{6.17}$$

As can be seen, the variance function is the statistical average of the second-order deviation of the signal from its mean at each time. Similarly, the discrete variance function is defined as follows:

$$\sigma(n) = E((x(w, n) - m(n))^2) = \sum_{i=-\infty}^{+\infty} (x(w_i, n) - m(n))^2 p_X(w_i, n) \tag{6.18}$$

A closer look at the equations presented earlier emphasizes the fact that while mean is the statistical (or ensemble) average of "$x(t)$," variance is nothing but statistical average of "$(x(t) - m(t))^2$." This statistical averaging can be extended to any general function "$g(x(t))$," namely,

$$\bar{g}(t) = E(g(x(t))) = \int_{-\infty}^{+\infty} g(x(t))p_X(t)dx(t) \tag{6.19}$$

Similarly, for the discrete processes, we have

$$\bar{g}(n) = E(g(x(w,n))) = \sum_{i=-\infty}^{+\infty} g(x(w_i,n))p_X(w_i,n) \tag{6.20}$$

Some other popular functions whose expectations are useful in practical applications are "moment functions." The moment of degree k is defined as $E(g(x(t)))$, where $g(x(t)) = x(t)^k$. As can be seen, the mean function is nothing but the moment of degree 1, and variance is closely related to the moment of degree 2. The moment of degree 2 is often considered as the statistical power of a signal.

6.4.2 Stationary and Ergodic Stochastic Processes

A subset of stochastic processes provides some practically useful characteristics. This family that is referred to as "stationary processes in wide sense" in which the mean and variance functions remain constant for all time, i.e., $m(t) = m_0$, and $\sigma(t) = \sigma_0$. In other words, even though the probability function $p_X(t)$ of such processes can change through time, the mean and variance of the process stay the same at all times. Such a simplifying assumption helps processing a number of practically useful signals. For instance, it is often the case that the mean and variance of signals such as ECG and EMG does not change at least during a rather large window of time. Such an observation allows calculation of mean and variance for only one time point because the assumption of stationarity in wide sense states that the mean and variance functions for all times will be the same.

A subset of wide sense stationary processes are "stationary in the strict sense" processes in which the probability function $p_X(t)$ is assumed to be independent of time. This means that if one finds the PDF for one time step, the same exact PDF can be used to describe all statistical characteristics of the process in all times. From the definition, one can see that while all strict sense stationary processes are also wide sense stationary, the opposite is not true. This means that the strict sense stationary assumption is a stronger assumption and therefore applicable to fewer real applications.

An interesting and very popular family of wide sense stationary processes is the set of wide sense stationary Gaussian processes. In such processes, since the PDF has only two parameters, mean and variance, once these two parameters are fixed in time, the PDF becomes the same for all time. This means that for Gaussian processes, strict sense and wide sense stationary concepts are the same. Since many processes can be approximated by some Gaussian process, such stationary Gaussian processes are extremely important in signal processing applications, especially biomedical signal and image processing. For instance, in almost all processing techniques used for analysis of EEG, ECG, and EMG, the processes are assumed to be stationary Gaussian. Hereafter, since strict and wide sense stationary Gaussian processes are the same; in referring to such processes, we only use the word stationary without mentioning the details.

So far we have made several simplifying assumptions to create stochastic formulations that are more applicable to practical image and signal processing applications. However, even with the assumption of stationarity, it is practically impossible to apply such formulations to some very important applications. At this point, we need to make another assumption to narrow down our focus further to obtain a more practically useful model of stochastic processes. The need and motivation for making more simplifying assumptions is as follows. Note that in real applications, the PDF is not known and must be estimated from the observed data. In order to obtain an estimate of the PDF or any statistical averages, we need to have access to several recordings of the process and then perform an ensemble averaging over these recordings to estimate the desired averages. However, in almost all applications, especially biomedical applications, very often only one signal reading is available. For instance, clinics and hospitals capture only one ECG recording from a patient. It is unreasonable to expect the clinics to collect a few hundred EEG recordings for each patient so that we conduct our ensemble averaging to calculate PDF!

From the earlier discussion, it is clear that in many practical applications, one recording is all we have, and, therefore, we need to calculate the averages such as mean and variance from only one recording. Statistically speaking, this is not feasible unless further assumptions are made. The assumption that helps us with such situations allows us to perform the averaging across time for only one recording and to treat these averages as our ensemble averages. The stationary processes in which the averages of any recording of the signal across time equal the ensemble averages are called "ergodic processes." Formally speaking, considering any outcome signal $x(w_i, t)$ recorded for an ergodic process, we have

$$\overline{g}(t) = E(g(x(t))) = \int_{-\infty}^{+\infty} g(x(w_i, t))dt \qquad (6.21)$$

Similarly, in discrete ergodic processes using only one recording of the stochastic process, $x(w_i, n)$, we can use the following relation to calculate all ensemble averages through averaging in time:

$$\overline{g}(n) = E(g(x(w, n))) = \sum_{n=-\infty}^{+\infty} g(x(w_i, n)) \qquad (6.22)$$

For ergodic processes, all averages such as mean and variance can be calculated using the aforementioned time averaging. Ergodicity is a practically useful assumption made in many biomedical signal and image processing applications, and unless indicated otherwise, all stochastic processes discussed in the book are assumed to be ergodic.

6.4.3 Correlation Functions and Power Spectra

In order to express the time patterns within a stochastic signal as well as the interrelations across two or more stochastic signals, we need to have some practically useful measures and functions. For instance, since almost all biomedical signals have some type of periodicity, it is extremely useful to explore such periodicities using techniques such as Fourier transform (FT). However, since these signals are stochastic, we cannot simply apply FT to one only recording of the signal. The approach we take in this section to address the aforementioned issue is rather simple; we construct meaningful determinist signals from a stochastic process and then process these representative determinist signals using the FT and other techniques. As we will see later in this chapter, these deterministic signals and measures are conceptually interesting and practically very meaningful. Even though the definition of these signals and measures can be described for nonstationary processes too, due to the fact that almost all biomedical applications processes and signals are assumed to be stationary, we focus only on stationary processes and specialize all definitions toward stationary processes.

The first function we discuss here is autocorrelation function. This function calculates the similarity of a signal to its shifted versions, i.e., it discovers the correlation and similarity between $x(t)$ and $x(t-\tau)$, where τ is the amount of shift. Specifically, the autocorrelation function, $r_{XX}(\tau)$, is defined as follows:

$$r_{XX}(\tau) = \int_{-\infty}^{+\infty} x(t)x(t-\tau)p_{XX}(x(t),x(t-\tau))dt \tag{6.23}$$

In the preceding equation, $p_{XX}(x(t), x(t-\tau))$ is the joint probability density function of $x(t)$ and $x(t-\tau)$. An interesting property of this function is its capability to detect periodicity in stochastically periodic signals. For such signals, whenever τ is a multiple of the period of the signal, the similarity between the signal and its shifted version exhibits a peak. This peak in the autocorrelation signal can be quantitatively captured and measured. In other words, a periodic autocorrelation signal not only reveals the periodicity of the stochastic process but also measures the main features of this periodicity such as the period of oscillation.

Another feature of the autocorrelation function deals with the value of τ at which the autocorrelation function reaches its maximum. A simple heuristic observation states that maximum similarly is gained when a signal is compared to itself (i.e., when there is zero shift). This argument explains why the maximum of the autocorrelation function always occurs at $\tau = 0$. The typical shapes of autocorrelation functions for periodic and nonperiodic processes are shown in Figure 6.2a and b.

Yet another interesting observation about the autocorrelation function deals with calculating this function for the white noise. From the definition of the white noise,

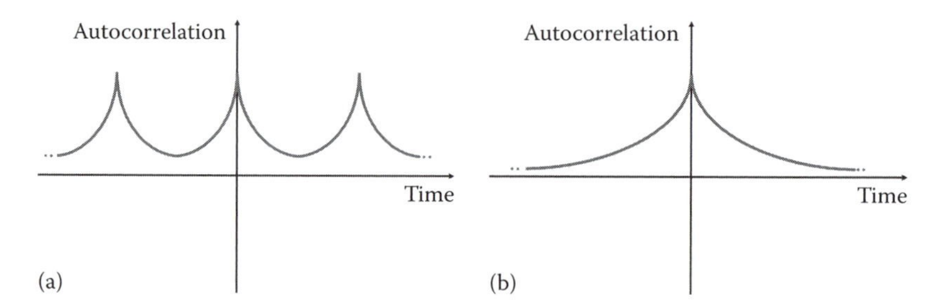

FIGURE 6.2 Typical shapes of autocorrelation function for (a) periodic and (b) nonperiodic signals.

we know that there is no dependence or correlation among random variables in consecutive times. This means that for any value $\tau \neq 0$, the autocorrelation function is 0. We also know that the similarity of a signal to itself is maximal. This means that the autocorrelation function for the white noise is indeed a spike (impulse) function that has a large value at the origin and 0 elsewhere.

The definition of the autocorrelation function for a discrete signal $x(n)$ is simply the same as the continuous case except for the substitution of the integral with a summation:

$$r_{XX}(m) = \sum_{n=-\infty}^{+\infty} x(n)x(n-m)p_{XX}(x(n), x(n-m)) \tag{6.24}$$

In the preceding equation, m identifies the amount of the shift in the discrete domain and $p_{XX}(x(n), x(n-m))$ is the joint probability density function of the random variables $x(n)$ and $x(n-m)$.

A natural and logical extension of the preceding functions is cross-correlation function. This function identifies any relation between a stochastic process $x(t)$ and the shifted version of another stochastic process $y(t)$, i.e., $y(t-\tau)$, as follows:

$$r_{XY}(\tau) = \int_{-\infty}^{+\infty} x(t)y(t-\tau)p_{XY}(x(t), y(t-\tau))dt \tag{6.25}$$

In the preceding equation, $p_{XY}(x(t), y(t-\tau))$ is the joint probability density function of random variables $x(t)$ and $y(t-\tau)$, and $r_{XY}(\tau)$ is the autocorrelation function between the two random variables $x(t)$ and $y(t-\tau)$.

The main application of this function is identifying potential cause-and-effect relationship between the random processes. As a trivial example, assume that we are to discover if there is a relationship between the blood pressure signal $y(t)$ and the ECG recordings of a patient, $x(t)$, measured an hour after the blood pressure was measured, i.e., $\tau = 1$ min. If the autocorrelation function showed a peak at $\tau = 1$ min, then one can claim that there might be some time-delayed relation between the blood pressure and the electrical activities of the heart muscles, i.e., ECG. Even though this trivial example may seem too simple and obvious, there are so many other factors, such as exercise and nutrition patterns whose potential effects on the function and activities of the heart are constantly investigated using the cross-correlation function.

The cross-correlation function for the discrete processes is defined as follows:

$$r_{XY}(m) = \sum_{n=-\infty}^{+\infty} x(n)y(n-m)p_{XY}(x(n), y(n-m)) \tag{6.26}$$

It is important to note that all autocorrelation and cross-correlation functions defined earlier, even though calculated from random variables, are indeed deterministic signals. This means that we can apply the FT on these signals and investigate the frequency contents of the underlying stochastic processes. The FT of the correlation signal is called power spectrum. For continuous stochastic processes, power spectrum is defined as follows:

$$R_{XX}(f) = FT\{r_{XX}(\tau)\} \tag{6.27}$$

and

$$R_{XY}(f) = FT\{r_{XY}(\tau)\} \tag{6.28}$$

Similarly, for the discrete stochastic processes, the power spectral functions are defined as follows:

$$R_{XX}(k) = FT\{r_{XX}(m)\} \tag{6.29}$$

and

$$R_{XY}(k) = FT\{r_{XY}(m)\} \tag{6.30}$$

For typical periodic signals, the overall shape of a power spectrum has two impulses located at positive and negative frequency of oscillation. The peak on the positive side is at the frequency of oscillation (one over the period of the signal), and the negative one is located simply at minus the frequency of oscillation.

An interesting power spectrum to study is that of the white noise. As discussed earlier, the autocorrelation function of the white noise is an impulse. We also know from the previous chapters that the FT of an impulse is a constant function that is flat in all frequencies. This flat shape is the reason the white noise is called "white." This analogy is originated in optics where the perception of each color is caused by an electromagnetic wave with a specific frequency, while white color, being a combination of all colors has all frequencies in it. Since the white noise's flat frequency spectrum has all frequencies in it, this noise is often referred to as the white noise.

The 2-D definitions for all concepts described previously are straightforward. In general, there are two approaches in biomedical signal and image processing. In the first approach, every signal is assumed to be deterministic and as a result, every measurement is directly used in Fourier, wavelet, and other types of analysis. Obviously, while the assumption made in this approach is not very realistic, the computational steps are simpler and straightforward. In the second approach, all signals are assumed to be stochastic processes, and, therefore, instead of applying the FT and other techniques directly on the measured signals, the secondary signals formed by concepts such as mean, variance, autocorrelation, and cross-correlation functions are used for Fourier and wavelet analysis. In this book, in order to cover the basic ideas of both approaches, we cover the concepts and applications from both approaches.

6.5 INTRODUCTION TO INFORMATION THEORY

Information theory is a field of study that investigates the mathematical formulation of "information." This theory is heavily used in signal and image processing, and as result, some fundamental concepts of this theory are covered next.

6.5.1 Entropy

The basic definition in information theory, i.e., entropy, is designed to measure the amount of information in a statement or variable. In order to reach to a suitable definition for information, let us start with an intuitive comparison of the information contained in the following three statements: (1) Earth is spherical, (2) humans have six legs, and (3) it is going to rain 40 days from today. The first statement, even though very true, has no surprise in it, and we gain no information from it. Obviously, no information is gained from the second statement, as we all know beforehand that this statement is false. The third statement, on the other hand, makes a prediction that may or may not be true.

From the preceding example, one can see that the basic measure of information is the degree of "surprise"; if the statement has obviously true or obviously false claims in it (e.g., $1 + 1 = 2$ or $1 + 4 = 10$), then there is no surprise or information in it. This suggests that the concept of probability can be used to form a potential measure of information. Assume that the probabilities of a random variable X with the outcomes x_i's are given as p_i's, where $i = 0, 1, 2, \ldots, N - 1$. Then one can suggest that the measure $1/p_i$ could be a measure of information. For this measure, when the probability of an incident gets smaller (and therefore we are more surprised), more information is gained. This measure has two problems associated with it. First, for zero probability, the information is calculated to be infinity. This is not what we expected as the information in an obviously wrong statement must be zero. The other problem deals with the outcome whose probability is one. For such a case, the calculated information is also one while we expect zero information from an obviously true statement.

In order to address at least one of the aforementioned issues, we can modify our information measure to "$\log(1/p_i)$." This modification ensures that for $p_i = 1$, the calculated information is indeed mapped to zero. However, the information calculated for an outcome with $p_i = 0$ is still infinity. In order to address this issue, we can further modify our measure to "$p_i \log(1/p_i)$." This measure gives zero information for outcomes with zero probability.

While the measure defined as "$p_i \log(1/p_i)$" correctly identifies the information of "each outcome," it fails to give an average amount of information for the random variable X as a whole. A logical approach to define such a measure is to add up the information measures of all N outcomes. This leads to the following measure, commonly referred to as entropy:

$$H(X) = \sum_{i=0}^{N-1} p_i \log\left(\frac{1}{p_i}\right) \tag{6.31}$$

The base in the preceding log function can be any number, but the most popular bases are "2," "e," and "10." Let us consider a random variable that is reduced to a deterministic signal, i.e., when for some $i = k$: $p_i = 0$ and for all other i's: $p_i = 0$. For such a case, from the earlier definition, we have $H(X) = 0$. This simply means that if one knows the outcome of a process beforehand (i.e., the k's outcome always happens), there is no surprise and therefore no information in the process. This is expected from a suitable measure of information, as discussed before.

The second observation deals with the other extreme case, i.e., when every outcome has the same probability. In such a case, we have $p_i = 1/N$, and, therefore, entropy is $H(X) = \log(N)$. One can easily prove that this is maximum possible entropy. In such random processes, we have no bias or guess before the outcome of the variable is identified. For instance, tossing a fair dice gives in general maximum information because no one can guess what number is going to show up on the dice beforehand, and, therefore, any outcome is very informative.

There are many other secondary definitions based on the basic idea of entropy. One of these measures is conditional entropy. Consider two random variables X and Y. Assume that we know the outcome of X statistically, i.e., based on the probabilities of the outcomes in X, we can expect what outcomes are happening more and what outcomes are less likely to happen. Knowing such information about X, now we want to discover how much information is gained when Y is revealed to us. For instance, if we already know that a patient has had a myocardial infarction (heart attack), how surprised we will be to know that there is a significant change in patient's blood pressure. Obviously, since we know that a heart attack has happened we are less surprised to hear that there have been some fluctuations in the blood pressure. The conditional entropy of Y given X identifies in average how much surprise is left in knowing Y, given that X has already happened. This measure is defined as follows:

$$H(Y \mid X) = \sum_{i=0}^{N-1} \sum_{i=0}^{M-1} p_{i,j} \log_2\left(\frac{1}{p_{j|i}}\right) \tag{6.32}$$

In the preceding equation, $p_{i,j}$ is the joint probability of the variables X and Y, and $p_{j|i}$ is the conditional probability of the variable Y given X.

Entropy plays an enormously important role in signal and image processing. As mentioned in the beginning of this chapter, in signal processing, entropy is considered as one of the complexity measures that distinguish simple signals from more sophisticated ones. The entropy of signals such as EEG and ECG has been used to detect or predict the occurrence of certain diseases. In most cases, a reduction in entropy is associated with a disease, and, therefore, most complex signals and systems are often considered normal in function.

6.5.2 Data Representation and Coding

A major application of coding and information theory is coding of information for compression purposes. In order to see this need more clearly, assume that you have used a transformation, such as wavelet or cosine transform, to reduce the redundancy on the transform level. The next step in compression is to decide how to represent and encode the surviving coefficients. In other words, the coefficients or values that can be real or integer numbers must be somehow coded using binary numbers. These binary numbers are then saved on electronic media, such as hard disk or CD. The question here is how to represent these coefficients (symbols) using binary numbers so that we minimize the storage space as much as possible. The data encoding is a major issue even if we attempt to save the images using the gray levels without using any transformations. The following example clarifies the issue:

Example 6.2

Assume that we have an image in which there are only five gray levels: 0, 1, 2, 3, and 4. The size of the image is 256 × 256. The frequencies of occurrence for these gray levels (i.e., probabilities of gray levels) are given as $p_0 = 0.05$, $p_1 = 0.03$, $p_2 = 0.05$, $p_3 = 0.07$, and $p_4 = 0.80$. A simple fixed-length binary code assignment would be assigning fixed-length binary codes to each gray level (symbol). For instance, with a fixed length of 3 bit, we can assign the following binary codes: $0 \rightarrow 000$, $1 \rightarrow 001$, $2 \rightarrow 010$, $3 \rightarrow 011$, and $4 \rightarrow 111$. As can be seen, 3 bit is used to store every gray level. For such an assignment and considering the frequency of occurrence of each gray level, the overall size of the space needed to save the image can be estimated as follows:

$$\begin{aligned}\text{Size of image} &= 256 \times 256 \times (3 \times 0.05 + 3 \times 0.03 + 3 \times 0.05 + 3 \times 0.07 + 3 \times 0.80) \\ &= 196{,}608\,\text{bit}\end{aligned}$$

Knowing that the number of bits allocated to each symbol is always three, one could have made the preceding calculation much easier. Now, let us explore if we can encode the gray levels as binary codes differently and reduce the total storage space needed. The problem with the fixed-length codes given earlier is ignoring the probability of each sample when assigning codes. We address this issue in our second encoding technique by giving longer codes to less probable symbols and shorter codes to more probable ones. For instance, consider the following codes: 0 → 110, 1 → 1110, 2 → 1010, 3 → 11110, and 4 → 00. For this code, the space needed to save the image is calculated as follows:

$$\text{Size of image} = 256 \times 256 \times (3 \times 0.05 + 4 \times 0.03 + 4 \times 0.05 + 5 \times 0.07 + 2 \times 0.80)$$
$$= 123{,}965\,\text{bit}$$

As can be seen, there is a significant decrease on the amount of space needed to save this image. Knowing that in biomedical applications, we need to store and transmit very many large medical images, the importance of using some optimal technique for binary representation of the biomedical data cannot be overestimated. Before describing the optimal technique for such an encoding and representation process, we have to add that in the literature of coding and information theory, in order to have a general criterion for the goodness of a code, a concept called the average length of the code, $\bar{L}$, is defined as follows:

$$\bar{L} = \sum_{i=0}^{M-1} p_i l_i \tag{6.33}$$

In the preceding equation, l_i and p_i are the length and probability of the ith codeword, respectively. This definition, unlike the total size used earlier, is independent of the size of the image or file before encoding. In addition, it is known that entropy in base 2 gives the theoretical limit on the average length of the best possible code. Therefore, it is desirable to compare the average code length of every code with the entropy and explore the quality of the obtained code compared to an optimal code. Such a measure is called "code rate" or "code efficiency" and is defined as follows:

$$R = \frac{H}{\bar{L}} \tag{6.34}$$

In comparison of two sets of codes using the code rate, the code with larger core rate (i.e., the core rate closer to one) provides a better code set.

6.5.3 Hoffman Coding

Hoffman coding is probably the best practical method of encoding the symbols with known probabilities. The basic idea of this method is very straightforward: Give longer codes to less probable symbols and shorter codes to more probable symbols. This way, in average, Hoffman code reduces the storage space for the lossless encoding of information. The practical steps in forming Hoffman codes can be described as follows:

Step 1: Take the two last probable gray levels.

Step 2: These two gray levels will be given the longest code word that differ only in one last bit.

Step 3: Combine these two gray levels into a single symbol and repeat Steps 1 to 3.

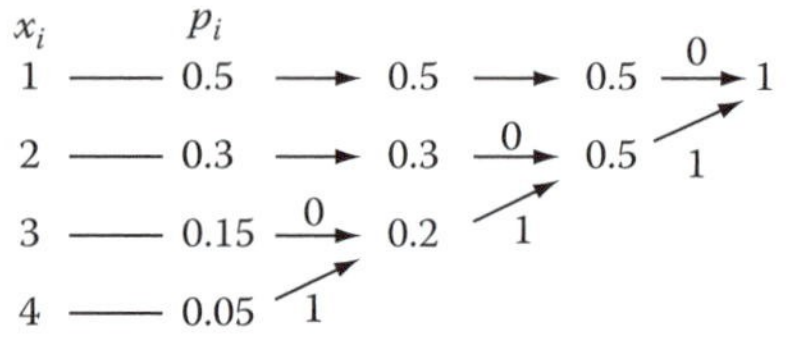

x_i	p_i			
1	0.5	0.5	0.5	0 → 1
2	0.3	0.3	0 → 0.5	1 ↗
3	0.15	0 → 0.2	1 ↗	
4	0.05	1 ↗		

FIGURE 6.3 Tree diagram for Hoffman coding.

The procedure for Hoffman coding can be more easily performed using a tree diagram. In the tree formation, first, the codes are listed in a column in a descending order according to their probabilities. Then, in a second column, the two least probable codes are combined with each other. The rest of the probabilities are copied to the second column. The same process is repeated on the new column until we reach a column with only one row (which has probability one). Then, 0's and 1's are assigned to each combination of probabilities in each transition from one column to another. As the last step, to form the code for a specific symbol or gray level, we start accumulating 0's and 1's encountered in a path from the last column of the tree toward the given code. This tree procedure is illustrated in the following example:

Example 6.3

An image has four gray levels {1, 2, 3, 4} with probabilities $p_1 = 0.5$, $p_2 = 0.3$, $p_3 = 0.15$, $p_4 = 0.05$. We design a Hoffman code for the image using a tree as shown in Figure 6.3.

Using the diagram, the resulting codes are $C(1) = 0$, $C(2) = 10$, $C(3) = 110$, and $C(4) = 111$. Remember that when assigning the codes using the tree diagram, we are moving backward, i.e., we start from the right-hand side and move toward the gray level in the left-hand side. Calculating the entropy and the average code length, we have $H = 1.6477$ and $\bar{L}(C) = 1.7$. This gives the code rate of $R = 96.92\%$. The reader can verify that the code rate for a fixed-length code with 2 bit is 82.38%. This shows the significant improvement gained by using Hoffman code.

The importance of Hoffman code in signal and image processing cannot be exaggerated. Compression technologies such as JPEG are all based on Hoffman coding. Without this compression method, the storage and communication of biomedical signals would have been practically impossible.

6.6 REGISTRATION OF IMAGES

In practical medical imaging applications, sometimes the images of the same tissue (e.g., the brain) are taken using different modalities such as MRI, CT, and PET. Knowing that each of these modalities provides certain types of information about the imaged tissues, it is important to coregister these images with each other. This allows the user to register the same objects in all images. For instance, image registration between MRI and CT of the head allows knowing the exact location of the objects such as the basal ganglia in both MRI and CT images.

Registration is important even when the images of the same tissue are taken at different times by the same modality or even by the same machine. It is often the case that the patient's exact position during the imaging acquisition changes from one set of measurement to another set of images captured at a different time. Moreover, the calibration of the imaging machines might be slightly different from one day to another. Therefore, such captured images need to be registered with each other using image processing methods.

There is another reason why image registration is a much needed process in imaging systems. It is often the case that when an image is generated by an imaging modality such as PET, the geometry of the produced image is a distorted version of the true geometry of the imaged tissue. For instance, it is often the case that some objects in the center are enlarged and some objects located toward the corners of the image are made smaller in size. In addition, it is rather usual to see that some or all of the imaged objects are tilted. In such cases, we need to use the available knowledge about the tissue to compensate for these distortions in the produced image and to form an image with the desired geometrical characteristics.

Returning to the typical use of image registration between two captured images, it is rather straightforward to note that image registration is simply creating a mathematical mapping between the pixel coordinates across a pair of images. This means that registration is nothing but forming a mapping T that maps the coordinates (x, y) in image I to the coordinates (x', y') in image I'. When coregistering the images taken by the same modality, since the physics governing the formation of both images is the same, the type of mapping T used for registration is often assumed to be linear. However, when registering the images captured by different modalities (e.g., registering MRI with PET images), the successful mapping functions are almost always nonlinear.

In the following, we discuss a general family of nonlinear mappings among images. Even though these mappings are nonlinear in their general formulation, they can be easily reduced to simple linear mappings. This mapping is very popular in biomedical image processing and is known to present reliable registration of modalities such as PET and MRI.

Consider a mapping T that maps the coordinates (x, y) in image I to the coordinates (x', y') in image I'. We define a nonlinear mapping using the following set of quadratic equations:

$$\begin{aligned} x' &= c_{11}x + c_{12}y + c_{13}xy + c_{14}x^2 + c_{15}y^2 \\ y' &= c_{21}x + c_{22}y + c_{23}xy + c_{24}x^2 + c_{25}y^2 \end{aligned} \tag{6.35}$$

In the preceding equation, any choice of the coefficients c_{ij}'s identifies a unique mapping T between the coordinates of the two images I and I'. It can be seen that if $c_{13} = c_{14} = c_{15} = c_{23} = c_{24} = c_{25} = 0$, the preceding mapping becomes a simple linear mapping between the two images.

In order to identify the mapping, all we need to do is to find the values of c_{ij}'s. This is often done using the coordinates of a set of "tie points" or "markers" in both images. In other words, we use the coordinates of a set of objects whose locations in both images are known to find the optimal mapping. The exact location of these tie points in both images are often visually identified by an expert. In registration of CT with other images, sometimes, certain markers (e.g., metal pins) are attached to the head that can be traced in all imaging systems. The coordinates of these points are then used to find c_{ij}'s, as described later.

As can be seen in Equation 6.35, the number of coefficients to be identified is 10. This means that 10 equations are needed to solve for all coefficients. Since each tie point provides two equations, altogether five tie points are required to uniquely identify the mapping. It is important to note that even though Equation 3.35 is nonlinear with respect to x and y, the equations are indeed linear with respect to c_{ij}'s. More specifically, after substituting for x, y, x', and y' with the coordinates of the tie points, the resulting set of equations is linear with respect to c_{ij}'s. This allows using simple matrix methods of solving for linear equations to find the coefficients.

If the number of the tie points is less than 5, it is a common practice to assume that some of the preceding coefficients are 0. This results in a simpler mapping between the two images. An example of this scenario is provided in the following.

Example 6.4

We are to coregister two images using three tie points. Having only three tie points means we can solve for only six coefficients. Hence, we apply a mapping as follows:

$$\begin{aligned} x' &= c_{11}x + c_{12}y + c_{14}x^2 \\ y' &= c_{21}x + c_{22}y + c_{25}y^2 \end{aligned} \tag{6.36}$$

Assume that the following tie points are given:

$$\begin{array}{ccc} I & \leftrightarrow & I' \\ (5,1) & & (4,3) \\ (10,3) & & (7,2) \\ (3,2) & & (5,2) \end{array}$$

This creates the following set of linear equations:

$$\begin{aligned} 4 &= 5c_{11} + c_{12} + 25c_{14} \\ 3 &= 5c_{21} + c_{22} + c_{25} \\ 7 &= 10c_{11} + 3c_{12} + 100c_{14} \\ 2 &= 10c_{21} + 3c_{22} + 9c_{25} \\ 5 &= 3c_{11} + 2c_{12} + 9c_{14} \\ 2 &= 3c_{21} + 2c_{22} + 4c_{25} \end{aligned} \tag{6.37}$$

As can be seen, the resulting set of equations is linear. One can rewrite these equations in the matrix form as follows:

$$\begin{bmatrix} 5 & 1 & 25 & 0 & 0 & 0 \\ 0 & 0 & 0 & 5 & 1 & 1 \\ 10 & 3 & 100 & 0 & 0 & 0 \\ 0 & 0 & 0 & 10 & 3 & 9 \\ 3 & 2 & 9 & 0 & 0 & 0 \\ 0 & 0 & 0 & 3 & 2 & 4 \end{bmatrix} \begin{bmatrix} c_{11} \\ c_{12} \\ c_{14} \\ c_{21} \\ c_{22} \\ c_{25} \end{bmatrix} = \begin{bmatrix} 4 \\ 3 \\ 7 \\ 2 \\ 5 \\ 2 \end{bmatrix} \tag{6.38}$$

The preceding equation can be solved using simpler matrix calculations, i.e., by multiplying both sides of the equation by the inverse of the square matrix on the left side of the equation, as follows:

$$\begin{bmatrix} c_{11} \\ c_{12} \\ c_{14} \\ c_{21} \\ c_{22} \\ c_{25} \end{bmatrix} = \begin{bmatrix} 5 & 1 & 25 & 0 & 0 & 0 \\ 0 & 0 & 0 & 5 & 1 & 1 \\ 10 & 3 & 100 & 0 & 0 & 0 \\ 0 & 0 & 0 & 10 & 3 & 9 \\ 3 & 2 & 9 & 0 & 0 & 0 \\ 0 & 0 & 0 & 3 & 2 & 4 \end{bmatrix}^{-1} \cdot \begin{bmatrix} 4 \\ 3 \\ 7 \\ 2 \\ 5 \\ 2 \end{bmatrix}$$

$$= \begin{bmatrix} 0.7368 \\ 1.6316 \\ -0.0526 \\ 0.3125 \\ 2.3438 \\ -0.9063 \end{bmatrix}$$

It is important to note that in mapping of the pixels from one image to another, we are using equations that give real numbers as the coordinates, while, in digital images, the coordinates need to be positive integers. This implies that the mapped coordinates have to be rounded up to the closest integer after mapping.

6.7 SUMMARY

In this chapter, a number of signal and image processing techniques were reviewed. These techniques included a number of methods for complexity analysis of signals and images, including fractal dimension and mobility measure. We also reviewed the cosine transform and its applications in signal and image processing. The theory of stochastic processes was briefly discussed in this chapter. The basic principles and applications of the coding and information theory were also reviewed. Finally, a brief description of the image registration methods was provided.

PROBLEMS

6.1 Read the image in the file "p_6_1.jpg" and save it as $f(x, y)$. This is the same MRI image used in Example 6.1. In this problem, we attempt to improve the compression quality by splitting the image into smaller subimages.

a. Split the image into subimages of 8 × 8, i.e., from the original images, form 64 subimages each capturing an 8 × 8 block of the image.
b. Calculate the discrete cosine transform of the subimages.
c. For each subimage, preserve the 16 DCT coefficients in the 4 × 4 matrix located on the top left corner of the DCT domain and set the rest of the coefficients to 0.
d. Calculate the IDCT of the resulting coefficients in Part "c" to reconstruct the subimages. Then, put the reconstructed subimage together to reform the entire image. Call this image $\hat{f}(x, y)$.
e. Assuming $N = 256$ as the dimension of the image in each coordinate, calculate the peak signal-to-noise ratio (PSNR) between the original image $f(x, y)$ and the reconstructed image $\hat{f}(x, y)$ as follows:

$$PSNR(f,\hat{f}) = \frac{256^2}{\sum_{i=0}^{N-1}\sum_{j=0}^{N-1}(f(x,y)-\hat{f}(x,y))^2} \tag{6.39}$$

f. Compare the PSNR value calculated in part "e" value with the PSNR resulting from the compression the entire image as one large block while reducing the size to one quarter of the original image. Has splitting the image into smaller blocks before compression improved the compression results?

6.2 Load the 1-D signal $x(t)$ given in the file "p_6_2.mat." This file contains 10 heartbeat signals. Five of these heartbeat time-series signals (denoted as Y1, Y2, etc.) are from five young subjects and the remaining signals (denoted as O1, O2, etc.) are from five elderly subjects (Courtesy of PhysioNet*).

a. Write MATLAB codes to calculate the Higuchi fractal dimension for all subjects. Average this measure across the young subjects and compare the resulting value with the average across the elderly subjects. Comment on the results.
b. Repeat the procedure in Part "a" for the complexity and mobility measures. Compare the measures in young and elderly subjects.

6.3 An image has five gray levels: 0, 1, 2, 3, and 4. From the frequency of occurrences calculated for each gray level over the entire image, the following probabilities have been obtained: $p_0 = 0.15$, $p_1 = 0.2$, $p_2 = 0.25$, $p_3 = 0.30$, and $p_4 = 0.2$.

a. Using the given probabilities, find the entropy of this image.
b. What distribution of probabilities for the given gray levels would provide maximum entropy? Find the value of this maximal entropy and compare it with the value obtained in part "a."

---

* Goldberger, A.L., Amaral, L.A.N., Glass, L., Hausdorff, J.M., Ivanov, P.Ch., Mark, R.G., Mietus, J.E., Moody, G.B., Peng, C.K., and Stanley, H.E. (2000, June 13). PhysioBank, PhysioToolkit, and PhysioNet: Components of a new research resource for complex physiologic signals. *Circulation* 101(23):e215–e220.

6.4 For the symbols of Problem 6.3,

a. Design a Hoffman code.
b. Calculate the code rate for this code.
c. Using code rate as the criterion, compare this code with a fixed-length code for these symbols.

6.5 The EEG signal captured under a fixed condition, i.e., having no stimulation at all or the same type of stimulation during the entire period of measurement, is often considered as an ergodic signal. A typical recording of EEG over a relatively long period of time is given in the file "p_6_5.mat".*

a. Calculate the mean of the stochastic process.
b. Calculate the variance of the stochastic process.
c. Assuming Gaussian distribution, find the PDF of the stochastic process.
d. Using the MATLAB command "`xcorr`", calculate an estimation of the autocorrelation function.
e. Using the correlation function estimated in part "c," estimate the power spectrum of the process.
f. Do you see any visible frequency(ies) in the power spectrum? Interpret your observations.

6.6 Load images in "p_6_6.mat." This file contains two images of the head that have been captured using different MRI machines. The first image is the same image used in Example 6.1. Another image has undergone a significant amount of distortion due to poor machine calibration. We are to register these images using a set of given tie points.

a. Show the images I and I'.
b. Use the following tie points to register the two images:

I	$\leftrightarrow$	I'
$(5,1)$		$(4,3)$
$(10,3)$		$(7,2)$
$(3,2)$		$(5,2)$

c. Show the resulting mapped image.

* Goldberger, A.L., Amaral, L.A.N., Glass, L., Hausdorff, J.M., Ivanov, P.Ch., Mark, R.G., Mietus, J.E., Moody, G.B., Peng, C.K., and Stanley, H.E. (2000, June 13). PhysioBank, PhysioToolkit, and PhysioNet: Components of a new research resource for complex physiologic signals. *Circulation* 101(23):e215–e220.

7 Clustering and Classification

7.1 INTRODUCTION AND OVERVIEW

This section is dedicated to clustering and classification techniques. The first issue to address is the exact definitions of "clustering" and "classification" and the comparison of the two processes. We start this section with the description of these concepts and their importance in biomedical signal and image processing. Then, we discuss several popular clustering and classification techniques including Bayesian methods, K-means, and neural networks.

7.2 CLUSTERING VERSUS CLASSIFICATION

In classification, one is provided with some examples from two or more groups of objects. For example, assume that in a study of cardiovascular diseases, features such as heart rate and cardiac output for a number of healthy persons as well as patients with some known diseases are available. This means that each example (i.e., a set of features taken from a person) is labeled either as healthy or as a particular disease. A classifier is then trained with the "labeled examples" to create a set of rules or mathematical model that can then look at the features captured from a new person and label the case as healthy or a particular disease. Since the set of examples provided to the classifier is used to tune and train the classifier, this set is also referred to as the "training set." Any other case (i.e., set of features captured from the patient) that has not been seen by the classifier (i.e., was not included in the training set) will then be used to "test" the quality of the classifier. In testing the classifier, the features from a person are provided to the trained classifier and the classifier is asked to predict a label for the case (i.e., predict if the case is healthy or a particular type of disease). Then, this prediction is compared with the true label of the case and if the two labels match, the classifier is said to have learned the concept. Often, in order to have a more reliable testing, a number of testing examples are used. The set of examples used to test the trained classifier is often referred to as testing set.

Since the labels for the examples in the training set are known, the training process followed to train a classifier is often called "supervised learning." This means that a "supervisor" has discovered the labels beforehand and provides these labels during the training process. The supervisor can also provide some labeled examples to be treated as the testing set.

Supervised training and classification are heavily used in biomedical sciences. In many applications, physicians can provide biomedical engineers with the previously diagnosed cases to be used for training and testing of a classifier. For example, many automated diagnostic systems for processing of MR images are available in which the system discovers the existence of different types of malignant and benign images. These systems are trained and tested with a number of previously diagnosed cases that radiologists have been provided by the designers of the automated system. Such automated systems, once reliably trained and tested, are capable of assisting physicians in processing and diagnostics of many cases in a very short period of time and, unlike physicians, are not susceptible to issues such as fatigue.

Clustering is a similar process but is often more difficult than classification. In clustering, the examples provided to the clustering method as the training set are not labeled; however, the clustering technique is asked not only to cluster (group) the data but also to provide a set of rules or mathematical equations to distinguish the groups from each other. At first glance, this task might seem unreasonable or even impossible, but as we show later in this chapter, clustering is even more natural and more useful in medical research. Next, a simple example is given that intuitively indicates the possibility and the need for clustering. The example is intentionally chosen to be nonbiomedical such that the importance and feasibility of clustering in all areas of signal processing is better portrayed.

Example 7.1

Assume that two features about a person are given: height and weight. Using these two features, every person can be represented as a point in a two-dimensional (2-D) space, as shown in Figure 7.1.

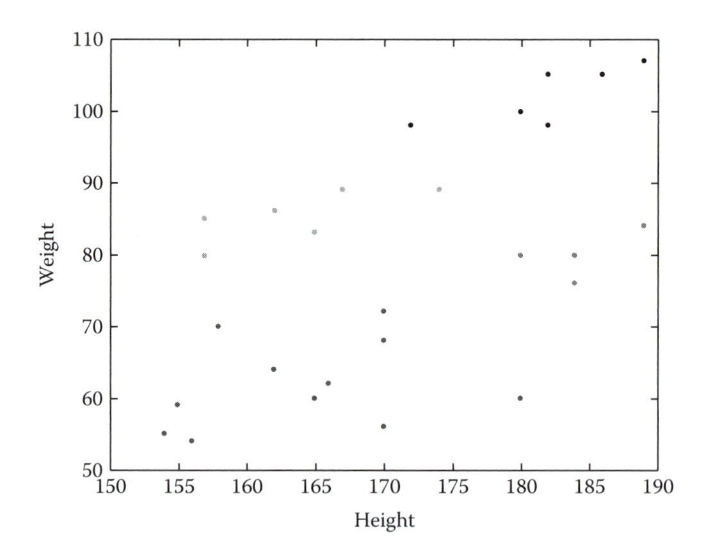

FIGURE 7.1 Two-dimensional feature space representing the weight and height of each person.

As can be seen, without any calculation and merely from observing the distribution of the points, one can see that we are dealing with four clusters (types) of persons, which can be defined as follows:

Cluster 1 (Red): People with small height (<170 cm) and small weight (<70 kg)
Cluster 2 (Yellow): People with small height (<170 cm) and high weight (>70 kg)
Cluster 3 (Green): People with high height (>170 m) and average weight (>70 and <90 kg)
Cluster 4 (Blue): People with high height (>170 m) and high weight (>90 kg)

Looking at health conditions of each cluster, one can see that people belonging to clusters 1 and 4 are more healthy than people in clusters 2 and 3. This means that while people in clusters 2 and 3 need to make some changes in their diet to become healthier, no particular recommendations might be made to the people in clusters 2 and 3. The clustering results as well as the dietary recommendations resulting from these clustering processes are rather intuitive but useful. This means that now the model can be used to analyze the examples that have not been seen by the clustering method. In other words, now that the clusters are formed, one can use the resulting rules to define clusters for assigning new examples to one of the groups. For example, in a classification process based on the resulting groups, a person whose height and weight are 180 cm and 82 kg, respectively, is mapped to cluster 4. Based on our intuitive analysis of cluster 4, people assigned to this cluster are rather healthy and no particular dietary recommendations are needed. It is important to note that this model was created without using any labeled examples, i.e., the training samples used to develop the model were not labeled by a supervisor.

As another biomedical example, consider the discovery of the genes that are involved in the biological pathways involved in a biological process. Essentially, this problem is often simplified to the identification and grouping of the genes that are activated and suppressed at the same time throughout the course of a biological process. In such studies, having no previous example, one simply finds the genes having similar patterns and groups them together as a cluster. When the clusters are formed, the clustering technique can extract some rules or mathematical methods to separate the clusters from each other. This type of learning in which no labeled examples are given and the method is designed to find the clusters without any supervision is called "unsupervised learning."

This chapter first introduces different methods of extracting useful features from signals and images and then presents some popular techniques for classification and clustering.

7.3 FEATURE EXTRACTION

The first step in both clustering and classification is finding the best features to represent an example (sample). For instance, in order to distinguish healthy people from the ones suffering from flu, one needs to collect relevant features such as temperature and blood pressure. The choice of the right features can dramatically affect the outcome of diagnosis. In general, there are two types of features that are often used in biomedical sciences that are discussed in the following text.

7.3.1 Biomedical and Biological Features

Biomedical and biological features, as defined in this book, are the features defined by the knowledge of biology or medicine available about the biological system under study. As the continuation of the previous example, when detecting flu, the most relevant feature proposed by physicians is the body temperature. In many medical applications, a number of features are proposed by the experts (e.g., physicians and biologists) that must be included in the classification of clustering process. In the following chapters, when discussing a number of physiological and biological systems, some important biomedical and biological features pertinent to those systems will be introduced.

Even though the importance of the features identified by the domain knowledge cannot be overestimated, there are a number of other important features that may not be defined in the medical knowledge base or even interpreted by the experts. We group these features as a second category.

7.3.2 Signal and Image Processing Features

In any field of study, there are many features of a quantity that may have not been identified or named by the experts but have the potential of improving the classification or clustering significantly. In biomedical signal and image analysis, some of these features are purely mathematical concepts that may not have a direct physiological or biomedical meaning for the users. As an example, consider the wavelet coefficients of a certain level of decomposition of a biomedical signal. While it may be difficult to find a direct and specific biomedical concept for such coefficients, they are known to be extremely useful features for clustering and classification of many important biomedical signals such as electroencephalogram (EEG) and electrocardiogram (ECG).

It has to be mentioned that some of the apparently pure signal and image processing features can be related to the biologically meaningful features. For example, in the detection of some diseases of the central nervous system (such as epilepsy) from EEG, physicians often count the number of signal peaks or spikes in a given period of time (e.g., a minute) and treat this number as an informative feature in the detection of the disease. It is clear that such a biomedical feature is very closely related to mathematical concepts such as the power of the signal in high frequency of the Fourier transform (FT). This example describes why one needs to study the biology and physiology of the system under study in order to devise mathematical features that best represent the qualitatively defined concepts quantitatively.

In this section, some of the most commonly used signal processing features often used in biomedical signal and image processing are briefly reviewed. Many transforms and computational concepts described in the previous chapters play important roles in extracting useful measures described in the following.

7.3.2.1 Signal Power in Frequency Bands

The high-frequency contents of a signal are often interpreted as a measure of rapid variation in the signal. Similarly, the contents of a signal at different frequency bands quantitatively express the features that are often vital for diagnosis of biomedical signals. For instance, in EEG (as will be described later), there are four important "waves" called alpha, beta, gamma, and delta that play central roles in the analysis of an EEG. These waves are nothing but variations at different frequencies and therefore can be easily extracted and measured using a filter designed in the frequency domain. Once a signal is filtered at a prespecified frequency range (using a band-pass filter), the power of the components passing through the filter describes how strong those particular frequencies are in the signal, for example, whether or not the prespecified waves exist in the recorded EEG.

7.3.2.2 Wavelet Measures

Wavelet transform (WT) provides a number of coefficients that decompose a signal at different scales (as discussed in Chapter 5). These features that are commonly used for classification and clustering of biomedical signals and images were discussed in Chapter 6.

7.3.2.3 Complexity Measures

As discussed in Chapter 6, complexity measures describe the sophisticated structure of biological systems quantitatively. For example, fractal dimension, as described in Chapter 6, is one of the most important complexity measures that expresses the complexity of a signal and is heavily used in biomedical signal processing techniques. Many biological systems are known to become less complex as they get older. For example, the study of the fractal dimension of EEGs taken from people belonging to different age groups indicates that as people get older, their fractal dimension decreases. This feature together with other complexity measures such as mobility, complexity, and entropy was described in Chapter 6.

7.3.2.4 Geometric Measures

Geometric features play an important role in image classification. Some of the main geometric features are described in the following.

Area: In almost all medical image classification applications, one needs to measure the size of the objects in an image. The main feature typically used for this is the area of the object. In image processing, the area of an object is often measured as the number of pixels inside the object. This means that after segmentation of the objects, the number of the pixels inside each closed region (object) indicates the size or area of the region. In processing of tumors, the area of the tumor in a 2-D image is considered as one of the most informative measures.

Perimeter: The evaluation of the perimeter of an object is often an essential part of any algorithm designed for biomedical image processing. Contour features such as perimeter allow distinguishing among the objects having the same area but different perimeter. For instance, two cell nuclei with the same area can have a very different contour shape; one can have a circular counter while the other might be a very long and narrow oval. Since the perimeter of the second cell is much more than that of the first one (while having the same area), the value of perimeter can be used as an informative image processing feature.

Compactness: While both area and perimeter are important features in image processing, it is often desirable to combine these two measures to create a rather unified size measure. This measure is called compactness and is defined as follows:

$$\text{Compactness} = \frac{\text{Perimeter}^2}{\text{Area}} \tag{7.1}$$

By dividing these two measures, compactness provides a feature that identifies the size of the perimeter for a given unit of area. The reason why perimeter appears in the equation as a squared order term is rather straightforward; the resulting measure is not supposed to have a unit. Compactness can easily distinguish between long and narrow oval-shaped objects that have large compactness values and circular objects that have small compactness values. Since many objects in biomedical images have oval and circular shapes (e.g., cells, nuclei, and tumors), features such as compactness are often considered as the main geometric measures during the classification process.

Major and minor axes: In order to express the dimension of the objects, it is a common practice to calculate the major axis of the object. The major axis is defined as the line connecting a pair of points located on the contour of the object whose distance from each other is maximal. In other words, in order to find the major axis, a pair of points on the contour is found whose distance from each other is more than any other pair of points on the contour. The line connecting these two points is the major axis. It is straightforward to see that the major axis of an oval is the line passing through both focal points. The length of the major axis is the largest dimension of the object that has physical and biological significance. The axis perpendicular to the major axis is called the minor axis. The minor axis of an oval is the smallest line connecting a pair of points on the contour. In a circle, any line passing though the center is both a major and a minor axis. The major and minor axes are important diagnostics features in cell image classification.

Eccentricity: An important feature called eccentricity is defined to evaluate the deviation of the object's shape from a symmetric circular shape. Eccentricity is defined as follows:

$$\text{Eccentricity} = \frac{\text{Length of Major Axis}}{\text{Length of Minor Axis}} \tag{7.2}$$

As can be seen, while the eccentricity of a circle is one, the eccentricity of an oval is always more than one. In addition, the larger this measure is, the less circular shape (and more linear) the object must be.

Fourier descriptors: An important feature of tumors and cells is the smoothness of the contour. This feature can be captured using measures called Fourier descriptors (FDs). The FDs are essentially the discrete Fourier transform (DFT) of the points on the contour of the object. Assume that the points $(x_0, y_0), (x_1, y_1), \ldots, (x_{K-1}, y_{K-1})$ are consecutive points forming the contour of the object. In order to form FDs, first, a sequence of complex numbers is formed as $z_i = x_i + y_i$, $i = 0, 1, \ldots, K-1$. Then, the

FD is simply defined as the DFT of the sequence z_i, $i = 0, 1,\ldots, K-1$. Plotting the magnitude of the FD would identify the existence of the high- and low-frequency variations on the contour. The small energy of the high-frequency coefficients shows that the contour is a smooth one. On the other hand, if the absolute value or energy of the high-frequency coefficients is large, the contour has many jumps and discontinuities. The energy of the FD coefficients is sometimes used directly as a feature in the classification process. This feature simply identifies the smoothness of the contour quantitatively.

FDs are also used for compression of the contour data. Specifically, if the high-frequency jitters are not of any significance, one can express the contour using only the low- and medium-frequency coefficients. This is an important technique that helps the storage of the contour information in applications such as cell image processing, where the large number of cells often prevents the storage of all detailed contour information.

Now that we know some of the practically important features in signal and image processing, we can start describing some of the fundamental techniques in clustering and classification.

7.4 K-MEANS: A SIMPLE CLUSTERING METHOD

K-means is one of the most popular techniques heavily used in biomedical signal and image analysis. In K-means, it is assumed that there are "K" groups of patterns in the data and the algorithm attempts to find the optimal clusters based on this assumption. Assume that n samples (patterns or examples) $x_0, x_1,\ldots, x_{n-1}$ are given and K-means is to be used to create K clusters from the data. Each of the clusters will have a cluster center, and each pattern will be assigned to one of the clusters. The way K-means works is rather simple: iteratively find the best centers of each cluster and then assign each pattern to the cluster whose center is the closet to the pattern.

The training of K-means method can be described in the following steps:

Step 0: Randomly initialize the centers $m_0, m_1,\ldots, m_{K-1}$.

Step 1: Find the distance of all samples $x_0, x_1,\ldots, x_{n-1}$ from all centers $m_0, m_1,\ldots, m_{K-1}$, i.e., for all $i = 0,\ldots, n-1$ and $j = 0,\ldots, K-1$ find

$$d_{ij}(x_i, m_j) = \left\| x_i - m_j \right\| = \left((x_{i1} - m_{j1})^2 + \cdots + (x_{ip} - m_{jp})^2 \right)^{\frac{1}{2}} \tag{7.3}$$

Step 2: Form clusters $j = 1, 2,\ldots, K-1$ by assigning each sample to the closet center, i.e., put together all examples whose distance to center j is minimal to form class j.

Step 3: Find the new centers by finding the sample that is the closet sample to the average of all samples in the class, i.e., new m_j is the average of all examples in class j.

Step 4: If during the last iteration, no example has changed its class, go to Step 5; otherwise, go to Step 2.
Step 5: Terminate process. The final clusters are the outputs of the algorithm.

The concept of K-means clustering is better described in the following simple visual example.

Example 7.2

In this example, without using any mathematics or calculations, we explore the mechanism of K-means clustering through a symbolic visual example. Consider the patterns given in Figure 7.2a. Each of the coordinates in Figure 7.2a is a feature, and each example is shown as a point. As can be visually perceived, there are three clusters of patterns.

Assuming $K = 3$, the centers of the three clusters must be randomly initialized in Step 0. In Figure 7.2b such a random initialization of the centers is shown. As can be seen, the initial centers randomly selected for two clusters on the right-hand side belong to the same cluster (the cluster on the far right). Such a choice, even though not the best initialization choice, will better exhibit the capabilities of K-means.

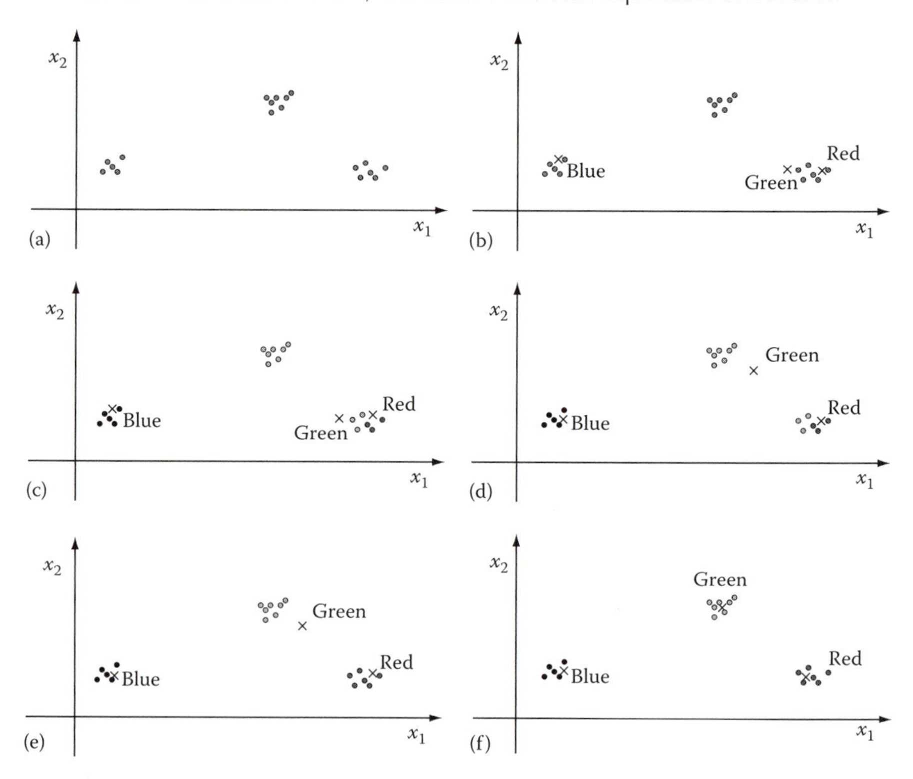

FIGURE 7.2 (a) The given patterns that naturally cluster as three linearly separable clusters. (b) Initialization of the cluster centers. (c) Assignment of examples to the initial clusters. (d) Calculation of the new cluster centers. (e) Assignment of examples to the clusters using the new cluster center. (f) Calculation of the new cluster centers.

In the next step, for each example in the feature space, we need to determine the cluster to which the example belongs to. This choice is simply made based on the proximity of the examples to the cluster centers. The results of this cluster assignment step are shown in Figure 7.2c.

Next, we need to average the members in each of the resulting cluster to find the new cluster centers and then reassign the samples to the clusters, this time using the new cluster centers. The new cluster centers are shown in Figure 7.2d. As can be seen, the centers of the clusters are now closer to the expected centers of the actual clusters. At the next iteration, we use the new cluster centers to assign every example to one of the three clusters. The results of this assignment are shown in Figure 7.2e. Finally, we calculate the new centers based on the clusters obtained in Figure 7.2e, which gives the cluster centers depicted in Figure 7.2f. At this point, the cluster centers are indeed in the center of actual clusters and repeating the process for extra iteration will not change the clusters. At this point, the algorithm has converged to the actual clusters, and, therefore, the iterations are terminated. This example shows how K-means can effectively cluster unlabeled data.

In MATLAB®, the command “k-means” is used to perform K-means clustering. We explore using MATLAB for K-means clustering in the following example.

Example 7.3

In this example, we first generate 40 random samples. Twenty samples in this pool are generated using a 2-D normal distribution centered at (1, 1), and the remaining 20 samples are from another normal distribution centered at (–1, –1). Then, a K-means algorithm is applied to cluster these samples into two clusters. The MATLAB codes for this example are as follows:

```
X=[randn(20,2) + 2.8 * ones(20,2);
randn(20,2)-2.8*ones(20,2)]
[cidx, ctrs] = kmeans(X, 2, 'dist','city', 'rep',5, 'disp',
   'final')
plot(X(cidx==1,1),X(cidx==1,2),'r.', ...
X(cidx==2,1),X(cidx==2,2), 'b.', ctrs(:,1),ctrs(:,2), 'kx');
```

In the preceding code, first, we use the command “randn” to generate 40 normally distributed random samples out of which 20 samples are around (1, 1) and the rest are centered at (–1, –1). Then, we use K-means algorithm to perform clustering of these samples and divide them into two clusters. Number “2” in k-means command reflects our desire to form two clusters for the data. The options “dist” and “sqEuclidean” specify the Euclidean distance as the distance measure for clustering. The rest of the code deals with the labeling of the samples in each cluster.

Figure 7.3 shows the result of clustering. Samples of one cluster are shown with red, and the samples belonging to the other class are graphed in blue color. We have also marked the center of each cluster by X’s. In this example, many points generated by the first random generator, centered at (1, 1), are correctly assigned to the “blue” cluster. However, some points closer to the origin, while generated by the random generator at (1, 1), may be assigned to the red group, which is mainly formed by the sample of the other normal distribution. This shows that even though K-means is a simple and rather fast algorithm, it has some limitations.

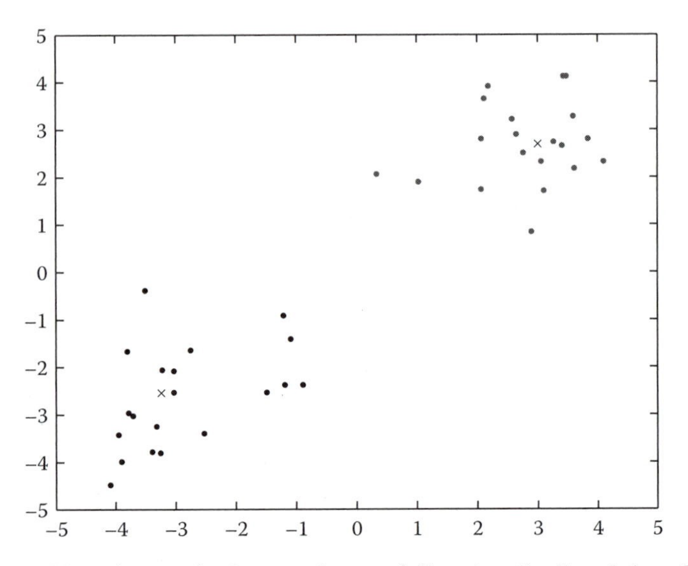

FIGURE 7.3 Clustering results for two classes of Gaussian distributed data. Samples of cluster 1 are shown in dark grey and samples of cluster 2 in light grey. The cluster centers are shown by ×'s.

7.5 BAYESIAN CLASSIFIER

One of the most popular methods in classification methods is the Bayesian classifier. Bayesian decision theory extracts some decision rules from the data and then evaluates the cost of these decisions. In Bayesian theory, it is assumed that we know the probability distribution of the involved classes. This is obviously a drawback for this technique because in many applications, these probabilities are not known. However, if a rather large sample of data is available, the probabilities can be estimated from data.

We describe the concepts and procedures of Bayesian theory with a simple example that deals with detecting tumor pixels in a digital image such as MRI. In such an application, we have two classes: a class of tumor pixels and a class of nontumor pixels. This means that in an image, each pixel belongs to one of the possible classes (states), tumor or nontumor. We denote by ω the state of the nature or simply the class of the sample. For tumor pixels, $\omega = \omega_1$, and for nontumor pixels, we set $\omega = \omega_2$.

An important concept, which is important in Bayesian theory, is "a priori probability." The concept of a priori probability in our simple example quantifies the probability of a pixel belonging to tumor or nontumor class. It is apparent that this probability for tumor pixels depends on the number of tumor pixels as well as the total number of all pixels (tumor and nontumor pixels). We denote a priori probability of the classes ω_1 and ω_2 as $P(\omega_1)$ and $P(\omega_2)$, respectively.

If we do not have any information other than a priori probability of each class and we are asked to make a decision about the class of a given pixel, we would simply choose the class whose a priori probability is larger, i.e., when $P(\omega_i) > P(\omega_j)$, we vote for ω_i. Note that such a decision, as long as a priori probabilities are known, does not depend on any observed data, and regardless of any observation in the features space, the decision is always made based on the previously known values of $P(\omega_1)$ and $P(\omega_2)$. Loosely speaking, such decisions are like predicting that a summer day is sunny based on the yearly statistics that identifies a fixed probability for summer days being sunny. Such a decision ignores any observation for some particular year. Even though this type of decision making based only on a priori probability can have a relatively high success rate in certain applications, it is blind to observations made from the system.

In many practical applications, however, the information contained in $P(\omega_i)$ probability measure is too limited to make a good decision. This is why we often use another variable to improve our decision about the class of the new samples. In the aforementioned example, assuming that the image to be processed is in color, the color of each pixel can be a suitable variable in helping us make a better classification decision. For each pixel, we have three color elements, r (the intensity of the red component), g (the intensity of the green component), and b (the intensity of the green component). Based on the class of the pixel (tumor or nontumor), the color elements will be in a specific range.

The color information then leads us to define a new probability called "class conditional probability." $P(r, g, b|\omega_1)$ is the class conditional probability of class 1, and $P(r, g, b|\omega_2)$ is the class conditional probability of class 2. For simplicity, we name the vector (r, g, b) as X. This reduces the notation for the class conditional probability to $P(X|\omega_i)$. The probability measure $P(X|\omega_i)$ quantifies the probability that the color of a pixel belonging to class ω_i be in the range of X. However, what we normally need to do for classification is rather the opposite of what we get from the class conditional probability, i.e., we are to determine the class of a selected pixel based on its color vector X. For instance, we know the color elements of a pixel and we intend to decide whether the pixel is a tumor or a nontumor pixel. This means that we need to determine the probabilities $P(\omega_i|X)$ as opposed to the conditional probabilities $P(X|\omega_i)$. The probability $P(\omega_i|X)$ quantifies the likelihood that a given pixel belongs to class ω_i, knowing that the color vector of the selected pixel is X. We call this probability "a posteriori probability." While it is often difficult to compute a posteriori probability directly, one can compute a posteriori probability using a priori and class conditional probabilities as follows:

$$P(\omega_i|X)P(X) = P(X|\omega_i)P(\omega_i) \quad (7.4)$$

Therefore,

$$P(\omega_i|X) = \frac{P(X|\omega_i)P(\omega_i)}{P(X)} \quad (7.5)$$

Practically, for any given pixel, we need to compute $P(\omega_i|X)$ for each of the classes i and then vote for the class whose a posteriori probability is the largest. Since $P(X)$ is the same for all classes, we can disregard this probability in the decision-making process and compare $P(X|\omega_i)P(\omega_i)$ terms with each other. For example, for the simple tumor example, the decision-making process becomes choosing ω_1 if

$$P(X|\omega_1)P(\omega_1) > P(X|\omega_2)P(\omega_2) \quad (7.6)$$

and ω_2 otherwise.

The simple Bayesian classification method, although straightforward and intuitive, may not be sophisticated enough to deal with real-world problems. In practice, simple Bayesian methods are often combined with some heuristic and domain-based knowledge to improve the classification results. One extension of the Bayesian classification method is achieved through the use of the concept of "loss function."

7.5.1 Loss Function

In many practical applications including medical diagnostics, it is often the case that some misclassifications are more costly than others. For instance, the cost of misclassifying a cancer sample as normal (healthy) is far more than misclassifying a normal sample as cancer. As a result, one would like to somehow incorporate the importance and impact of each decision directly in the classification algorithm.

Loss functions are used to give different weights to different classification mistakes. Assuming the two-category classification, such as in the simple example discussed earlier, there will be two types of acts: α_1 and α_2. Now, let us define $\lambda(\alpha_i|\omega_j)$ as the loss when action α_i is taken, while the true state of the nature is ω_j. Using the loss functions $\lambda(\alpha_i|\omega_j)$, $i = 1, 2, j = 1, 2$ $(i \neq j)$, a new risk function for each action can be defined to improve the decision criteria and incorporate the relative importance of each misclassification in the decision process. This risk function can be defined as follows:

$$R(\alpha_i|X) = \lambda(\alpha_i|\omega_1)P(\omega_1|X) + \lambda(\alpha_i|\omega_2)P(\omega_2|X) \tag{7.7}$$

The best decision is then made based on these risk functions. For instance, if $R(\alpha_1|X) < R(\alpha_2|X)$, α_1 will be the action.

Example 7.4

Figure 7.4 shows two categories forming a 2-D dataset. The data for each category are Gaussian distributed. We intend to use Bayesian decision rule to find a decision boundary between the two categories.

To do this, we need to estimate probability function for each category. Since we know that probability functions of these two categories are Gaussian, all we need to do is to compute the sample mean and sample variance of each category to obtain the probability density functions (PDFs). Calculating the sample means and sample variances of these two categories, we have

$$\mu_1 = \begin{bmatrix} 4 \\ 4 \end{bmatrix} \quad \mu_2 = \begin{bmatrix} -1 \\ 4 \end{bmatrix} \quad \Sigma_1 = \begin{bmatrix} 1/2 & 0 \\ 0 & 1/2 \end{bmatrix} \quad \Sigma_2 = \begin{bmatrix} 1/2 & 0 \\ 0 & 1/2 \end{bmatrix}$$

Using Equation 7.4, the optimal decision boundary can be obtained as follows:

$$P(X|\omega_1)P(\omega_1) = P(X|\omega_2)P(\omega_2) \tag{7.8}$$

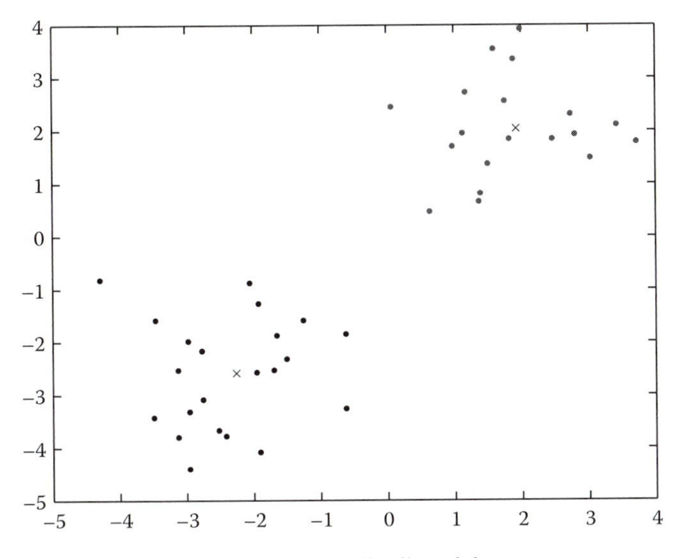

FIGURE 7.4 Two categories of 2-D Gaussian distributed data.

Assuming that we have equal a priori probabilities, i.e., $P(\omega_1) = P(\omega_2)$, Equation 7.6 will be simplified to

$$P(X|\omega_1) = P(X|\omega_2) \tag{7.9}$$

Now, for Gaussian distributions,

$$p(X) = \frac{1}{(2\pi)^{d/2}|\Sigma|^{1/2}} \exp\left[-\frac{1}{2}(X-\mu)^t \Sigma^{-1}(X-\mu)\right] \tag{7.10}$$

By substitution of Equation 7.8 in Equation 7.7 and using "ln" function for both sides of Equation 7.7, we have

$$(X-\mu_1)^t \Sigma_1^{-1}(X-\mu_1) - \frac{1}{2}\ln|\Sigma_1| = (X-\mu_2)^t \Sigma_2^{-1}(X-\mu_2) - \frac{1}{2}\ln|\Sigma_2| \tag{7.11}$$

The reason for applying the logarithm function on is to reduce exponential equations to a simpler form. Since in this example, variances are assumed to be equal, i.e., $\Sigma_1 = \Sigma_2$, these terms can be eliminated from two sides of Equation 7.9. Using the values of μ_1, μ_2, Σ_1, and Σ_2 of the samples shown in Figure 7.5 and solving Equation 7.9 for the point where the two distributions intersect, X_1, we obtain this value as $X_1 = 8/3$. This means that when a new sample is measured, the comparison of the features of the new sample with X_1 will identify the class the sample belongs to.

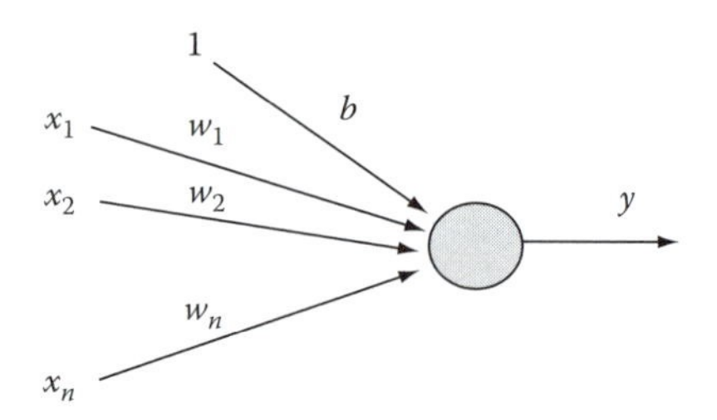

FIGURE 7.5 Structure of a perceptron.

7.6 MAXIMUM LIKELIHOOD METHOD

One of the main problems in pattern recognition is parameter estimation of the probability functions. Maximum likelihood estimation (MLE) is one of the most popular methods to address this problem. Methods based on MLEs often provide better convergence properties as the number of training samples increases.

As mentioned previously, in order to form the Bayesian decision equations, the class conditional probabilities are needed. Since in practice, the knowledge of these probabilities is not available, efficient techniques are employed to estimate these probabilities. Assume that the type or family of the PDF $p(X|\omega_i)$, for example, Gaussian, is known, one can determine the parameters of this probability function.

Suppose that there are c classes in a given pattern classification problem. Also, assume that the n sample $x_1,\ldots, x_n$ created by one of the classes (according to the PDF of that class) are collected in a set D. Note that we do not know which class this set of observed data belongs to and we are to use the MLE to predict which one of these classes c is more likely to have generated the data. We assume that the samples in D are independent and identically distributed (i.i.d.). As mentioned before, we are assuming that the PDFs, i.e., $p(X|\theta_i)$'s for $i = 1, 2,\ldots, c$, have a known parametric form, and, therefore, we only need to determine the parameter vector θ that uniquely identifies the PDF of one of the classes. Then, knowing that the samples are independent, we can describe the probability of obtaining the sample set D assuming that the parameters are θ as follows:

$$p(D|\theta) = \prod_{k=1}^{n} p(X_k|\theta) \tag{7.12}$$

We call $p(D|\theta)$ the likelihood of θ because this probability identifies the likelihood of obtaining the samples in D given that the estimated parameter set θ is a suitable one. The MLE is simply an estimation method that finds the set of parameters that maximizes the likelihood function $p(D|\theta)$. In other words, the maximum likelihood function results in a probability function that is more likely to produce the observed data. Note that since we do not know the true set of parameters, all we can obtain is an estimation of these values through methods such as maximum likelihood. As such, we denote by $\hat{\theta}$ the MLE of θ, which maximizes $p(D|\theta)$.

Once again and due to the multiplicative nature Equation 7.10 that defines the likelihood function, instead of optimizing the likelihood function $p(D|\theta)$ directly, we often use the log of this function. Using Equation 7.10, we obtain a new function $l(\theta)$ defined as follows:

$$l(\theta) = \sum_{k=1}^{n} \ln p(X_k|\theta) \tag{7.13}$$

This function is often referred to as the log likelihood function. Next, in order to obtain the best estimation, $\hat{\theta}$, we need to see how the log likelihood function can be maximized. A simple approach is to utilize the gradient of this log likelihood function to find $\hat{\theta}$ that maximizes $l(\theta)$. Calculating the gradient of the likelihood function in terms of θ, we have

$$\nabla_\theta l = \sum_{k=1}^{n} \nabla_\theta \ln p(X_k|\theta) \tag{7.14}$$

Next, all we have to do is to set $\nabla_\theta l$ equal to zero to find $\hat{\theta}$, i.e., our best estimation of parameters would be the value θ that satisfies the equation $\nabla_\theta l = 0$. The exact form of this equation evidently depends on the exact form of the probability functions $p(X_k|\theta)$'s. For many practical choices of $p(X_k|\theta)$, the equation $\nabla_\theta l = 0$ becomes too complicated to be solved manually, and, therefore, computational software such as MATLAB would be needed to find the maximum likelihood estimation $\hat{\theta}$.

Example 7.5

In this example, we show how to perform MLE in MATLAB. In MATLAB, one can utilize the command "mle" to estimate the parameters assuming a certain probability distribution. As can be seen in the following code, we first produce a vector of 400 normally distributed random samples. In the command "mle", we need to determine the form of the distribution under which the data are produced and what "mle" estimates are the set of parameters for the chosen distribution form. There are some other commands in MATLAB that apply "mle" estimator to estimate parameters of some popular distributions such as binomial, exponential, gamma, etc. The following code shows the command "binofit" that uses "mle" estimator to estimate parameters of binomial distribution and "expfit" that estimates parameters of the exponential distribution.

```
x1=randn(1,400);
mle(normal,x1);
r=binornd(100,.9);
[phat,pci]=binofit(r,100);
lifetimes= exprnd(700,100,1);
[muhat,muci]= expfit(lifetimes);
```

It is important to note that, in practice, the type of distribution function producing the data is unknown. In the previous example, even though we have produced that data using a Gaussian distribution, we attempt to find the best parameters for some other distributions, because in order to emulate real problems, we must assume that no knowledge of the true distribution is available.

With MLE giving us the most likely PDFs for classes, one can then use methods such as Bayesian classifiers to perform classification. However, as previously mentioned, for most sophisticated problems, one may need to use more sophisticated classifiers such neural networks, as discussed in the following.

7.7 NEURAL NETWORKS

Even though maximum likelihood and other statistical methods prove to be effective techniques in rather simple problems, they may not provide the best solutions for more complex problems. In addition, the need to make an assumption on the type of the distribution function producing data, as explained earlier, is another disadvantage of such methods.

In practice, methods such as neural networks are preferred in more sophisticated problems. Neural networks are computational methods directly inspired by the formation and function of biological neural structures. Just like the biological neural structures, artificial neural networks are simply a formation of artificial neurons that learn patterns directly from examples. These methods are distribution free, which means no assumptions are made on the type of the data distribution. In addition, due to the nonlinear nature of the method, neural networks are capable of solving complex nonlinear classification problems that cannot be addressed by simple statistical methods. Neural networks are composed of a number of neurons that are connected through some "weights." Since the structure and the function of each neuron is known, in order to train a neural network, one needs to use the given training examples to find the best values of the weights. Once the weights are found, the neural network is uniquely defined and can be used for classification and modeling.

Despite all capabilities listed for neural networks, the reader needs to be warned not to use neural networks for certain types of applications. For example, neural networks require many training examples to learn a pattern, and if, for the problem to be addressed, sufficient number of examples are not available, neural networks may not be the best solutions. This is due to the fact that neural networks can easily fit any training data and if the training dataset is too small to be a good representative of the problem, neural networks are simply overfitting the training examples without learning the true patterns.

There are many families of neural networks, but, here, we focus on the most popular one, which is the family of multilayer sigmoid neural networks. These structures are supervised classification methods that can theoretically model any complex system to any desired accuracy. We start describing these structures with a simple single-neuron structure known as a perceptron.

7.7.1 PERCEPTRON

Perceptrons are nothing but simple emulation of the biological neurons. These classifiers, as the simplest forms of neural networks, have a simple but effective learning procedure. More specifically, given that the classes can be separated by straight lines, perceptrons can always provide the correct classifiers. Figure 7.5 shows the structure of a simple perceptron. Just as in a biological neuron that receives some inputs from the neighboring neurons and produces an output, a perceptron has a number of inputs and one output. As can be seen, an extra input, called bias, is added to the regular inputs. As discussed in more detail later in this chapter, even though the value of this input is constant, the insertion of the bias input helps improve the classification performance.

As can be seen in Figure 7.5, there is a weight associated with the connection between any of the inputs x_i's and the output of the neuron. The strength of each connection is described by a weight w_i, and the weight of the bias input is denoted by b. The total effect of the inputs on the perceptron is given as the weighted summation of the inputs:

$$y_0 = b + \sum_i x_i w_i \tag{7.15}$$

Then, the output of the perceptron is calculated based on y_0 as follows:

$$y = \begin{cases} 1 & \text{if } y_0 > T \\ 0 & \text{if } -T < y_0 < T \\ -1 & \text{if } y_0 < -T \end{cases} \tag{7.16}$$

where T is a threshold value that is often set by the user.

The thresholding process shown in Equation 7.14 is exactly what is happening in biological neurons, i.e., if the total excitation of the neighboring neurons is more than a threshold value, the neuron fires. The choice of the threshold value T is rather arbitrary, but when this value is chosen, it is fixed throughout training and testing processes. It has to be mentioned that perceptrons can be designed to accept or produce binary (0 or 1), bipolar (1 and −1), or even real values. The earlier formulation, i.e., bipolar, can be easily modified to create binary and real-valued models too.

As briefly mentioned earlier, besides the regular inputs to a perceptron, which are the features of the samples, it is often necessary to add another input, which is always set to a constant such as 1. This input, which is called bias, is needed to produce better separation among the classes of patterns. Knowing that bias is always set to 1, it is evident that no new information is added to the network by adding the bias, but a new term is added to the summation terms in y_0. In addition, the weight connecting this constant input to the perceptron needs to be updated as any other weights in the system.

Next, we discuss the training of a perceptron. Note that the main goal of training a perceptron is to teach the perceptron how to classify each input pattern and determine the particular class the pattern belongs to. In other words, training is nothing but to adjust the weights of the perceptron to make it produce 1 if the sample belongs to a particular class and −1 if the sample does not belong to this class. A perceptron first initializes the weights of the network by random numbers and then uses an iterative technique for updating of the weights, i.e., when encountering an example, the values of the weights are iteratively adjusted to produce the correct or better classification. Specifically, assume that for a sample $\boldsymbol{x}_j = (x_{j1}, x_{j2},\ldots, x_{jn})$ the true target output is t. We use this knowledge to update the weights. Assume that with the old (current) values of the weights, the estimated output for $\boldsymbol{x}_j$ is y. Then, if $y = t$, then the old values of weights are fine and no real update is needed. Otherwise, the old values of the weights are updated as follows:

$$\begin{aligned} w_i(new) &= w_i(old) + tx_{ji} \\ b(new) &= b(old) + t \end{aligned} \tag{7.17}$$

where
  x_{ji} is the ith element of the sample vector $\boldsymbol{x}_j$
  $w_i(new)$ is the new value of the weight w_i

The training process is continued until the exposure of the network can correctly classify all examples in the training set. In order to train a neural network of any type, it is often the case that the network must be exposed to all training quite a few times. Each cycle of exposing the network to all training examples is called an epoch.

The learning process described in the following can result to rather oscillatory results in consecutive epochs. In other words, each time an example is used for training, the weights are significantly changed to accommodate that particular example, but as soon as the next example is used for training, the weights are very much changed in favor of the new example. The same scenario is repeated in the consecutive epochs, and, therefore, the values of weights oscillate among some sets that accommodate particular examples. In order to address this issue, instead of the learning equations of Equation 7.15, the following learning criteria are used:

$$\begin{aligned} w_i(new) &= w_i(old) + \alpha t x_{ji} \\ b(new) &= b(old) + \alpha t \end{aligned} \tag{7.18}$$

In the preceding equations, $0 < \alpha < 1$ is called the learning rate. The fact that the learning rate is less than one, each time a new example is used for training, instead of adjusting the weights completely to accommodate that training example as we did in the previous training scheme, the weights are adjusted only to some degree that depends on the exact value of α. Choosing α to be a number close to 0.1 or so would effectively eliminate the unwanted oscillations in the weight values.

Before providing an example for perceptron, we focus on the perceptron's resulting classifier. A closer look at the formulation of perceptron reveals that a perceptron splits the feature space into three subspaces. For instance, assuming 2-D inputs, a trained perceptron produces two separating lines. These two lines split the space into three regions: a positive region (in which all examples belongs to the class under study), a negative region (in which none of the examples belongs to the class under study), and a dead zone. One of these separating lines that separates the positive region from the dead formulates the positive region as follows:

$$w_1x_1 + w_2x_2 + b > T \tag{7.19}$$

The other one separates the negative region from the dead zone and forms the negative region as follows:

$$w_1x_1 + w_2x_2 + b < -T \tag{7.20}$$

Next, we make two observations in the preceding formulations. First, note that the earlier description of the positive and negative regions further describes the need for bias. If $T = 0$, i.e., no bias, all border lines pass through the origin. This significantly limits the capability of the method to find an optimal separation between classes. In other words, adding bias to a network effectively increases the capabilities of the network in separating the classes. The second observation justifies the statement made earlier about the perceptron. As mentioned previously, a perceptron can create correct classification only when the classes are linearly separable. From the preceding formulation, it can be seen that in a perceptron the boundary between the classes is a line (2-D space), plane (three-dimensional [3-D] space), or hyperplane (four-dimensional [4-D] space or higher dimensions). All these boundaries are linear and therefore cannot separate classes that are only nonlinearly separable. For nonlinearly separable spaces, as we will see later, networks more sophisticated than a perceptron are required.

As mentioned earlier, the perceptron algorithm can be simply modified for bipolar, binary, and real-valued input and output vectors. The following example describes a problem with binary inputs and binary outputs.

Example 7.6

A typical demonstration example for perceptron is using perceptron to model the logical "OR" function. Assuming two inputs for the OR function, the output is 1 if any of the inputs is 1; otherwise, when both inputs are 0, the output of the function is 0. Augmenting the input space by adding the bias input, the perceptron will have three inputs. Then, the training set for the perceptron will be as follows. For inputs $(x_1, x_2, b) = (1, 1, 1)$, $(x_1, x_2, b) = (1, 0, 1)$, and $(x_1, x_2, b) = (0, 1, 1)$, the target value will be $t = 1$, and for the input $(x_1, x_2, b) = (0, 0, 1)$, the output will be $t = 0$.

In training the perceptron, we assume $\alpha = 1$ and $\theta = 0.2$. Table 7.1 shows the training steps for this perceptron. In each step, we change the weights of network based on the learning rate and the output of the network. Training continues until for a complete epoch, no weight is changing its value. In last training step, where there is no change in weights, the final weights are $w_1 = 2$, $w_2 = 2$, and $w_3 = -1$. Therefore, the positive

TABLE 7.1
Training of Perceptron

Input					Target	Weight			Weights		
x_1	x_2	b	y_0	Output	Value	Changes			w_1	w_2	w_3
1	1	1	0	0	1	1	1	1	1	1	1
1	0	1	1	1	1	0	0	0	1	1	1
0	1	1	1	1	1	0	0	0	1	1	1
0	0	1	0	0	−1	0	0	−1	1	1	−1
1	1	1	1	1	1	0	0	0	1	1	−1
1	0	1	0	0	1	1	0	1	2	1	2
0	1	1	3	1	1	0	0	0	2	1	2
0	0	1	2	1	−1	0	0	−1	2	1	1
1	1	1	4	1	1	0	0	0	2	1	1
1	0	1	3	1	1	0	0	0	2	1	1
0	1	1	2	1	1	0	0	0	2	1	1
0	0	1	1	1	−1	0	0	−1	2	1	0
1	1	1	3	1	1	0	0	0	2	1	0
1	0	1	2	1	1	0	0	0	2	1	0
0	1	1	1	1	1	0	0	0	2	1	0
0	0	1	0	0	−1	0	0	−1	2	1	−1
1	1	1	2	1	1	0	0	0	2	1	−1
1	0	1	1	1	1	0	0	0	2	1	−1
0	1	1	0	0	1	0	1	1	2	2	1
0	0	1	1	1	−1	0	0	−1	2	2	0
1	1	1	4	1	1	0	0	0	2	2	0
1	0	1	2	1	1	0	0	0	2	2	0
0	1	1	2	1	1	0	0	0	2	2	0
0	0	1	0	0	−1	0	0	−1	2	2	−1
1	1	1	3	1	1	0	0	0	2	2	−1
1	0	1	1	1	1	0	0	0	2	2	−1
0	1	1	1	1	1	0	0	0	2	2	−1
0	0	1	−1	−1	−1	0	0	0	2	2	−1

response line will be $2x_1 + 2x_2 - 1 > 0.2$, or simply $x_1 + x_2 > 0.6$, and the negative response line becomes $2x_1 + 2x_2 - 1 < -0.2$ or $x_1 + x_2 < 0.4$.

In MATLAB, the command "`newp`" is used to create a perceptron network. This command is as follows:

```
net = newp(PR,S)
```

where

`PR` is a vector identifying the range of the input elements (i.e., min and max of each input)

`S` is the number of perceptrons (neurons)

Next, we solve the problem discussed in Example 7.6 using MATLAB.

Example 7.7

In this example, we solve the OR gate problem using MATLAB. First, we define a perceptron net as `net = newp([0 1; -2 2],1)`. Next, we define the input values `P = [0 0 1 1; 0 1 0 1]` and target values `T = [0 1 1 1]` and then apply the "train" command to train the network with the specified input and target (output) values. And finally, using "sim" command, we simulate the network and compare the predicted output values generated by the trained network against the true target values. The complete code has been shown as follows:

```
net= newp([0 1; -2 2],1);
P = [0 0 1 1; 0 1 0 1];
T = [0 1 1 1];
net = train(net, P,T);
Y = sim(net, P)
```

7.7.2 Sigmoid Neural Networks

For a few decades, it was experimentally believed that single-layer neural networks such as perceptron have certain limitations that prevent the use of these methods for real-world problems. One such limitation was the observation made about the perceptron that such structures cannot separate patterns that are not linearly separable. But after a few decades, multilayer sigmoid neural networks were proposed to solve the problems of single-layer neural networks. Simply put, it turned out that with multiple layers of perceptrons and other types of neurons, any complex pattern, linear or nonlinear, can be effectively classified. Figure 7.6 shows a multilayer backpropagation neural network.

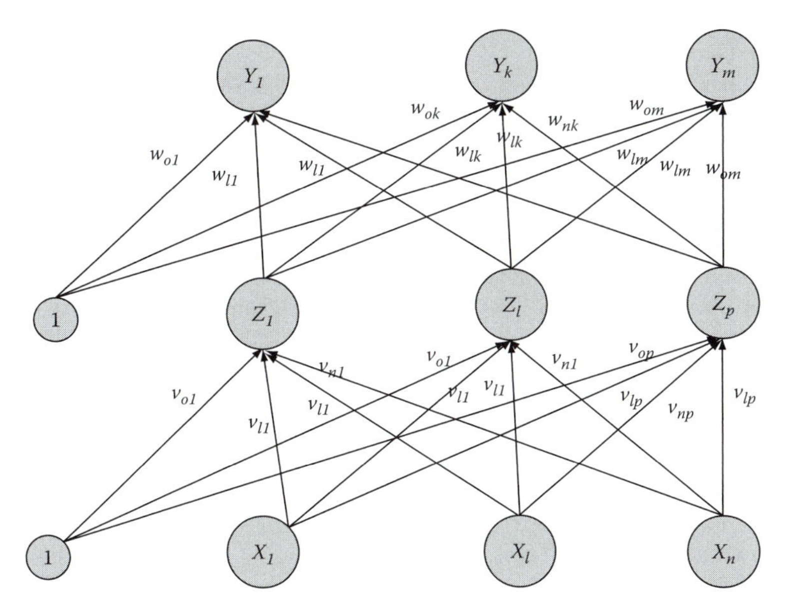

FIGURE 7.6 Typical multilayer sigmoid neural network with one hidden layer.

A multilayer sigmoid neural network always has one input layer (**X** units) that has as many neurons as there are inputs to the network. Similarly, there is always an output layer (**Y** or **T** units) that has as many outputs as the number of outputs of the networks. Such structures can have an arbitrary number of hidden layers (**Z** units) between the input and output layers. Each of these hidden layers can have an arbitrary number of neurons. The number of hidden layers and the number of neurons in each layer are to the most part chosen experimentally through a process of trial and error. Even though paradigms such as computational learning theory have attempted to create rules for setting the optimal number of hidden layers and the number of neurons in each hidden layer, these numbers are often set in such a way to avoid the overcomplexity of the network and, at the same time, provide a powerful function to estimate complex problems.

Backpropagation neural networks, another name given to multilayer sigmoid neural networks, are among the most popular types of the neural networks used in real applications. In reality, backpropagation as defined later is merely one method of training sigmoid neural networks, but since this algorithm is almost always used for training these structures, in many books, multilayer sigmoid neural networks are also called backpropagation neural networks. Another common name that is often mistakenly used to describe multilayer sigmoid neural networks is multilayer perceptrons. As we will see later on, the type of neurons used in multilayer sigmoid neural networks are continuous-output neurons and not perceptrons that are discrete neurons.

7.7.2.1 Activation Function

In perceptron, the activation function was a simple thresholding process, i.e., if the weighted sum of input is less than a certain threshold value, the output is set to some value, and if the weighted sum is less than the threshold, a different value is introduced as the output of the neuron. This threshold effect simply makes the perceptron a discrete neuron, i.e., the output value is not continuous and belongs to a discrete set. As briefly mentioned before, the activation functions and neurons used in multilayer sigmoid neural networks are continuous, differentiable, and monotonically increasing. These characteristics for the activation functions are needed to guarantee that the network and its elements (e.g., neurons outputs) are all differentiable. As we will see in this section, almost all training methods used for multilayer sigmoid neural networks apply partial derivatives of the neurons, layers, and final output. In addition, it is often preferred to have the activation functions whose derivates can be computed easily.

One of the most popular activation functions is binary sigmoid function (also referred to as "logsig"):

$$f_1(x) = \frac{1}{1+\exp(-x)} \tag{7.21}$$

which gives the derivate $f_1'(x)$ as follows:

$$f_1'(x) = f_1(x)[1 - f_1(x)] \tag{7.22}$$

Two other popular sigmoid activation functions that are often used for bipolar and real-valued outputs are "atan" and "tansig" activation functions defined as follows:

$$f(x) = \frac{2}{\pi}\tan^{-1}(\sigma x) \tag{7.23}$$

and

$$f(x) = \tanh(\sigma x) \tag{7.24}$$

As can be seen, these two functions create numbers between −1 and 1 as their output, and that is why they are called bipolar activation functions.

7.7.2.2 Backpropagation Algorithm

In this section, we explain backpropagation algorithm. As in the perceptron, first, the weights of the network are initialized by randomly generated numbers. Backpropagation algorithm then updates the weights of the neural network through the propagation of error from the output backward to the neurons in the hidden and input layers. Backpropagation algorithm has four main stages as follows: (1) calculation of the output based on the current weights of network and the input patterns, (2) calculation of the error between the true target output and the predicted output, (3) backpropagation of the associated error to the previous layers, and finally, (4) adjustment of the weights according the backpropagated error. As can be seen, in steps 2 and 3 of backpropagation, each input units receives an input signal and transmits this input signal to hidden layer units. Then, each hidden layer unit computes its activation and sends it to the output units. For simplicity, from this point on, we assume that the network has only one hidden layer but the same algorithm can be easily extended to the networks for more than one hidden layer.

First, the output of the network must be computed. For output unit k, the weighted sum of the inputs (from hidden layers) can be calculated as follows:

$$y_{0k} = w_{ok} + \sum_j z_j w_{jk} \tag{7.25}$$

Then, the output of this output node, y_k, is calculated as follows:

$$y_k = f(y_{0k}) \tag{7.26}$$

Next, the output of each output node y_k and the corresponding target value t_k are used to compute the associated error for that pattern (example). This error, δ_k, is calculated as follows:

$$\delta_k = t_k - y_k \tag{7.27}$$

These errors in output units are then distributed back to the units of hidden layer and are also used to update the weights between hidden layer units and output layer units. In order to see how this is done, note that for the neurons in the hidden layers we have

$$z_{0j} = v_{oj} + \sum_i x_i v_{ij} \tag{7.28}$$

and

$$z_j = f(z_{0j}) \tag{7.29}$$

where

v_{ij}s are the weights ending at the hidden unit j
v_{oj} is the bias weight of the hidden unit j
z_{0j} is the weighted sum of the inputs entering the hidden node j
z_j is the output of the hidden node j

The updating of the weights v_{ij}s and v_{oj} is then performed as follows:

$$v_{ij}(t+1) = v_{ij}(t) + \alpha\delta_j x_i \tag{7.30}$$

$$v_{0j}(t+1) = v_{0j}(t) + \alpha\delta_j \tag{7.31}$$

In the preceding equations, α is the learning rate as defined for the perceptron. Note the role δ_j plays in the updating of v_{ij}s and v_{oj}. This role described why the algorithm is named as backpropagation; the error of the output layer is for updating of the weights of the hidden layer. The same process is used to update the weights between input units and any other hidden layer units. The training process continues until either the total error at the output is not improving or a prespecified maximum number of iterations have been passed.

7.7.2.3 Momentum

While training a neural network, the training algorithm often encounters a noisy sample. Algorithms such as backpropagation are often misled by the noisy data and change the weights according to the noisy or even wrong data. The noisy data also cause the training process to take much longer to reach the desired set of parameters. This problem encourages us to, instead of updating weights only based on new sample, consider the momentum of the previous values of weight in updating the weights. If the previous examples (that are less noisy) are pushing weights in the right direction, the momentum of the previous samples can somehow avoid the undesirable effects of the noisy data on the weights.

In order to use momentum in backpropagation algorithm, we must consider weights from one or more previous training patterns. For example, in the simplest manner, the weights of steps t and $t-1$ are considered in updating of the weights in step $t+1$, i.e.,

$$w_{jk}(t+1) = w_{jk}(t) + \alpha\delta_k z_j + \mu\left[w_{jk}(t) - w_{jk}(t-1)\right] \tag{7.32}$$

$$v_{ij}(t+1) = v_{ij(t)} + \alpha\delta_j x_i + \mu\left[v_{ij}(t) - v_{ij}(t-1)\right] \tag{7.33}$$

where μ is the momentum parameter and is in the range from 0 to 1. The larger μ is used, the more robust the training algorithm becomes. By adjusting the value of the momentum parameter, μ, large weight adjustment can be achieved, and, at the same time, the convergence of weights to desired values can be expedited.

7.7.3 MATLAB® for Neural Networks

Since not meaningful, backpropagation example is short enough to be handled manually; at this point, we start describing the use of MATLAB for training of multilayer sigmoid feedforward neural networks.

Example 7.8

In this example, we show how to use neural network toolbox of MATLAB to create and train a backpropagation network. The simplest method of using MATLAB capabilities in forming neural networks is using the command "`nntool`". This command opens a dialog box for neural network toolbox. Figure 7.7 shows this dialog box.

As it can be seen in Figure 7.7, by clicking on "New Network," one can open a new window in which we can create and train a new network. Figure 7.8 shows this window. In this window, we can determine the type of the network. For example, addressed here, we select our network as a feedforward backpropagation network

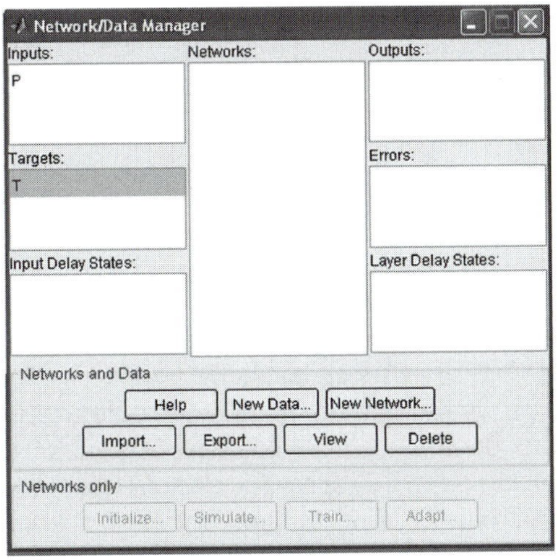

FIGURE 7.7 Neural network dialog box.

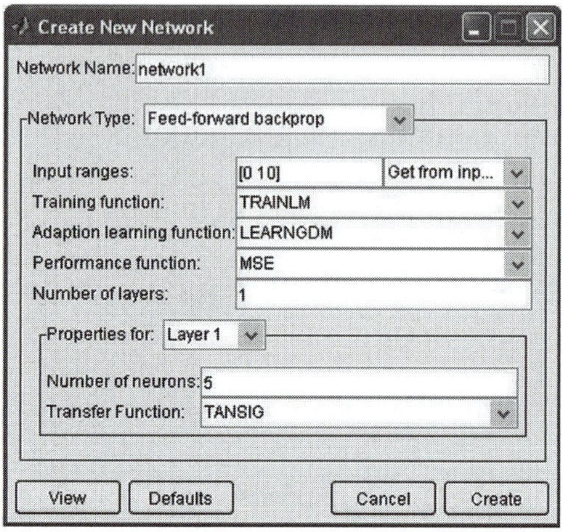

FIGURE 7.8 Neural network window for designing network parameters.

and select that input range as the interval between 0 and 10. In addition, we can select how many layers are desired for our network. In this example, we select one hidden layer and the number of neurons in this hidden layer is chosen as five.

After setting features of the network, we return to the main window (Figure 7.7) and use "Import" option to select the input and target files. At this point, the network is ready to be trained.

7.8 SUMMARY

In this section, different methods of classification and clustering were discussed. The main clustering method covered, K-means, was described using visual, numeric, and MATLAB examples. Statistical classification methods, including Bayesian decision method and MLE were explained using both numerical and MATLAB examples. Different types of neural networks were also explained. Perceptron and multilayer sigmoid neural networks were described in detail.

PROBLEMS

7.1 Load the file named "p_7_1.mat." This synthetic dataset contains 400 2-D samples from four classes. At this point, assume that the data are not labeled, i.e., we do not know the class of the data points.

a. Perform clustering with K-means initializing the clusters to (0, 0), (0, 1), (1, 0), and (1, 1). Stop the iterations after 50 iterations. Plot the position of center of each cluster in 2-D space for all iterations.
b. Repeat part "a," but, this time, initialize the clusters to (0.5, 0.5), (0.5, 0), (0, 0.5), and (0, 0). Stop the iterations after 50 iterations. Plot the position of center of each cluster in 2-D space for all iterations.
c. Repeat part "a," but, this time, initialize the clusters to some random number. Stop the iterations after 50 iterations. Plot the position of center of each cluster in 2-D space for all iterations.

d. Now, assume we know that data points are created by Gaussian random generators as follows: the first 100 data points centered at (1, 1), the second 100 data points centered at (1, 0), the third 100 data points at (0, 1), and the last 100 points at (0, 0). With that in mind, compare the results of the last three parts and comment on the sensitivity of the K-means clustering technique to the initialization and the convergence rate to the final cluster centers.

7.2 We are to use a perceptron to model logical "AND" function (gate) with two inputs. The output of an AND gate is 1 only if both inputs are 1. Form the training set and manually train the perceptron. Assume the learning rate of 0.5 and initialize the weights as follows: $w_1 = 1$, $w_1 = -1$, and $w_1 = 1$. Use binary inputs and binary outputs.

7.3 Repeat Problem 7.2 to model the logical "NOR" function. The output of a NOR gate is 1 only if both inputs are 0. Form the training set and manually train the perceptron. Assume the learning rate of 0.5 and initialize the weights as follows: $w1 = 1$, $w1 = -1$, and $w1 = 1$. Use binary inputs and binary output.

7.4 Prove that perceptron cannot be trained to model "XOR" gate. The output of a XOR gate is 1 only if both inputs have different values, i.e., if one input is 0, the other one must be 1 to have 1 as the output. Inability of perceptron is a historical observation that changed the direction of the field of neural networks.

7.5 Two conditional probability functions $P(x|\omega_1)$ and $P(x|\omega_2)$ are given as follows:

$$p_1(x) = \frac{1}{\sqrt{2\pi}} \exp\left[-\frac{(x-1)^2}{2}\right] \tag{7.34}$$

and

$$p_2(x) = A\exp\left(-|x|\right) \tag{7.35}$$

a. Find the value of A.
b. Assuming that $P(\omega_1) = P(\omega_2)$, find the border (in terms of x) for the Bayesian decision.
c. If the observation $x = 0.5$ is made, according the Bayesian classifier designed in part "b," which class does this sample belong to?

7.6 A set of observation, generated by an unknown probability function, is given as follows:

8.5, 7.2, 12.6, 11.1, 8.4, 9.4, 10.3, 6.5.

Consider the following probability functions:

$$p_1(x) = \frac{1}{\sqrt{2\pi}} \exp\left[-\frac{(x-1)^2}{2}\right] \tag{7.36}$$

and

$$p_1(x) = \frac{1}{\sqrt{2\pi}} \exp\left[-\frac{(x-10)^2}{2}\right] \tag{7.37}$$

If we are to choose between the preceding PDFs, use MLE to identify the functions that best approximate the unknown distribution.

7.7 Load the file "p_7_7.mat." This synthetic dataset contains a set of samples generated by an unknown distribution.

a. Assume that the data are generated by a Gaussian distribution and use MATLAB to find its parameters.
b. Assume that the data are generated by a binomial distribution and use MATLAB to find its parameters.
c. Assume that the data are generated by an exponential distribution and use MATLAB to find its parameters.
d. Comparing the results of the preceding three parts, which distribution is more likely to have produced that data?

7.8 Load the file "p_7_8.mat." This synthetic dataset contains the input and output of a system to be modeled using neural networks. There are two classes identified as 1 and −1. The data have been split into two sets: training and testing.

a. Use MATLAB and the training data to create a three-layer sigmoid neural network as a classifier of the data. Assume there are two hidden neurons and choose a suitable learning rate.
b. Simulate the trained neural network against both the training and testing data and compare the accuracy on the neural model on these two sets.
c. Repeat parts "a" and "b" assuming ten hidden neurons in the hidden layer and compare the results with those of part "b."

7.9 In this problem, we are to develop a simple classifier to extract some measures from the heartbeat signals and predict whether the person whose heartbeat is recorded is young or elderly. Read the file p_7_9.mat. This is the same set of data used in Problem 6.2.* This file contains 10 heartbeat signals. Ten heartbeat time-series signals (denoted as Y1, Y2, etc.) are from five young subjects and five elderly subjects (denoted as O1, O2, etc.).

a. Calculate the following measures for each signal: complexity, mobility, and Higuchi fractal dimension.
b. Assuming that the distribution of all measures within the same group (old or young) is Gaussian, use MLE to estimate these distributions.
c. Using the resulting probabilities, design a Bayesian classifier and evaluate the performance of the resulting classifier.

REFERENCE

Goldberger, A.L., Amaral, L.A.N., Glass, L., Hausdorff, J.M., Ivanov, P.Ch., Mark, R.G., Mietus, J.E., Moody, G.B., Peng, C.K., and Stanley, H.E. (2000, June 13). PhysioBank, PhysioToolkit, and PhysioNet: Components of a new research resource for complex physiologic signals. *Circulation* 101(23):e215–e220. [Circulation Electronic Pages; http://circ.ahajournals.org/cgi/content/full/101/23/e215].

* From Goldberger et al. (2000).

Part II

Processing of Biomedical Signals

8 Electric Activities of the Cell

8.1 INTRODUCTION AND OVERVIEW

The electric activities of the cell constitute a major physical property of the cell that allows a wide spectrum of functionalities such as messaging, cellular communications, timing of cellular activities, and even regulation of practically all biological systems. The same electric properties of the cell are exploited for a number of biomedical signal measurements and imaging. Due to the importance of the cell's electric activities, we briefly explore these properties in this chapter.

It was not until the second half of the twentieth century that the theoretical explanation for electric potentials of the biological cells, in particular cellular membrane potential, was described by Alan Lloyd Hodgkin and Andrew Fielding Huxley.

We start this chapter with the description of the chemical activities of the ions and biological fluids and then formulate the mathematical formulation of the mechanism under which these ions create a potential difference across the cell membrane.

8.2 ION TRANSPORT IN BIOLOGICAL CELLS

All animal tissues, such as muscles, nerves, and bones, are made up of individual cells. These cells have liquids both outside the cell, which are called extracellular fluid, and inside the cell, which are called intracellular fluid. The intracellular fluid is also called the cell plasma. All biological liquids are mostly water with various molecules, atoms, and ions suspended. The intracellular volume is separated from the extracellular fluid by a cell membrane.

The cell membrane is constructed of a bimolecular lipid layer in between monomolecular protein layers on either side. A diagram of the cell membrane construction is outlined in Figure 8.1. The cell membrane is semipermeable to small molecules and ions. This means that only certain atoms, molecules, and ions are capable of passing through the membrane.

Both the intracellular liquid and the extracellular fluid contain organic and inorganic molecules. All salts and acidic and alkaline chemical compositions when dissolved in water form electrically charged elements called ions. All the dissolved charged atoms or molecular structures are distributed in the bodily liquids with different concentrations for the intracellular liquid and the extracellular liquid. These concentrations are not constant, nor are they the same for all cells. The concentrations mentioned later in this chapter are averages for one particular species. Other molecular chains are also dissolved, but not all molecules separate out into ions,

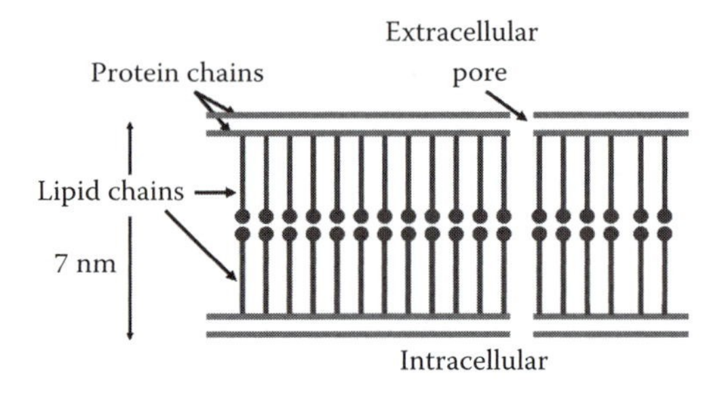

FIGURE 8.1 Molecular model of the cell membrane.

e.g., proteins and sugars. This is due to the fact that since water is a dipole, it will dissolve other dipoles as well as ions.

The cell membrane has permanent openings that will allow small ions to move in and out of the cell freely. This type of ion migration across the membrane constitutes passive ion control. In passive control, the charge gradient across the membrane pushes or pulls some ions inside or outside. In other words, the passive controls include the narrowing and widening of certain channels in the cell membrane through electric and chemical stimuli.

The membrane also has channels that can control the volume of ions it allows to pass through. The active control of ion migration across the cell membrane includes linking ions to molecular carriers that will pull the ions through the membrane. An example of this mechanism is the sodium–potassium pump that trades sodium against potassium by a chemically mediated process of active transportation.

The cellular metabolism also creates ions through the oxidation of carbohydrates. This oxidation results in bicarbonate in addition to energy that the cell uses to steer and fuel the cellular processes.

In order to describe the electric communication between cells, all the electric phenomena surrounding the cell membrane will be discussed next.

8.2.1 Transmembrane Potential

We start this section with a brief discussion on the formation of a static electric potential due to the presence of various ions with different concentrations on both sides of the cell membrane.

In general, if a solution is released next to pure water in the same reservoir, the diffusion of atoms, molecules, and ions will eventually result in a homogeneous concentration throughout the reservoir. If the solution is released in the same reservoir separated by a semipermeable membrane that has a different permeability for positive ions than for negative ions or different permeability based on size of molecules and ions, a concentration gradient will occur. An example of this process in biological cells is schematically illustrated in Figure 8.2 for a typical cell.

As shown in Figure 8.2, both intra- and extracellular fluids contain the following ions: sodium (Na^+), potassium (K^+), chlorine (Cl^-), and various small amounts of other positive ions, called cations, and negative ions, called anions. Some examples of the anions are amino acids, certain peptides, and hydrochloric

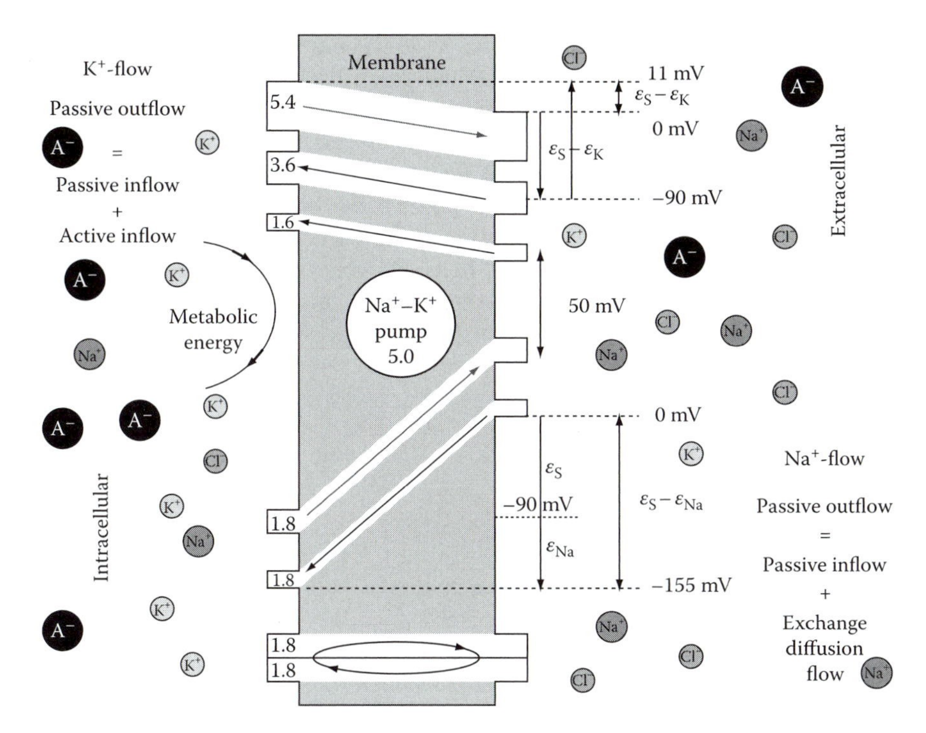

FIGURE 8.2 Na, K, and Cl ions together with other residual ions control the cell potentials. The value ε_s represents the steady-state membrane potential (ε_m). The ion flows are in picomoles per cm^2 per second [pM/cm^2s].

acid (which includes bicarbonate, HCO_3^-). The bicarbonate is a crucial part of the pH balance in the cells.

The ions will be separated by the semipermeable cell membrane that, as mentioned earlier, maintains a relatively stable concentration gradient for each of the respective ions. Since there are different concentrations of positive and negative ions on both sides of the membrane, the membrane acts as a capacitor with a resulting electric potential. The capacitive membrane potential is described as follows:

$$dV = \frac{dQ}{C} \tag{8.1}$$

where

the constant C is the capacitance
dV is the electric potential gradient of the cell membrane (the capacitor)
dQ is the differential element of the charge residing in the membrane

The resulting charge can be related to the equivalent sum of ions, n, and the valence, Z, of the respective ions on either side of the membrane as follows:

$$Q = nZe \tag{8.2}$$

In the preceding equation, the electron charge, e, is equal to -1.6022×10^{-19} C. In the equation, the only charges under consideration are within a cell-layer thickness distance from the cell membrane, approximately 1 μm thickness. The existence of these charges will produce a diffuse current across the membrane that causes a secondary electric potential across the membrane. In equilibrium, the electric potential, V, generated by the surplus of either the positive or negative ions on one side of the membrane will produce an electric potential that will counteract the free diffusion, and a steady state is formed with a constant voltage. In steady state, the ion potential resulting from both the sodium and the chlorine gradients are equal to each other due to the fact that there is no ion current under complete steady-state conditions, and there is a full electrochemical balance in ion concentrations dictated by the individual electric potential gradients, i.e.,

$$\frac{[Na]_e}{[Na]_i} = \frac{[Cl]_i}{[Cl]_e} \tag{8.3}$$

The square brackets indicate concentrations, while the subscripts "i" and "e" represent intra- and extracellular conditions, respectively.

This steady state is called the Donnan equilibrium of the ion concentrations for the cell at rest. The total absence of ion movement makes the time frame for the Donnan equilibrium to reach steady state over a period of greater than a quarter of an hour. For every ion, the Donnan equilibrium results to the following equilibrium potential for that ion:

$$\varepsilon_{m,ION} = \frac{KT}{q} \ln \frac{[ION]_e}{[ION]_i} \tag{8.4}$$

where

K is the Boltzmann's constant
T is temperature in Kelvin
q is the charge

At the room temperature, we have $KT/q = 26\,\text{mV}$. In the previous equation, $[ION]_e$ represents the concentration of the ion and $[ION]_i$ denotes the external concentration of the same ion. As shown in the previous equation, the membrane potential is always assumed to be the potential difference from the intracellular side to the extracellular side. The transmembrane voltage created by each ion is called the Nernst voltage for that ion.

As previously mentioned, the physical basis of these electric potential differences is the presence of ion channels and pumps within the cellular membrane. The static potential is not solely determined by one single ion but by a variety of ions. Each ion will make a contribution that is a function of the respective concentration gradients. In general, the actual membrane potential is not merely the sum of the Nernst potentials of all individual ions involved.

TABLE 8.1
Some Sample Ion Concentrations, Their Relative Permeability with Respect to That of Potassium, and Their Respective Nernst Potentials for Each Ion

Ion	Intracellular Ion Concentration [mM]	Extracellular Ion Concentration [nM]	Relative Permeability [–]	Nernst Potential [mV]
K^+	155	4	1	−97.5
Na^+	12	145	0.04	66.4
Cl^-	4	120	0.45	−90.7

A^- represents assorted cations and A^+ stands for assorted anions.

The potassium ion is the smallest of the intra- and extracellular ions, and the membrane is fully permeable to potassium. The chlorine ion is larger than the potassium ion and has a slightly lower permeability. The sodium ion is the largest of them all, and the membrane has the highest resistance to passage by the sodium ion. This is shown in Table 8.1.

A closer look at the transmembrane potentials for individual ions reveals that the permeability of potassium is large and the membrane potential is a small negative number (−7.5 mV), while the permeability of the sodium is small and the membrane potential is a large positive number (+156.4 mV).

As can be seen from the definition of the Nernst potentials, the main factor in maintaining the Nernst potentials the same of each ion is ensuring that the concentration of the intercellular and extracellular fluids for each ion are constant. As mentioned earlier, the sodium–potassium pump has a central role in maintaining the concentration of the ions therefore maintaining the transmembrane voltage. This pump essentially exchanges potassium for sodium from extra- to intracellular fluid in a 2:3 ratio, respectively.

The sodium and potassium concentrations resulting from the active Na–P pumps determine the membrane potential. The chlorine effect, although secondary to potassium and sodium, is often incorporated in the determination of the overall potential. The following equation, called the Goldman equation, is often used to calculate the overall equilibrium membrane potential incorporating sodium, potassium, and chlorine ions:

$$V_m = \frac{KT}{q}\ln\left(\frac{P_{K^+}[K^+]_e + P_{Na^+}[Na^+]_e + P_{Cl^-}[Cl^-]_i}{P_{K^+}[K^+]_i + P_{Na^+}[Na^+]_i + P_{Cl^-}[Cl^-]_e}\right) \tag{8.5}$$

where V_m is the overall steady-state equilibrium potential across the membrane calculated as the extracellular potential minus the intracellular potential.

The Goldman equilibrium describes the steady-state equilibrium for a cell under the conditions that the sodium and chlorine current are equal to each other and are not 0. The overall rest potential is different for different specialized cells, but it is always negative. For instance, the muscle has a rest transmembrane potential of approximately −90 mV, and the nerve axon has on average a transmembrane potential of −70 mV.

8.3 ELECTRIC CHARACTERISTICS OF CELL MEMBRANE

Considering the fact that the cell membrane has charges on either side and that there is an ion current flowing through the membrane, the cell membrane can be regarded as an electric circuit. As with any electric conductor, there will be electric resistance and capacitance to identify. One can also consider the Nernst potential as a battery in the cell membrane circuit. These electric characteristics allow modeling the cellular activities using its equivalent electronic circuits.

We start this section by defining the membrane resistance.

8.3.1 Membrane Resistance

The membrane forms a resistance for each of the ions passing through it. The membrane resistance is defined as the inverse of the conductance, which, in this case, represents the ease with which the ions can pass through the channels in the membrane. The conductance is in fact a function of the ion concentration and the ion flow. If the conductance for one individual ion channel is G_i, the total resistance of the membrane of one single cell involves all the N individual channels summarized as follows:

$$G = \sum_{N} G_i \tag{8.6}$$

The conductance is related to the permeability but is not interchangeable. Since the resistance, R, is defined as the reciprocal of the conductance, the value can now be recalculated as

$$R = \frac{1}{G} = \frac{1}{\sum_{i=1}^{N} G_i} \tag{8.7}$$

Equation 8.7 equates to a set of parallel channel resistors in a cell circuit. The unit for resistance is Ohm (Ω).

8.3.2 Membrane Capacitance

As mentioned earlier, the fact that there are ions dissolved in the intra- and extracellular liquid lined up on either side of the membrane makes the membrane a capacitor. The charges are separated by the thickness of the membrane, which is only a few molecular chains thick and is in the order of 7.5 nm.

The capacitance is defined in Equation 8.1. Generally speaking, the capacitance of a typical cell membrane is relatively high. This is due to the fact that the thickness of the cell membrane is very small while the area of the membrane is relatively large. For muscle cells and neurons, the capacitance is in the order of 1 μF/cm^2, which is indeed a large number per unit area.

With an electric potential of −90 mV, the field intensities are also relatively high. The charges responsible for this potential are only the ions within 0.8 nm distance from the membrane. Any ions removed farther than 0.8 nm from the membrane are typically assumed to have no immediate impact on the potential.

8.3.3 Cell Membrane's Equivalent Electric Circuit

Combining all the electric properties of the cell membrane, i.e., resistance, capacitance, and electromotive force, one can achieve the electric equivalent circuit for the cell membrane as shown in Figure 8.3.

All circuit theory rules, such as the Kirchhoff laws, can be applied to this circuit. For instance, at any time, the sum of all currents to one junction needs to be 0 since there cannot be accumulation of charges. In addition, when adding all electric potentials in a loop, the summation must be 0.

The resulting circuit can be used to calculate the flow of each of the ion pumps knowing the Nernst potentials as well as the channel resistances for all neurons. This circuit, besides being used to calculate the currents, will help us develop a more important model of the membrane called Hodgkin–Huxley model, as discussed later in this chapter.

8.3.4 Action Potential

As discussed earlier, the cell will try to maintain a gradient of ions across its membrane, which in turn maintains a certain electric potential across the membrane. However, this condition describes the steady-state situation when the cell

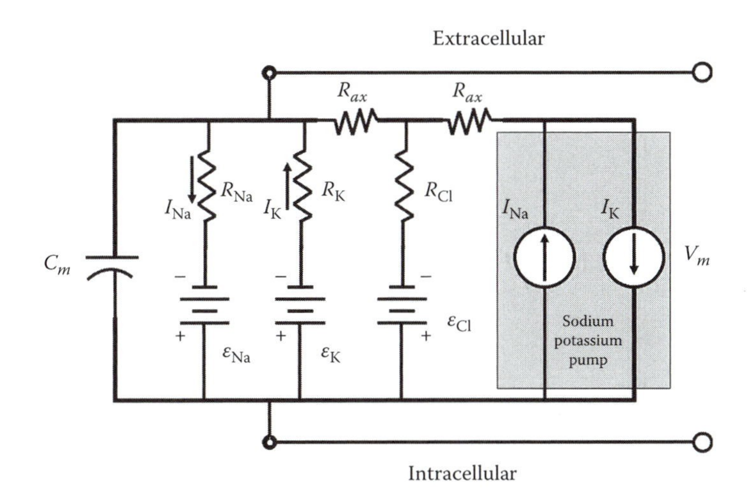

FIGURE 8.3 Combining all the electric properties of resistance, capacitance, and electromotive force presents the electric equivalent circuit for the cell membrane.

is at rest. Certain cells such as muscle and nerve cells are excitable cells in which the permeability of the membrane can be altered under the influence of external conditions. The permeability of the cell for chlorine ions has a relatively insignificant role in adjusting the cell potential due to the small size of these ions. On the other hand, the pores in the membrane that let sodium and potassium ions through can widen and/or change their polarity to allow a greater or smaller flow of these ions through.

The external change in conditions that change the permeability of the membrane is often referred to as a stimulus. In general, the stimulus can be an electric excitation from another source, either a neighboring cell or an extremity of the cell itself that is sensitive to a particular change in environment, for example, temperature, pressure, or light.

The process of the formation of an action potential can be described in simple words without any mathematical formulation. As the cell is stimulated by an external factor, the rising potential difference across the cell membrane (due to the stimuli) initially activates and opens a large number of sodium ion channels. The opening of the sodium channels, or equivalently the sharp increase in the permeability or conductance of the membrane for the sodium ions, causes an avalanche that sharply increases the sodium influx. This process that makes the inside of the cell more positive is called depolarization. The changes in permeability of the sodium channels are shown in Figure 8.4. The reason this stage is called depolarization is the fact that in the rest condition preceding depolarization, the cell potential is negative and the depolarization changes the polarity of the voltage across the membrane. The depolarization potential has specific values for specific cell types. However, this potential is always positive and ranges from +30 to +60 mV.

The depolarization stage continues until the maximum positive potential is reached after which the cell starts a stage called "repolarization." Specifically, at the end of depolarization stage, the positive potential opens a number of potassium channels that allow the potassium ions residing inside the cell leave the cell. This process reduces the potential difference continuously. At a certain point in time, so many potassium ions

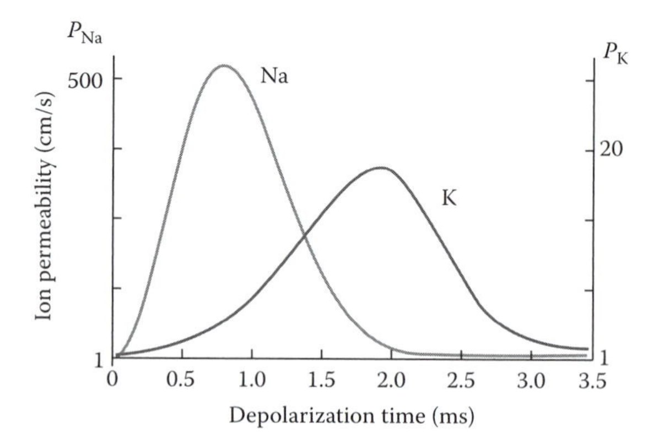

FIGURE 8.4 Sodium conduction is the first ion conduction that is increased, followed by the potassium ion flow with a slight delay.

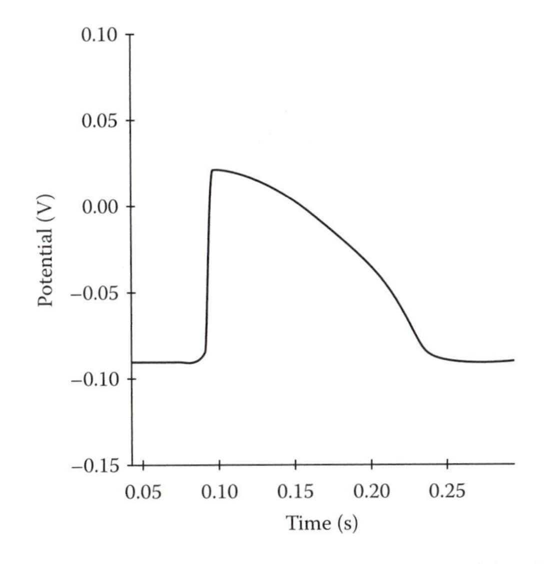

FIGURE 8.5 Typical action potential. (Courtesy of Steve Knisley, PhD, Departments of Biomedical Engineering and Medicine, Adjunct Professor of Applied and Materials Sciences, University of North Carolina at Chapel Hill and North Carolina State University, Chapel Hill, NC.)

have left the cell that the potential difference becomes negative, i.e., the cell repolarizes. The changes in permeability of the sodium channels are also shown in Figure 8.4.

A cycle of depolarization and repolarization processes causes the cell potential to undergo a pulse-form variation, which is called an action potential. A typical action potential is shown in Figure 8.5. Action potentials are means neurons and other cell types use to communicate with each other. There are several types of cells, and the action potential in each cell type has its own specifications and details.

After the repolarization process, the cell undergoes a short phase called the absolute refractory period in which no other stimuli can stimulate the cell. This absolute refractory period lasts for approximately 1 ms. During this period, the cell membrane does not respond to any stimulus no matter how strong these stimuli might be. After this absolute refractory period follows a relative refractory period, which will allow a stimulus to initiate a depolarization, however, at a higher threshold.

Both depolarization and repolarization processes first happen locally. This means that, at first, the stimulus initiates a change in the membrane potential locally, but then, the local changes stimulate the neighboring sections of the membrane, thus causing the membrane potential change to spread.

As mentioned before, an action potential starts with the occurrence of some external stimuli. The only condition for a stimulus to excite the cell is that it needs to exceed a certain threshold to instigate the cell to open its pores (i.e., sodium ion channels). In other words, a minimum positive potential is needed to depolarize the membrane.

The characteristic action potentials that are often used to study this phenomenon are observed in nerve cells (neurons). The action potentials observed in neurons are the means of communication and messaging among the neighboring neurons forming a network. In other words, nerve cells are specialized to receive and transmit these types of impulses (action potentials) to communicate information from one location to the next by stimulating the train of neighboring cells. Transmission of action potentials among the neurons provides complex functions such as the control and cognitive capabilities of the human brain.

Now that we reviewed the process of action potential formation on the qualitative level, next we use an electric model of the cell to describe action potentials using a set of differential equations.

8.4 HODGKIN–HUXLEY MODEL

In 1952, A.L. Hodgkin and A.F. Huxley published their findings on the ion flow through the giant squid axon membrane and described the theoretical principle of the action potential. The Hodgkin–Huxley model is essentially a detailed version of the circuit shown in Figure 8.3. We start describing this model from the steady-state condition. Under steady state, sodium ions (Na^+) act as the primary cation in the extracellular fluid, while the potassium ions (K^+) play the role of the primary cation in the intracellular fluid, and chlorine can be considered as the primary extracellular anion. This combination with the fixed concentration of the ions makes the cell maintain an equilibrium potential. Additional anions and cations play rather insignificant roles and are not included in the model. Table 8.1 shows the ion concentrations and the rest potentials that are associated with the various equilibrium concentrations.

When, due to an external stimuli, a change occurs in the electric potential of the membrane, V_m, there will be a current associated with that change. Since the membrane can be considered as a capacitor, I, in addition to the ion flow, I_i,

$$I = C_m \frac{dV_m}{dt} + I_i \tag{8.8}$$

The ion current itself is the result of sodium and potassium ion flow, I_{Na^+} and I_{K^+}, respectively. The effect of other ions such as chlorine is also included in the model as a leakage current, I_l. With these assumptions, we can calculate the total ion flow, I_i, as follows:

$$I_i = I_{Na^+} + I_{K^+} + I_l \tag{8.9}$$

Now, notice that the sodium current is the result of the sodium conductance times the difference between the membrane potential and the sodium potential itself:

$$I_{Na^+} = G_{Na^+}(V_m - \varepsilon_{Na^+}) \tag{8.10}$$

Similarly, the ion current of potassium can be summarized as follows:

$$I_{K^+} = G_{K^+}(V_m - \varepsilon_{K^+}) \tag{8.11}$$

Since the leak current is the overall effect of various ions, no definite claims can be made about the conductance. It is often more desirable to use the average leak resistance instead:

$$I_l = G_l(V_m - \varepsilon_l) = \frac{(V_m - \varepsilon_l)}{R_l} \tag{8.12}$$

Combining all the aforementioned conditions for the depolarization and ion currents gives

$$I = G_{Na^+}(V_m - \varepsilon_{Na^+}) + G_{K^+}(V_m - \varepsilon_{K^+}) + G_l(V_m - \varepsilon_l) + C_m \frac{dV_m}{dt} \tag{8.13}$$

The timing of the ion conductance changes is vital in creating an action potential. The sodium conduction is the first ion conduction that is initiated, followed by the potassium ion flow at a slight delay. This was illustrated in Figure 8.4. The conductance for the sodium and the potassium ions requires further clarification since as can be estimated from Figure 8.4, these parameters are both time dependent and voltage dependent. The time and voltage dependency of these two factors provides the delayed peaks in ion concentrations shown in Figure 8.4.

Hodgkin and Huxley derived the following empirical relationships for the sodium conductance:

$$G_{Na^+}(t) = G_{Na^+}^{Max} m(t)^3 h(t) \tag{8.14}$$

In the preceding relation, $G_{Na^+}^{Max}$ is the maximum (peak) conductance, and time functions $m(t)$ and $h(t)$ are defined by the following experimentally designed differential equations:

$$\frac{dm(t)}{dt} = 0.1 \frac{-V_m + 25}{\left(e^{\frac{-V_m+25}{10}} - 1\right)}(1 - m(t)) - 4e^{\frac{-V_m}{18}} m(t) \tag{8.15}$$

and

$$\frac{dh(t)}{dt} = 0.07e^{\frac{V}{20}}(1 - h(t)) - \frac{1}{e^{\frac{-V_m+30}{10}} - 1} h(t) \tag{8.16}$$

Similarly, the potassium conductance is described in the Hodgkin–Huxley model as follows:

$$G_{K^+}(t) = G_{K^+}^{Max} n(t)^4 \tag{8.17}$$

In the preceding relation, $G_{K^+}^{Max}$ is the maximum (peak) conductance, and the time function $n(t)$ is calculated by the following experimentally designed differential equation:

$$\frac{dn(t)}{dt} = 0.01\frac{-V_m+10}{\left(e^{\frac{-V_m+10}{10}}-1\right)}(1-n(t)) - 0.125e^{\frac{-V_m}{80}}n(t) \tag{8.18}$$

The Hodgkin–Huxley model, described earlier, is known to provide one of the most reliable estimations of the electric activities of the cell. The exact set of parameters and constants depend on the exact cell to be modeled. This model is heavily used in modeling of the electric activities of single neurons as well as the communications among biological neural networks.

Knowing the mechanism of action potentials both on qualitative and quantitative levels, now we are ready to discuss how these electric activities are captured using electrodes.

8.5 ELECTRIC DATA ACQUISITION

Action potentials can be measured with the help of conductors called electrodes. Such electrodes can be placed in contact with the cell membrane, inside the cell, or even at the surface of the organ that envelops the sources of action potentials. All biological media have an ample supply of ions throughout the entire tissue to conduct the currents resulting from electric potentials anywhere in the tissue. Electrodes measure the potential of every point in the tissue against a ground electrode or even a conveniently chosen reference point on the body itself.

In experimental as well as research setups, the cellular potential is often measured by a microelectrode such as popular needle electrodes. In such cases, the relative electric potential of the inside of the cell with respect to the outside can be measured as negative values at first (during the rest period) but then flip to a positive values during depolarization. In a clinical setting, due to the cost as well as the intensive nature of such electrode, this type of measurements is rarely used. A typical needle electrode is shown in Figure 8.6.

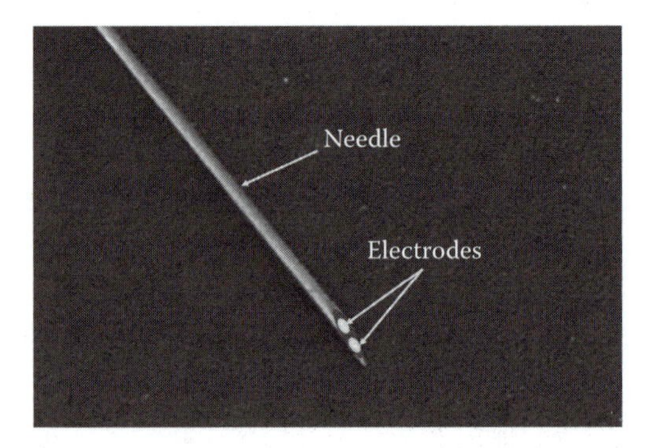

FIGURE 8.6 Needle electrode.

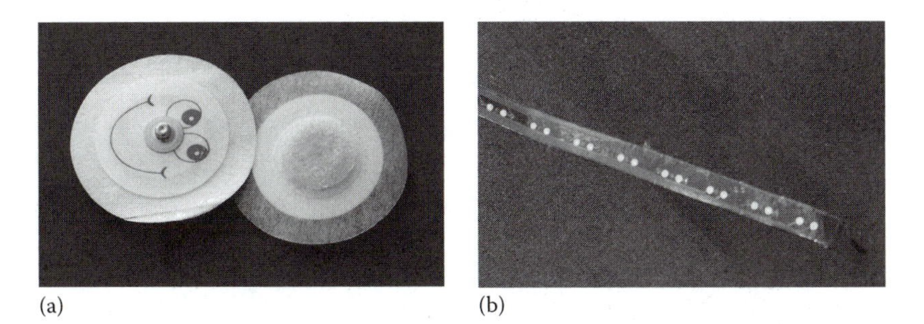

(a) (b)

FIGURE 8.7 Two representative types of surface electrodes: (a) metal electrode with conductive gel, commonly used to record heart depolarization potentials on the skin and (b) strip electrode with eight bipolar electrodes (16 electrodes).

In the clinical setting, one usually needs to measure the depolarization in close proximity to the source but still from the outer surface only. Two different kinds of typical surface electrodes are shown in Figure 8.7. The electric activity of individual cells can manifest itself on the skin surface as surface potentials. These surface potentials are in fact the culmination of all cellular depolarizations that occur at the exact same time everywhere in the body. In our description of high-level signals such as EEG and EMG, we will discuss how these signals are measured and analyzed. As can be guessed, the interpretation of these surface potentials presents a serious challenge for various reasons. One of the challenges is the fact that the signals measured at the skin surface are created by many cells and therefore do not say much about the individual cells that might be the target of the study. Furthermore, the conductivity of the various tissues involved in the formation of the measured signals is not uniform and ranges from perfect conductors such as blood to almost perfect insulators such as the air in the lungs. In other words, because of the mathematically unknown shape of the conduction distribution inside the body, the reverse problem of finding the source that belongs to a measured signal distribution can be a complicated challenge.

8.5.1 Propagation of Electric Potential as a Wave

The initial depolarization of a section of membrane induces a depolarization in the directly adjacent membrane due to the fact that the depolarization in this case by definition exceeds the threshold potential. The depolarization propagates along the length of the membrane, which suggests that the spread of action potential in a cell can be considered as a wave propagation phenomenon. In order to see this clearly, consider the schematic structure of a typical neuron shown in Figure 8.8. As can be seen, a neuron is composed of a cell body (soma), the dendrites, and the axon. When the dendrites sense the external stimuli influence, the soma is depolarized, and this depolarization effect propagates through the axon. Once the depolarization reached the other end of the axon, the connectors at the end of the axon stimulate the dendrites of the other neurons.

Now assume that, as shown in Figure 8.9, an electrode is placed at point outside the neuron observing the propagation of the depolarization wave through the axon.

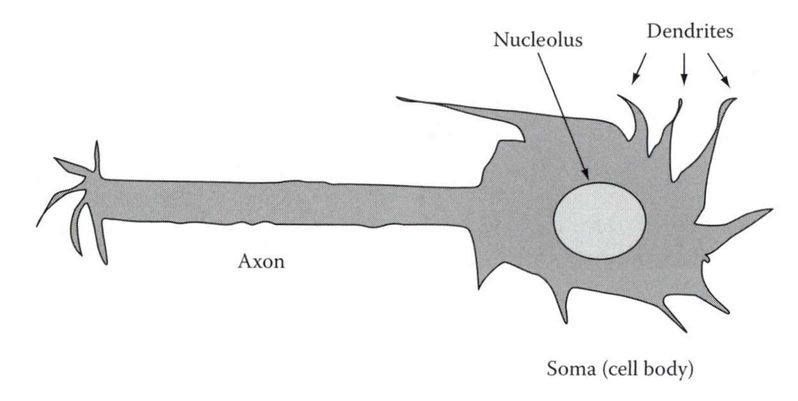

FIGURE 8.8 Schematic diagram of a nerve cell (neuron).

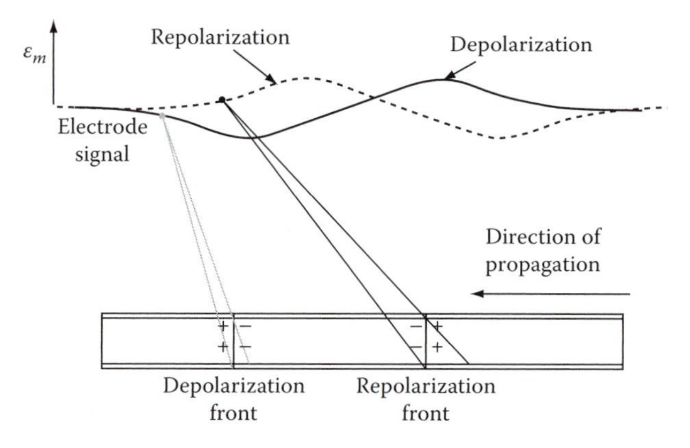

FIGURE 8.9 Propagation of action potential in an axon.

The electric activities of the neuron, i.e., the depolarization waves, move from part of the axon to another. As can be seen, every compartment of the axon depolarizes and repolarizes consequently. This causes the electrode to record the wave patterns shown in Figure 8.9.

The distance separating the depolarization front and the repolarization front are determined by the duration of the action potential and the speed of propagation of the signal along the axon membrane. For instance, if the depolarization takes 1 ms and the propagation velocity is 2 m/s, the distance traveled by the wave along the axon will equal 2 mm.

8.6 SOME PRACTICAL CONSIDERATIONS ON BIOMEDICAL ELECTRODES

In recording of the cell electric signals, two issues will determine the accuracy of the recorded signal and the usefulness of drawing conclusions based on this information: the contact surface and the electrode compatibility.

When electrodes are placed on the skin surface, the following practical issues have to be taken into consideration. The skin's outer surface, the epidermis, is a mixture of live and dead cells. Dead cells do not properly conduct electricity since the dead cells have no cytoplasm and no charge carriers as such. In addition, the skin may excrete fat, which is also a poor conductor. Sweating, on the other hand, improves conduction because of the salt content, i.e., the ions Na^+, K^+, and Cl^-. These issues can be handled by typical skin preparation and treatments such as degreasing of the skin and exfoliating the skin.

Degreasing the skin can lower the skin–electrode impedance by a factor of 30, and applying a conducting impedance matching layer between the electrode and the skin can lower the impedance by approximately a factor of 60. Exfoliation will result in impedance lowering by a factor of 250. All measures combined can bring the transfer impedance down by a factor of approximately 2000.

In addition to the epidermis, the dermis can form a capacitive element. This capacitance is formed by the poor conduction conditions of the epidermis, the abundant supply of ions in the dermis, and the ample supply of free electrons in the electrode. This means that the transfer impedance is not just resistive but also capacitive. There can be a small contribution of inductive impedance based on the underlying tissue structure.

An ideal electrode needs to be easy to apply and maintain electric stability to ensure reproducible measurement. In addition, an electrode needs to be able to conduct an alternating signal; this does not imply that it needs to be able to measure a steady-state potential.

Additional considerations are that electrodes need to be made of metals that will not dissolve, e.g., gold, silver, or platinum. The electrodes will require a large surface area to limit current density in addition to a connection to a high-impedance amplifier input to curb total current.

8.7 SUMMARY

In this chapter, we described the electrochemical phenomena causing action potentials as well as cell membrane potential. We also presented a mathematical model of the cell membrane's electric activities called Hodgkin–Huxley model. This model is often used to relate the intercellular and extracellular ion concentrations to the overall cell membrane as well as action potentials. Finally, we briefly reviewed the structure and applications of some commonly used biomedical electrodes.

PROBLEMS

8.1 Import the data in the file "p_8_1.xls" in MATLAB® and plot the signal. In order to do so, use File/Import Data ... on the main MATLAB menu and follow the steps in loading and naming of the data. The file contains the data from a surface electrode measuring a nerve impulse. Sample frequency 1000 Hz.*

a. Use discrete Fourier transform (DFT) to describe the signals in the frequency domain. Determine the dominant frequency.
b. Measure the duration of an entire pulse and comment on the results.

* N.M. Maurits, PhD, Department of Clinical Neurophysiology, Groningen University Medical Center (GUMC), Groningen, the Netherlands.

8.2 Import the data in the file "p_8_2.xls" in MATLAB and plot the signals. These are several signals recorded from a single cell in different places along the cell. Sample frequency 1000 Hz.*

a. Repeat the calculations in parts "a" and "b" of Problem 8.1 on the recordings I and II.

b. Repeat the calculations in parts "a" and "b" of Problem 8.1 on the recordings II and III and compare the data from different locations.

* N.M. Maurits, PhD, Department of Clinical Neurophysiology, Groningen University Medical Center (GUMC), Groningen, the Netherlands.

9 Electrocardiogram

9.1 INTRODUCTION AND OVERVIEW

Electrocardiogram (ECG) is the most commonly used biomedical signal in clinical diagnostics of the heart. The word "electrocardiogram" is a combination of three words: electro, pertaining to electric signal; cardio, which translates into heart; and gram, which stands for recording. The recording of the electric activity of the heart is called ECG.

A cardiac muscle contraction is a direct result of the cellular electric excitation described by the ECG. The depolarization initiates the shortening of each individual muscle cell. The electric activation of each cell is an indication of the functioning of that cell. Therefore, the ECG is the result of depolarization of the heart muscle in a controlled repetitive fashion. By tracking the process of electric depolarization of the cardiac muscle cells, an impression of the heart's functionality can be formed and used to recognize regions in the heart structure that are not functioning to specifications and may require medical attention. Any deviation from the typical ECG observed in the recorded electric depolarization signal is analyzed and classified as a certain cardiac disorder.

The principal concepts of the biological cell and the electric potential across the cell membrane were discussed in Chapter 8. In this chapter, first, the function of the heart as a pump will be discussed. Then, in order to fully understand the electric signals generated by the heart with respect to each contraction, some basic phenomena involved in the contraction process will be described. Finally, the formation, measurement, and processing of ECG will be discussed.

9.2 FUNCTION AND STRUCTURE OF THE HEART

The heart is the structure comprised of cardiac muscles that are responsible for circulating blood through the body. The anatomy and conduction system of the heart is outlined in Figure 9.1. The heart has four major functions: collecting the blood that needs to be refined from all parts of the body (through veins), pumping this collected blood to the lungs, collecting the refined blood from the lungs, and pumping the refined blood back to all parts of the body.

As can be seen in Figure 9.1, the heart has four chambers: two atria and two ventricles. The atria work in unison and so do the ventricles. The atrium is separated from the venous system by a valve so that flow is only possible in one direction. The superior vena cava and the inferior vena cava lead into the right atrium in combination with the coronary sinus, while the pulmonary veins supply the left atrium. When the atrium contracts, it pumps the retained blood into the ventricle that is separated by a valve as well. The valve only allows flow from the atrium to the ventricle and not in the opposite direction. This valve is called the atrioventricular valve.

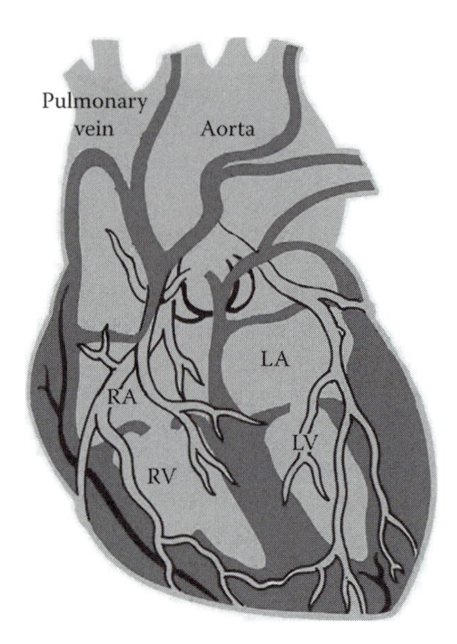

FIGURE 9.1 Function and structure of the heart.

The atrioventricular valve between the right atrium and the right ventricle is also called the tricuspid valve because of the three-leaf structure. The left atrium and left ventricle have the bicuspid valve, or mitral valve, that separates the two chambers.

The ventricle expands when it is filled with the pressure generated by the blood flow from the atrium. The ventricle contracts out of sync with the atrium as the result of an electric delay line between the excitation of the atrium and the ventricle. The ventricle pumps the blood into an artery, which again is separated from the ventricle by a one-way valve. The left ventricle pumps blood into the aorta, which is separated from the ventricle by the aortic valve to prevent backflow. The aorta supplies the refined blood to the body. The right ventricle squeezes the blood that needs refining into the arteria pulmonalis, separated by the pulmonary valve. The arteria pulmonalis feeds into the lung circulation.

A schematic representation of the blood circulation provided by the heart is illustrated in Figure 9.2.

The wall of the atrium and the ventricle consists of three main layers. Moving from the inside outward, the inner lining of the heart wall is called the endocardium; it consists of a single cell layer of flat, thin endothelial cells. The second layer is the myocardium; it is the main muscle of the ventricle. The epicardium is the outside lining of the ventricular wall; it consists of a single cell layer made up of flat cells. The left and right ventricles are separated by the septum, which is also a three-layer structure with endocardium, myocardium, and epicardium. The entire heart is suspended in the pericardial sack, which provides free movement in the area of the chest in between the lungs on the left side of the body.

The main functionalities of the heart are provided by the structure and characteristics of the cardiac muscle to be described next.

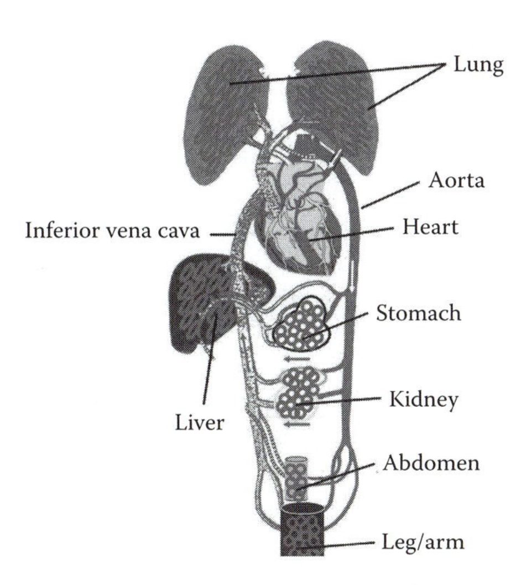

FIGURE 9.2 Relative locations of the elementary components in the circulation mechanism of the heart.

9.2.1 Cardiac Muscle

The main function of the cardiac muscle can be summarized as follows. An action potential that causes the heart muscle cells to contract reduces the atrial and ventricular volume, respectively. This results in an increase in pressure, leading to an outflow through the valve when the pressure before the valve exceeds the pressure behind the valve. This process provides the pressure changes to open and close the valves and therefore perform the pumping role of the heart. The contraction part of the heart is called the systole. Each systolic period is followed by a rest period, which is called the diastole.

In order to see how these contractions are provided by the cardiac muscle, we need to study the characteristics of cardiac muscles more closely. As a smooth muscle type tissue, the cardiac muscle is a hollow muscle that is designed to force blood into a tube to fill the body. The cardiac muscle has many of the typical properties of other muscle cells, except for the fact that cardiac muscle fibers are not excited all at once by one motoneuron. One major difference between skeletal muscle and heart muscle is with regard to the duration of the action potential. The cardiac muscle has a considerably longer depolarization and repolarization period. The longer depolarization period (several hundred milliseconds versus only a few milliseconds for skeletal muscle) ensures the maximum contraction from one single impulse. The longer repolarization period in the cardiac muscle ensures that there will be no immediate overlap in contractions.

An important fact about the function of the cardiac muscle is that the depolarization period is a function of the frequency in which the cardiac muscle receives the initiation pulses. During this time and the subsequent repolarization period, theoretically, no new depolarization can be initiated. However, both the depolarization and the repolarization period are subject to shortening if the demand is there. The higher the repetition rate becomes, a shorter depolarization period is achieved. This is another fact differentiating the cardiac muscle from skeletal muscle. This characteristic of cardiac muscle allows the heart to adapt the state of physical exercise.

The remarkable difference with skeletal muscle in organizational structure is the presence of a wire mesh of excitable cells: nodal tissue, running through the cardiac muscle tissue. This network of excitable cells is in charge of control and adjustment of the heartbeat and is further described in the next section.

9.2.2 Cardiac Excitation Process

The nodal cells are located in the heart. They initiate, synchronize, and regulate the heart contractions by generating periodic action potentials. The network of these cells is shown in Figure 9.3.

The nodal cells in the heart do not possess a rest potential but have a constant ion leak. The persistent ion leak eventually causes these nodal cells to depolarize spontaneously at regular intervals when the cell membrane potential exceeds a certain threshold. The nodal cells will also produce a repolarization after each depolarization. All the nodal cells are linked together electrically, such that any nodal cell can start the depolarization process. There is however an order of depolarization, i.e., some cells depolarize faster than others, giving the fastest cell always the upper hand. If, however, the faster cells are damaged, the slower cells will take the lead.

These nodal cells are organized in two general groups: the sinoatrial node (S-A node) and atrioventricular node (A-V node). These two nodes are called natural pacemakers. The S-A node, which is the main pacemaker of the heart, stimulates the atria and the A-V node in turn and, after a delay, stimulates the ventricles. The electric delay between the activation of the S-A and A-V nodes is created by the propagation of electric impulses via the bundle of tissues between the two nodes. This delay gives the atrium time to empty out into the ventricle, and the contraction of the atrium is followed in due time by the contraction of the ventricle to obtain maximum pumping efficiency. The functions as well as the location of each of these nodes are further described as follows.

The S-A node is located in the wall of the hollow vein, on the upper side on the border with the right atrium. This is the primary nodal tissue, i.e., pacemaker,

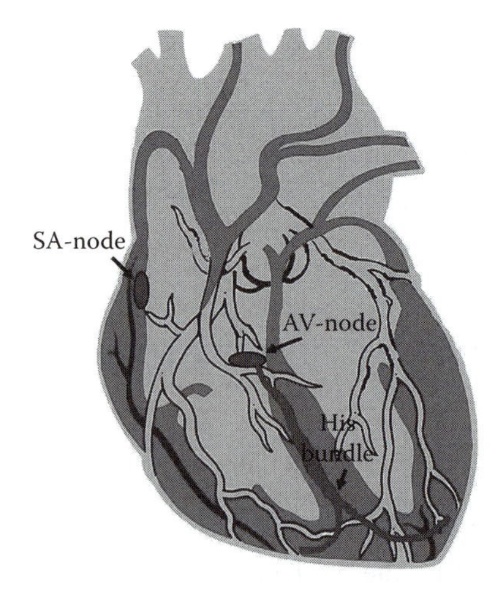

FIGURE 9.3 Location of natural pacemakers and conduction system of the heart.

producing impulses in a regular fashion to excite the atrium first, before trickling down to the ventricle through the A-V node. The S-A node is tunable by hormonal and parasympathetic nerve impulses.

The A-V node is positioned in the part of the septum close to the base of the heart, i.e., the border between the atria and the ventricles, just above a section called the annulus fibrosus. The annulus fibrosus is a connective tissue that separates the atria from the ventricles and is an electric insulator. The A-V node is also under the endocardium of the right atrium. This node not only generates impulses under stimulus from the atrial depolarization but also has a depolarization sequence of its own since it is constructed of nodal tissue as well. The depolarization rate of the A-V node is generally slower than that of the S-A node. The impulse generated by the A-V node is conducted through a bundle of nodal cells called the His bundle that branch into multiple branches of conducting fibers that carry the depolarization impulse to the apex of the heart, the bottom of the heart, farthest away from the outlet valves of the ventricle, which are at the base of the atrium again. The branches of fibers spreading out from the His bundle are called Purkinje fibers. The A-V node has a range of cells with different depolarization speeds. The cells of the A-V node farthest from the His bundle are the fastest depolarizing, and the lower ones are closer to the contact with the His bundle. The His bundle acts solely as conductor of electric pulses. There are many terminal points of the Purkinje fibers at the apex of the heart, ensuring a massive contractile motion at the tip. The polarization propagation speed is approximately 0.5 m/s for the cardiac muscle tissue, while the propagation speed for the His bundle is approximately 2 m/s.

As mentioned earlier, the cardiac muscle is different from most other cells; in the fact, that the cells themselves pass the depolarization signal on to only certain neighboring cells. All cardiac muscle cells in turn are connected to each other by a conducting cell wall section, the intercalated disk. The intercalated disk conduction is illustrated in Figure 9.4. The intercalated disk transmits the depolarization wave to the adjacent cell, and this cell will respond as long as it is not in the repolarization phase. The fact that the cells themselves pass the depolarization signal on to only certain neighboring cell is of crucial importance for the understanding of how an ECG is formed at the electrodes.

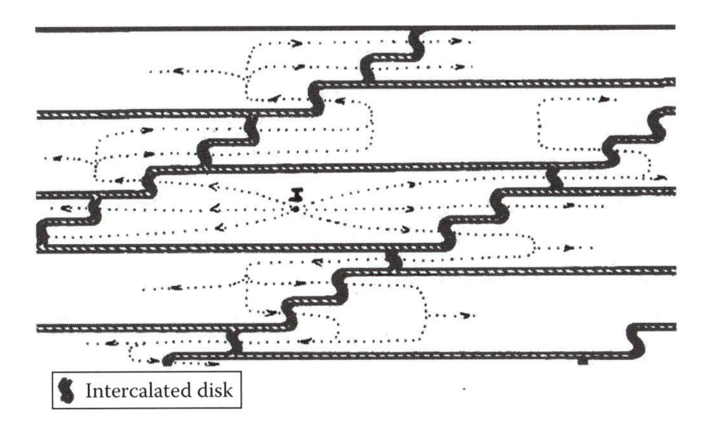

FIGURE 9.4 Intercalated disks in the electric excitation mechanism of the heart.

If all cells are successfully excited at the apex of the heart, the migration of electric excitation wave front through the intercalated disks will provide a smooth depolarization. This depolarization front moves homogeneously upward toward the base of the heart, and as a result, the blood is effectively forced out off the ventricle with maximum efficiency. This description of the heart activity assumes a healthy normal working heart. Detectable deviations in the depolarization wave front will elicit any abnormalities in the ejection sequence and are therefore an integral part of diagnosing the proper functioning of the pump action of the heart.

Now that we have familiarized ourselves with the structure as well as the mechanical and electric activities of the heart, we are ready to describe ECG.

9.3 ELECTROCARDIOGRAM: SIGNAL OF CARDIOVASCULAR SYSTEM

The depolarization and repolarization process during each heart cycle generates local electric potential differences, which can be measured on the skin using electronic recording equipment. This group of signals, called ECG, constitutes the most informative clinical signal commonly used in the diagnosis of the cardiovascular system.

9.3.1 Origin of ECG

The ECG represents the repetitive electric depolarization and repolarization pattern of the heart muscle. The schematic form of one period of the ECG is illustrated in Figure 9.5a, and a typical healthy ECG signal is shown in Figure 9.5b.* The ECG is characterized by five peaks, represented by the letters P, Q, R, S, T, and sometimes followed by a sixth peak, the U wave. The P wave is the result of the depolarization of the atrium, while the remaining waves are caused by the ventricle.

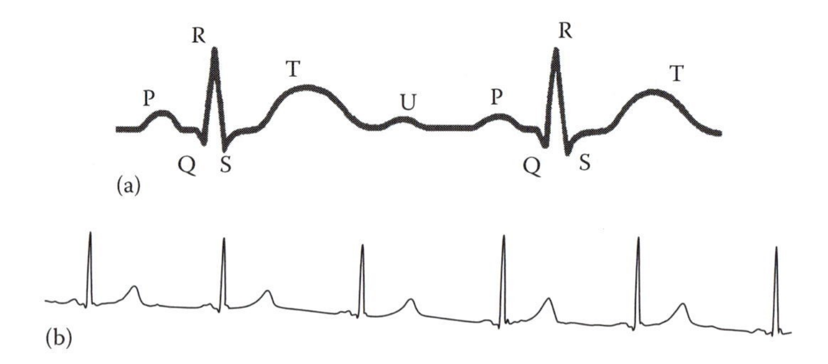

FIGURE 9.5 (a) Characteristic wave in one cycle of a normal ECG and (b) a healthy ECG.

* All ECG recordings in the main body of this chapter were provided by Dr. Laszlo Littmann of the Carolinas Medical Center, Charlotte, NC.

The electrocardiography made its introduction through the pioneering efforts of the Dutch scientist Willem Einthoven in 1903. He used a galvanometer to design a way to record the action potentials. He also introduced the markers P, Q, R, S, and T on the standard ECG. The initial ECGs were recorded directly on paper and, in fact, still are in many clinical cardiac electrophysiology laboratories. The galvanometer was directly coupled to an ink pen. This way, a voltage leading to a deflection of the galvanometer would move or direct the pen over the paper. Each individual electrode had its own galvanometer and separate ink pen. This method still stands as the gold standard for analog recordings. However, nowadays, as described later, the electrodes are connected to amplifiers and filters.

As mentioned earlier and shown in Figure 9.6, the P wave is caused by the depolarization of the atrium. The initial recording of the P wave lasts for approximately 90 ms and is usually not much greater than 2.5×10^{-4} V. The depolarization of the atrium during the P wave causes the atrium to contract and fill the ventricle. The transition of the atrial depolarization to the A-V node is usually not detected, and the A-V node itself is too small and too far from the electrodes on the outside of the body that it will not register either. The quiet time between the P wave and the QRS complex is often used as a reference line.

The QRS complex lasts for approximately 80 ms and has amplitude of about 1 mV. The QRS complex shows the depolarization of the septum (the wall separating the left and right ventricle) and the conduction through the Purkinje fibers. The final piece of information in the QRS complex is the depolarization of the ventricular wall from the inside to the outside and from the bottom to the top. The repolarization takes place from the outside to the inside and has the opposite polarity of the depolarization. The repolarization effects show up in the ECG electrode as a pulse called T wave.

The repolarization wave of the atrium will not be recorded under normal recording conditions. It is extremely weak and it will fall in the middle of the depolarization account that represents the ventricular contraction excitation, the QRS complex. During repolarization, the atrium relaxes and fills back up. The repolarization can be distinguished from the depolarization in the cardiac action potential from the

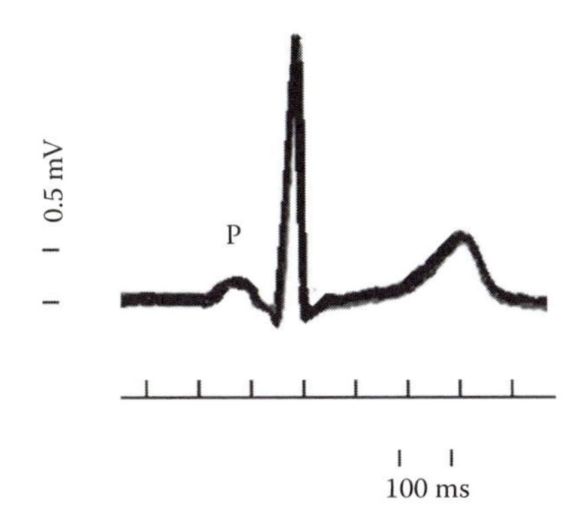

FIGURE 9.6 Timing of all important waves of ECG, in particular P wave, are shown that further identifies when and why these waves are formed.

fact that the repolarization wave front is significantly longer in time duration than the depolarization wave front. The repolarization also has a much smoother action potential gradient, which incorporates a smaller gradient in the time derivative of the cell membrane potential.

The ventricular repolarization is represented in the T wave of the ECG signal. The T wave has a smaller amplitude than the QRS complex. If present, the U peak also represents a portion of the ventricular repolarization.

Because of the electric nature of the heart muscle, the depolarization and the repolarization are separated by a relatively long time period. As a result, in the electric recording of the heart activity, the expected triphasic action potential phenomenon will never be seen.

9.3.2 ECG Electrode Placement

The ECG is not measured directly on the heart itself but on the exterior of the body. Various internationally accepted electrode placements are in existence, which are described next.

The oldest standard of ECG measurement is a three-point extremities recording on the arms and one leg, which is essentially the same as the original Einthoven electrode placement. The recording uses three bipolar measurements that are as follows: recording I is between left (L) and right (R) arm, i.e., $V_L - V_R$; recording II is between left leg (F, for foot) and right arm, i.e., $V_F - V_R$; and recording III is between left leg and left arm, i.e., $V_F - V_L$. This standard ECG configuration for the electrode placement is illustrated in Figure 9.7.

Another popular electrode placement arrangement is outlined in Figure 9.8. A scrolling curve on the chest outlines the electrode placement starting from the right, with one electrode on either side of the sternum and three more electrodes

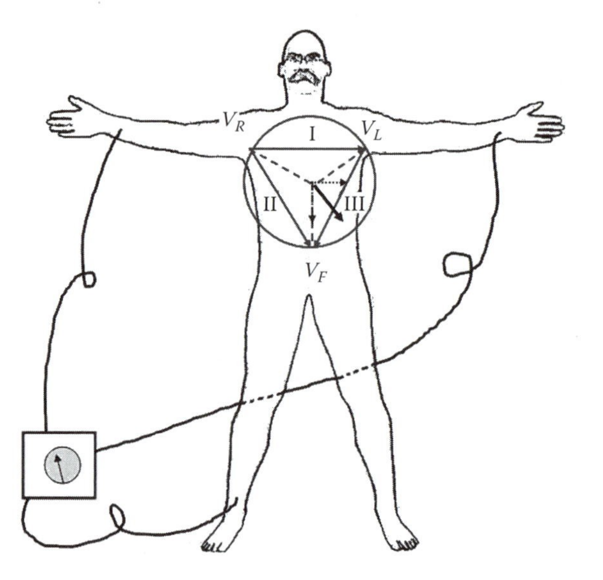

FIGURE 9.7 Traditional electrode configuration as proposed by Einthoven.

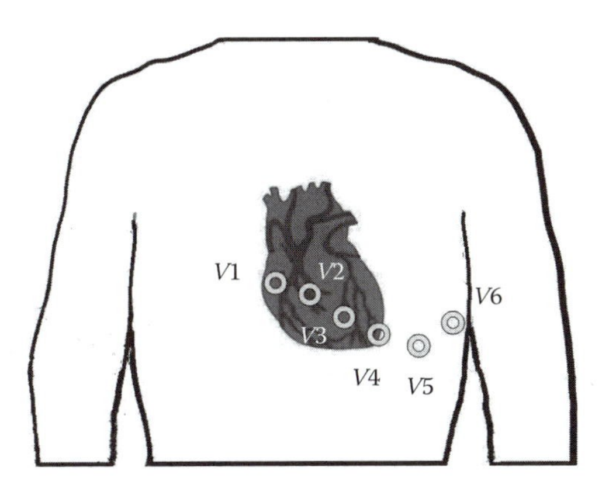

FIGURE 9.8 Chest electrode configuration in the Wilson placement.

trailing along the left side of the sternum at the fifth rib with the sixth electrode underneath the armpit on the sixth rib. This electrode placement using six electrodes is called *V*1–*V*6. These six electrodes are added to the ones at the three extremities. This ECG standard is called the Wilson placement. As can be seen, in this standard, the electrode placements follow the outline of the heart from top to bottom.

In the Wilson placement, due to the symmetry of the left and right heart as well as the synchronicity between the left and the right sides, some of the depolarization effects will cancel each other out. Specifically, since one event (electric pulse wave) can be moving away from the electrode while another event is moving toward the electrode, the electric field vectors would nullify each other, which is a source of information on its own. Even in an event where the two waves do not cancel each other, the resulting recordings will be an indication of a problem in the depolarization pattern providing invaluable diagnostic information.

It was later found by Goldberger that the sensitivity of the measurements can be improved by uncoupling the extremity at which the signal is desired and making the differential measurement with other electrodes. The uncoupling of each of the individual recordings gives the following augmented recordings:

$$aV_R = V_R - \frac{V_L + V_F}{2} = \frac{2V_R - V_L - V_F}{2} \tag{9.1}$$

$$aV_L = V_L - \frac{V_R + V_F}{3} = \frac{2V_L - V_R - V_F}{2} \tag{9.2}$$

$$aV_F = V_F - \frac{V_R + V_L}{2} = \frac{2V_F - V_R - V_L}{2} \tag{9.3}$$

Combining all the previous measurements gives a total of three electrodes on the extremities (Einthoven), six on the chest (Wilson placement), and the three uncoupled recordings introduced by Goldberger, creating a total of 12 recordings that are typically obtained during a routine cardiac examination.

In general, all electric recordings are made in differential amplifier mode. In differential amplification, the electric potential difference signal measured between two points is amplified, and, therefore, the common signal components that will be recorded on both electrodes simultaneously will be filtered out. This process is called common-mode rejection. Since various noise sources will have an identical impact on the recorded electric activity on electrodes, by measuring the difference between the electrodes, i.e., common-mode rejection, the noise is simply eliminated.

In general, the 12 recording protocol is the standard mode of operation. However, other minimally invasive electrode placement techniques involve the use of a spring-loaded catheter placed inside the left ventricle with multiple strands of electrode wires. Each strand can have 16 electrodes, and there can be 16 strands deployed. These strands will press against the endocardial wall and record an array of simultaneous measurements in close proximity to the depolarizing cells. This type of measurement is usually reserved for research purposes and for cases that are difficult to diagnose by standard procedures.

More accurate measurements can be made with the help of coronary electrode placement and ventricular electrode placement through insertion of a catheter equipped with electrodes. Most catheters have two or three electrodes on a single catheter, and several catheters can be inserted simultaneously.

9.3.3 Modeling and Representation of ECG

Einthoven introduced the concept that electric activity of the heart can be described by a single current dipole with a resulting three-dimensional (3-D) rotating field vector, called the heart vector. The concept of the heart vector is illustrated in Figure 9.7, where all the recordings at a 120° angle difference with each other are combined to give the geometrical projection in one resultant direction. The heart vector represents the magnitude and the direction of the dipole moment caused by the current dipole, which is the cumulative polarization and repolarization ion flow across the cardiac cells.

The main postulate in the forming and analysis of the heart vectors is that the electric activity of the heart at any time can be described by the heart vector. In order to provide a geometry that simplifies the calculations of the heart vector, the human body is considered as a sphere with the source of the heart vector located at the center. In this geometry, even though the two arms and the left leg all protrude from the sphere, they are assumed to be in one plane and at equal distances from the center. In forming the heart vectors, it is also assumed that the electric conduction is homogeneous and isotropic over the sphere.

At first glance, it seems that each of the arm and leg recordings I, II, and II described for the Einthoven placement contributes some additional information on the magnitude and direction of the heart vector. However, the three recordings are not truly independent, since applying Kirchhoff rule gives

$$V_{II} = V_I + V_{III} \tag{9.4}$$

This indicates a direct dependence between the three recordings, stating that these three measurements are only in a single two-dimensional (2-D) plane and therefore fail to reveal the whole depolarization story. As can be seen, in order to address this issue, one can include more electrode recordings in forming the heart vector. For instance, including both the Winston and Goldman electrode placements will provide a 3-D heart vector.

9.3.4 Periodicity of ECG: Heart Rate

The leading ECG feature deciphering the hemodynamic phenomena is the frequency of relaxation and contraction of the heart muscle, i.e., the pulse or heart rate. As mentioned before, a complete heart cycle is started by the atrial contraction, associated with the pulse represented by the P wave. After the atrial contraction, the ventricular contraction occurs, which is preceded by the QRS complex marking the systole. The cycle ends with rest in which both atria and ventricles are in relaxed state or diastole. This rest state then leads to atrial contraction and repeat of the cycle. The repetition of this entire cycle makes ECG and all other heart signals periodic. As mentioned in Part I of the book, the most informative measure in periodic signal is the frequency of the variations. This is why the heart rate is the most indicative measure of the cardiovascular system.

In an average person, the heart rate is approximately 75 beats per minute, which yields a period of 0.8 s on the ECG. The various stages of the contraction are spread out over this period in the following sequence. The atrial contraction in this case lasts approximately 0.1 s, followed by a ventricular contraction that lasts 0.3 s, with an end pause of 0.4 s. This means the atrial diastole lasts 0.7 s in this example, and the ventricular diastole lasts 0.5 s.

The heart rate is sensitive to internal and external stimuli that can increase or decrease the heart rate. Two different types of mechanisms that can affect the heart rate can be distinguished: intrinsic and extrinsic. The intrinsic mechanisms are due to the changes (e.g., stretching) in the S-A node, which directly alters the heart rate. Another intrinsic effect is temperature, which can affect the heart rate both in an upward and downward direction depending on raised or lowered temperature, respectively. The extrinsic regulatory mechanism includes both parasympathetic and sympathetic nervous systems. These autonomic nerve systems affect the release of acetylcholine or noradrenaline–adrenaline that changes the heart rate. The parasympathetic and orthosympathetic nervous system affects the heart rate through the nervi vagi. The final and most well-known mechanism in heart rate control is the hormone adrenaline released by the adrenal glands, which increases the heart rate for the fight-or-flight reaction.

Various deviations in the typical heart rhythm are often caused by either impulse generation malfunctioning or conduction distortion. The activation in the atria may be fully irregular and chaotic, producing irregular fluctuations in the baseline. As a consequence, the ventricular rate becomes rapid and irregular, even though the QRS contour may still look normal. This electric phenomenon is referred to as atrial fibrillation (AF). When the electric disturbance is confined to the ventricles, the resulting disease is referred to as ventricular arrhythmias.

9.4 CARDIOVASCULAR DISEASES AND ECG

These deviations from the normal functionality of the cardiovascular system are associated with certain pathological conditions, which can be either genetic or due to malfunctions such as infections, lack of oxygen, and obstruction of blood vessels that supply blood to the heart itself. In this section, some of the main cardiovascular diseases are briefly introduced and the changes in ECG and related diseases are discussed. This brief discussion of cardiovascular diseases will allow us to devise computational methods for the processing of ECG that can detect abnormalities in their early stages.

9.4.1 Atrial Fibrillation

AF is one of the most common arrhythmias that occur as a result of rheumatic disease, infections (such as pericarditis), atherosclerotic disease, or hyperthyroidism. These conditions caused by AF are not as life threatening as some of the ventricular arrhythmias but provide an increased risk for stroke. Physical symptoms include palpitations, dizziness, and shortness of breath. Some people having AF never notice any sign of discomfort.

AF has a very rapid and chaotic ECG. AF results in rhythms of 150–220 beats per minute. The most prominent feature of the ECG of AF is an abnormal RR interval, while the ventricular rates are generally faster than of a healthy heart.

AF is also characterized by the lack of P wave in the ECG, or the P wave is very small and does not precede the relatively regular-looking QRS complex. Figure 9.9 shows an example of a typical AF ECG that was captured using the Wilson

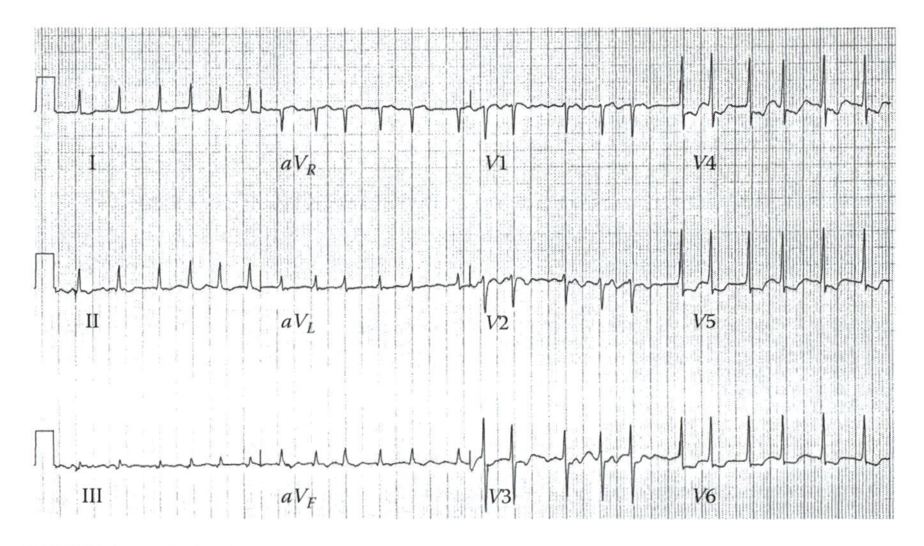

FIGURE 9.9 Atrial fibrillation ECG using the Wilson placement combined with augmented Einthoven electrode recording, giving a total of nine recordings. The calibration block at the beginning of each recording is 200 ms wide.

placement combined with augmented Einthoven electrode recording, giving a total of nine recordings. One of the standard chart recordings are given by the augments Einthoven recordings aV_R, aV_L, and aV_F, combined with the Wilson recording $V1$ through $V6$.

9.4.2 Ventricular Arrhythmias

In ventricular arrhythmias, ventricular activation does not originate in the A-V node. Moreover, the arrhythmia does not proceed in the ventricles in a normal way. In a normal heart in which the activation proceeds to the ventricles along the conduction system, the inner walls of the ventricles are activated almost simultaneously, and the activation front proceeds mainly radially toward the outer walls. As a result, the QRS complex of a healthy heart is of relatively short duration. In ventricular arrhythmias, however, since either the ventricular conduction system is broken or the ventricular activation starts far from the A-V node, it takes a longer time for the activation front to proceed throughout the ventricular muscle. This results to longer QRS complex. The criterion for normal ventricular activation requires the QRS interval to be shorter than 0.1 s. A QRS interval lasting longer than 0.1 s indicates abnormal ventricular activation. One example of ventricular arrhythmia is illustrated in Figure 9.10.

Another characteristic of ventricular disturbance is the premature ventricular contraction. A premature ventricular contraction is one that occurs abnormally early. If the origin of the disturbance is in the ventricular muscle, the QRS complex has a very abnormal form and lasts longer than 0.1 s. Usually the P wave is not associated with it. The arrhythmogenic complex produced by this supraventricular arrhythmia lasts less than 0.1 s.

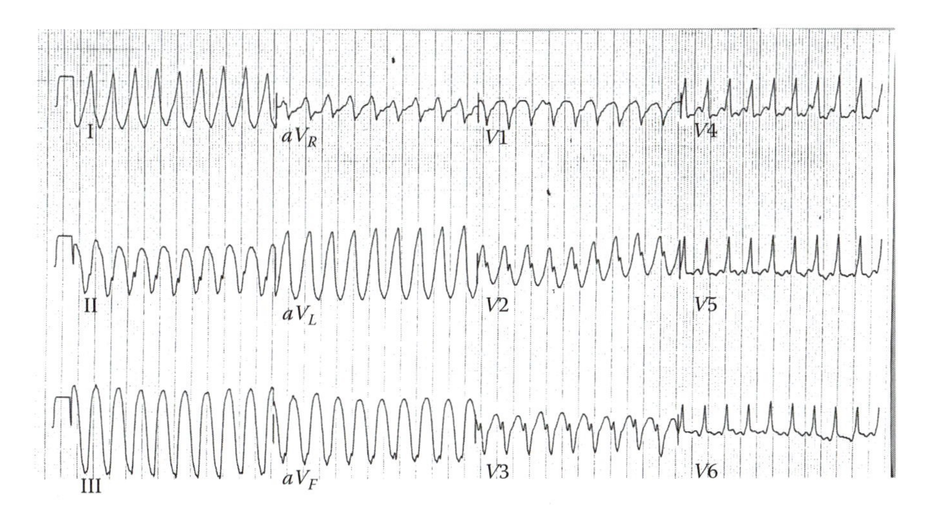

FIGURE 9.10 ECG of a characteristic VT using the Wilson placement combined with augmented Einthoven electrode recording, giving a total of nine recordings. The calibration block at the beginning of each recording is 200 ms wide.

9.4.3 Ventricular Tachycardia

A rhythm of ventricular origin may be a consequence of a slower conduction in ischemic ventricular muscle that leads to circular activation (reentry). This results in the activation of ventricular muscles at a high rate (over 120 beats per minute), causing rapid and wide QRS complexes. Such an arrhythmia is called ventricular tachycardia (VT).

VT is often a consequence of ischemia and myocardial infarction. The main change in ECG that indicates the occurrence of VT is the very fast heart rate that can be easily detected in the Fourier domain using discrete Fourier transform, or DFT.

9.4.4 Ventricular Fibrillation

When ventricular depolarization occurs chaotically, the situation is called ventricular fibrillation. This is reflected in the ECG, which demonstrates coarse irregular undulations without QRS complex. The cause of fibrillation is the establishment of multiple reentry loops usually involving diseased heart muscle. In this type of arrhythmia, the contraction of the ventricular muscle is also irregular, and, therefore, the timing is ineffective at pumping blood. The lack of blood circulation leads to almost immediate loss of consciousness and even death within minutes. The ventricular fibrillation may be stopped with an external defibrillator pulse and appropriate medication.

9.4.5 Myocardial Infarction

If a coronary artery is occluded, the transport of oxygen to the cardiac muscle is decreased, causing an oxygen debt in the muscle, which is called ischemia. Ischemia causes changes in the resting potential and in the repolarization of the muscle cells. This abnormality is observed in ECG as changes in the shape of the T wave. If the oxygen transport is terminated in a certain area, the heart muscle dies in that region. This is called a myocardial infarction or heart attack. After a blockage in the blood vessels supplying the heart muscle with oxygen and nutrients, the muscle cells in the region are severely compromised. Some cells may die while others will suffer severe damage, all resulting in a decreased ability to conduct impulses by generating its own depolarization. The dead cells will eventually be replaced by collagen since the heart does not have the ability to regenerate.

An infarct area is electrically silent since it has lost its excitability. According to the solid angle theorem described in Chapter 8, the loss of this outward dipole is equivalent to an electric force pointing inward. With this principle, it is possible to locate the infarction. The compromised cells will generate an action potential in a much slower fashion, causing a localized delay in the depolarization wave front. If this delay is enough to emerge at the time that healthy cells have already been repolarized, a subsequent delayed depolarization wave front may pass through the region of the heart that had just contracted. This generates a chaotic electric pattern and a disorganized contraction agreement.

Figure 9.11 shows nine sections of a recording in combined Einthoven and Wilson electrode placement of an inferior myocardial infarction. A heart attack can result in various deviating ECG patterns. In many heart attack cases, due to the existence of

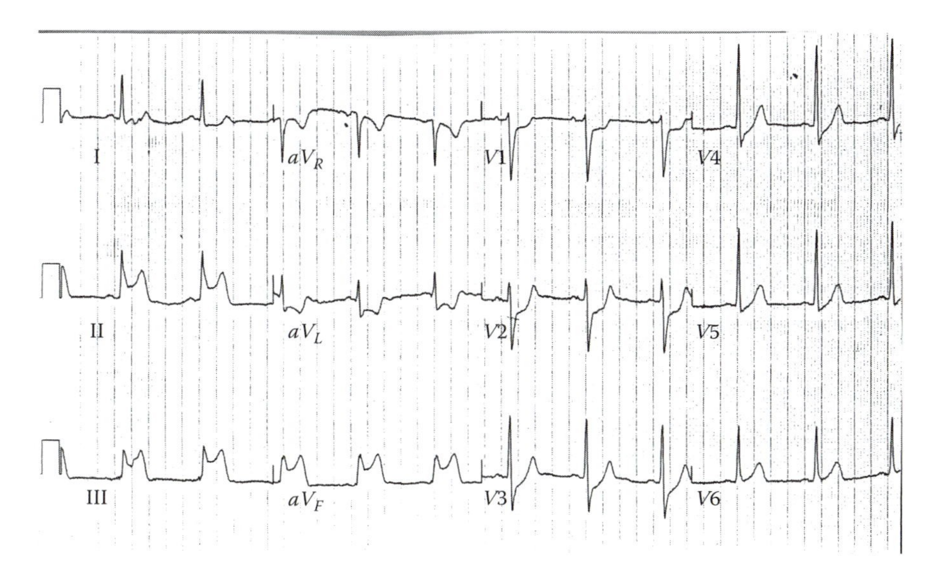

FIGURE 9.11 ECG recording of an inferior myocardial infarction using the Wilson placement combined with augmented Einthoven electrode recording, giving a total of nine recordings. The calibration block at the beginning of each recording is 200 ms wide.

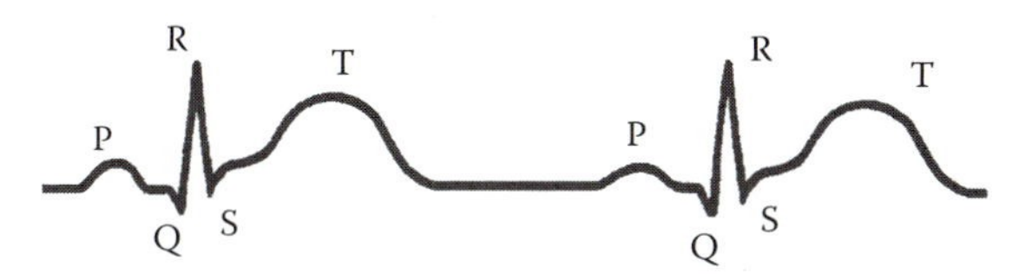

FIGURE 9.12 Schematic illustration of ST elevation during myocardial infarction.

the dying cells in the heart muscle, there will be no significant dip between the QRS complex and the T wave. The period between the S part and the T wave will also seem continuous. This is referred to as ST elevation. Figure 9.12 illustrates the effect of dying cells on the ST potential. The ST elevation is one of the most recognizable indicators of myocardial infarction.

9.4.6 Atrial Flutter

When the heart rate is sufficiently elevated so that the isoelectric interval between the end of T and beginning of P disappears, the arrhythmia is called atrial flutter. The origin is also believed to involve a reentrant atrial pathway. The frequency of these fluctuations is between 220 and 300 beats per minute. The A-V node and thereafter the ventricles are generally activated every second or every third atrial impulse (2:1 or 3:1 heart block).

9.4.7 Cardiac Reentry

Under certain conditions, the electric depolarization can conduct back into the atrium from where it immediately conducts over the His bundle back into the ventricles.

Another frequent form of reentry is a short circuit in the Purkinje fibers at the end of His bundle. The signal traveling through the His bundle does not conduct through one of the branches in one direction but will allow conduction in the opposite direction, providing a secondary activation of the ventricles through the healthy His branch. Cardiac reentry is one of the main causes of ventricular arrhythmias.

9.4.8 Atrioventricular Block

As mentioned earlier, the A-V node is slower than the S-A node, and, as a result of various illnesses, the conduction from S-A node to A-V node can be interrupted. This is called AV block. Under these circumstances, the atria will contract faster than the ventricles and the pump function will be severely compromised. As discussed earlier, if the P wave precedes the QRS complex with a PR interval of 0.12 s, the AV conduction is normal. If the PR interval is fixed but shorter than normal, either the origin of the impulse is closer to the ventricles or the AV conduction is utilizing an (abnormal) bypass tract leading to preexcitation of the ventricles. The latter is called the Wolff–Parkinson–White (WPW) syndrome and is discussed later. The PR interval may also be variable, such as in a wandering atrial pacemaker and multifocal atrial tachycardia. An example of the ECG recorded during a third-degree AV block is shown in Figure 9.13.

Based on the specific condition of the block, different types of AV blocks are defined. The conduction system defects producing a third-degree AV block may arise at different locations.

9.4.8.1 Main Types of AV Block

The A-V node can suffer several types of damages that are also referred to the heart block. The main five gradations of heart block that can be distinguished are as

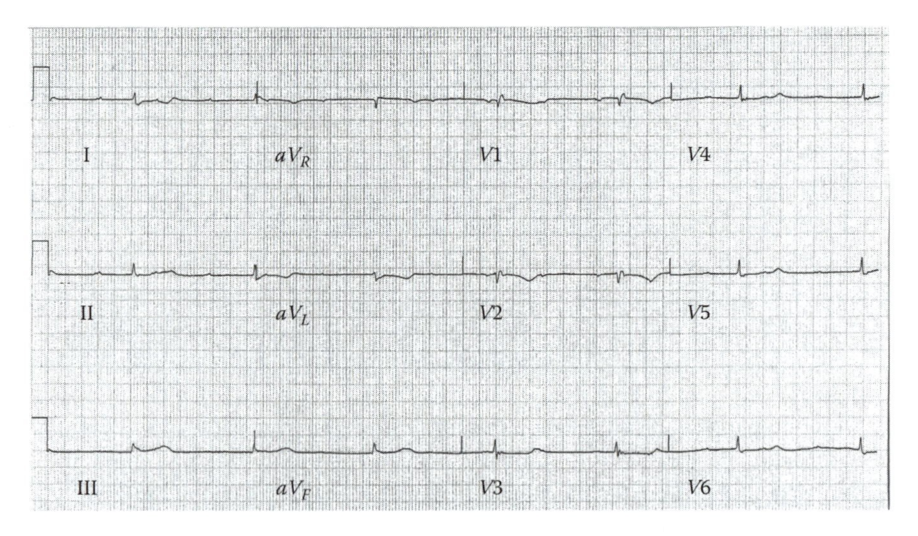

FIGURE 9.13 Third-degree AV block recorded by augmented recording of standard Einthoven electrode placement combined with six-electrode Wilson chest electrode placement.

follows: first- and second-degree block, bundle-branch block, right-bundle-branch block (RBBB), and left-bundle-branch block (LBBB).

In first-degree block, the conduction in the A-V node is still present but has depreciated severely, resulting in a significant delay. In such cases, the QRS complex is consistently preceded by the P wave but the PR interval is prolonged by over 0.2 s. This phenomenon is recognized by an elongated PR interval, which defines the time between the atrial depolarization and the onset of QRS complex.

When the internal conduction has degenerated to the point that only one out of every two or three action potentials passes through, this is defined as second-degree block. Second-degree block is shown in the ECG as an excessive number of P nodes but frequently lacking QRS complexes. If the PR interval progressively lengthens, leading finally to the total disfiguring of a QRS complex, the second-degree block is called a Wenkebach phenomenon.

Third-degree (or total) AV block is shown as a complete lack of synchronicity between the P wave and the QRS complex, i.e., the most severe grade of heart block is the result of a nonconducting A-V node in which the atrium and the ventricle depolarize and contract independent of each other. Bundle-branch block denotes a conduction defect in either of the bundle branches or in either of the left bundle branches. If both bundle branches demonstrate a block simultaneously, the progress of activation from the atria to the ventricles is completely inhibited, and this is regarded as third-degree AV block. The consequence of left or right-bundle-branch block is such that, activation of the ventricle must await initiation by the opposite ventricle. After this, activation proceeds entirely on a cell-to-cell basis. The absence of involvement of the conduction system, which initiates early activity of many sites, results in a much slower activation process along normal pathways. The consequence is a bizarre-shaped QRS complex with abnormally long duration. The ECG changes in connection with bundle-branch block associated with an acute myocardial infarction are illustrated in Figure 9.14.

Another related block is the RBBB. If the right bundle branch is defective to the point that electric impulse cannot travel through it to the right ventricle, activation will reach the right ventricle by excitation from the left ventricle. The depolarization now travels first through the septal and right ventricular muscle. This progress is,

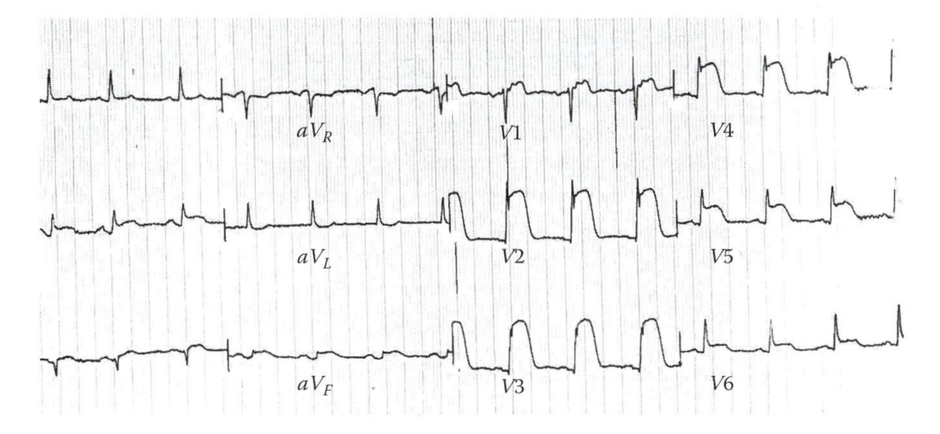

FIGURE 9.14 ECG of acute myocardial infarction and associated bundle-branch block.

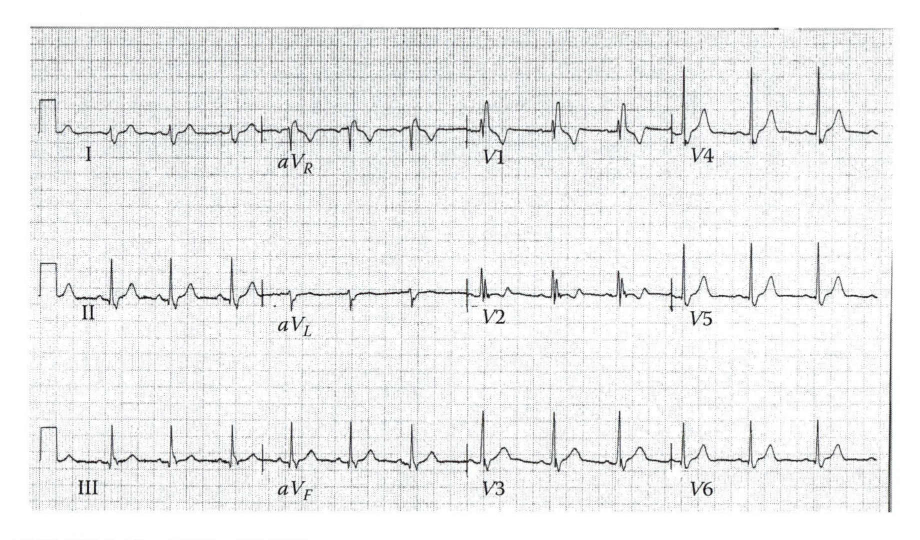

FIGURE 9.15 ECG of RBBB.

of course, slower through the conduction system and leads to a QRS complex wider than 0.1 s. Often, the criterion for the duration of QRS complex in RBBB and LBBB is that the duration of QRS needs to exceed 0.12 s. In RBBB, activation of the right ventricle is delayed to the point that it can be seen following the activation of the left ventricle. At this point, activation of the left ventricle still takes place as normal. RBBB causes an abnormal QRS heart vector and points toward the right ventricle. This is seen in the lead I recording of the ECG as a broadened S wave. Another typical manifestation of RBBB is frequently observed in lead V_1 as a double R wave, called an RSR' complex. Figure 9.15 shows a representative ECG of an RBBB.

The situation in LBBB is similar, but activation proceeds in a direction opposite to that found in RBBB. Again, the duration criterion of the QRS complex for complete block is in excess of 0.12 s. The abnormal sites of pulse initiation in the left ventricle make the heart vector progress at a slower rate and larger loop radius, resulting to a broad and tall R wave. This effect is usually observed in leads I, aV_L, V_5, or even V_6. Figure 9.16 shows a representative ECG of an LBBB.

As discussed earlier, when the break in conduction only manifests itself in either one of the ventricles, this indicates the conduction lost is in the His bundle. In this case, the ventricle that has been disconnected is excited through the intercalated disks connecting the left and right ventricles. The disconnected ventricle will depolarize later than the one that is still connected. As a result, the QRS complex widens. Sometimes the left and right depolarizations are far enough apart for the ECG to show two separate QRS complexes in direct sequence.

A related type of block, called WPW Syndrome, will be discussed next.

9.4.9 Wolf–Parkinson–White Syndrome

Technically, the ventricles and atria are supposed to be electrically isolated from each other. However, sometimes there may be a small amount of conduction passing

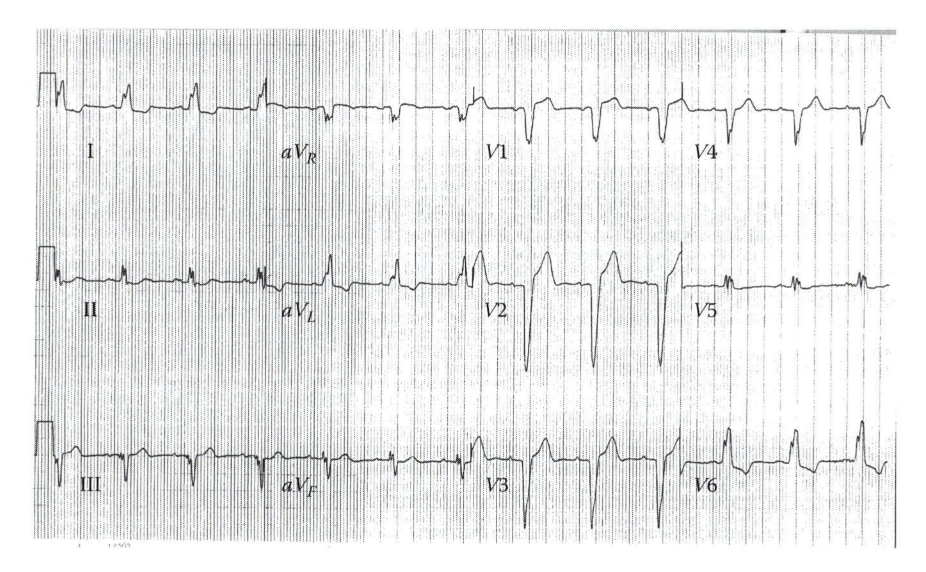

FIGURE 9.16 ECG of LBBB.

directly from the atrium to the ventricle. In this situation, the A-V node is effectively circumvented, and the delay introduced by the A-V node and His bundle combination is no longer able to hold the ventricular contraction off until the ventricle is filled by the atria. The QRS will follow directly on the down slope of the P wave. Meanwhile, the A-V-node stimulus will still proceed and depolarize in sequence with the "shortened" atrium–ventricle passage. This will lengthen the QRS complex, making it terminate at the originally expected time period as during a normal ECG recording.

One cause for a broad QRS complex that exceeds the 0.12 s duration may be the WPW syndrome. The cause of the WPW syndrome is the passage of activation from the atrium directly to the ventricular muscle via an abnormal route. This bypass is called the bundle of Kent, which bypasses the AV junctions. This results in an activation of the ventricular muscle before normal activation reaches the ventricular muscle via the conduction system. This process is called preexcitation, and the specific ECG depends on the respective location of the accessory pathway. In WPW syndrome, the time interval from the P wave to the R wave is normal. The QRS complex in this case has an earlier-than-normal sharp onset called the delta wave. The premature ventricular excitation manifesting the delta wave results in a shortening of the PQ time. An illustration of the impact on the conduction pattern during WPW syndrome given in Figure 9.17.

9.4.10 Extrasystole

Both chemical and mechanical stimuli can trigger spontaneous depolarization of a single cardiac cell, which translates to the conduction of activation to the neighboring cells. The only difference between this type of disease and normal heart is the resulting excitation that can be caused by any cell located at any location in the heart muscle. This random pulse generation is called an ectopic stimulus. In this situation, the P wave is often missing in its entirety for the QRS complex.

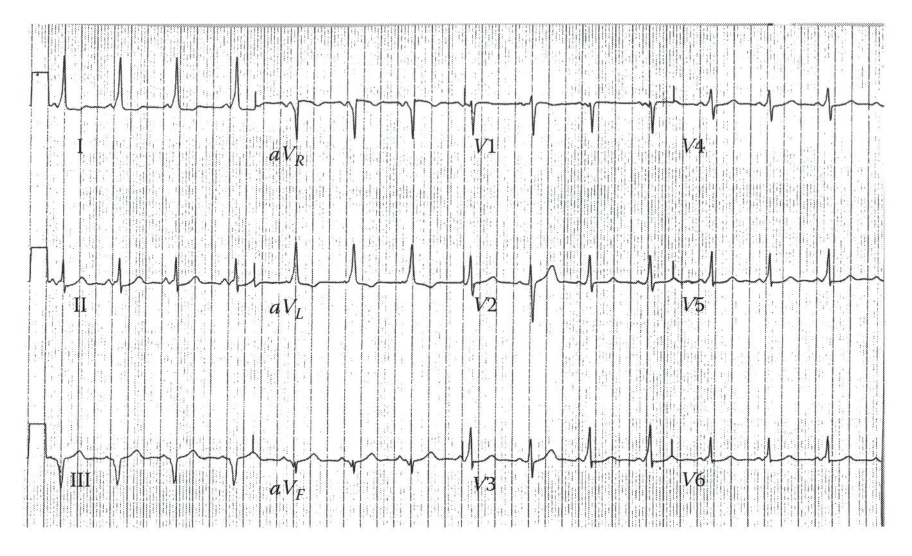

FIGURE 9.17 ECG of WPW syndrome.

9.5 PROCESSING AND FEATURE EXTRACTION OF ECG

The interpretation of the recorded ECG is often based on a physician's experience. The physician's decision is typically based on the previously mentioned "time-based criteria" described for the ECG of the diseased cases. Such criteria are often rooted in the physiology of the cardiovascular system and are very well understood by the physicians.

While the computer-aided diagnostic systems commonly used in many clinical electrocardiography clinics utilize all the time-based criteria mentioned earlier, they also use the typical signal processing and pattern recognition measures and techniques for diagnostics.

It has been reported that the computer-aided interpretation of characteristic patterns found in ECG provides better than 90% accuracy of recognizing the underlying electric and hemodynamic causes and factors for appropriate treatment. For majority of the diagnostic interpretations, it is either the measurement of time intervals (i.e., time-based criteria) that provides an insight in the underlying causes, or the altered shapes of the actual waveform that reveal the underlying causes of the hemodynamic complications. The purely signal processing measures and methods capture small changes in ECG that may go unnoticed by the human eyes. It is also important to note that even for measuring time-based criteria, the computer-aided systems can provide a more reliable and accurate measurement and description of the time-based measures such as the duration of the heart cycle. More specifically, the signal processing techniques can more accurately calculate the time intervals and analyze the resulting numbers.

Some of the main feature extraction and signal processing methods, including the extraction of the time-based features mentioned earlier for some specific diseases will be discussed next.

9.5.1 Time-Domain Analysis

As discussed earlier, the most significant time-domain feature in the ECG is the duration of the heart cycle. The heart cycle duration is frequently derived by measuring the time span from one R wave to the next. Other features are essentially the duration of each wave (i.e., the duration of QRS complex) and the time separation among the waves (e.g., the time interval between T and P waves, i.e., TP interval). Two specific time features are further described in the following.

An important time domain feature is the duration of QRS complex as described earlier. Generally, the QRS complex is identified by the characteristic shape and relative stable time constant in the pattern. Another feature of interest is the time interval between the T wave and the subsequent P wave. The importance of this measure shows the separation between two important events, i.e., the pulse rate of the sinus node, which is expressed in the P wave, and the repolarization phenomenon that is the origin of the T wave.

9.5.2 Frequency-Domain Analysis

In any ECG waveform, the QRS complex is well localized as the high-frequency region. The P and T waves are mainly the low-frequency components. The ST segment in the ECG is time restricted with mostly low-frequency content.

The normal ECG and the deviating ECG often have significantly different frequency contents. Since the normal heart rate is in the range of 60–100 beats per minute, the fibrillation can exceed 200 beats per minute. In addition to the frequency differences, the depolarization and repolarization ramps also change under diseased conditions, requiring a much wider frequency bandwidth to describe each different phenomenon.

The standard ECG can be described by the first eight harmonics of the heart rate in the Fourier domain. This provides a basic representation as shown in Figure 9.18. Figure 9.18a shows the nine-electrode recording for a normal ECG as shown in Figure 9.5, and Figure 9.14b illustrates the superposition of the first eight harmonics reconstructing the ECG from Figure 9.3. Any minor high-frequency deviation from the normal ECG often creates variations in the ECG that requires a much larger number of harmonics to describe the frequency-domain features of the ECG. As a rule of thumb, a frequency analysis should span no less than the frequency range of 0–100 Hz for an apparently normal ECG. Arrhythmias may require a frequency analysis up to 200 Hz. However, entering even higher-frequency spectra, the spectrum will be dominated by noise and will not contribute additional information.

An important disease that is often detected in the frequency domain is sinus tachycardia. A sinus rhythm of higher than 100 beats per minute is called sinus tachycardia. Similar conditions often occur as a physiological response to physical exercise or physical stress, but, in diseased cases, the condition results from congestive heart failure. More specifically, if the sinus rhythm is irregular such that the longest PP or RR intervals exceed the shortest interval by 0.16 s, the situation is diagnosed as sinus arrhythmia. This condition is very common in all age groups but

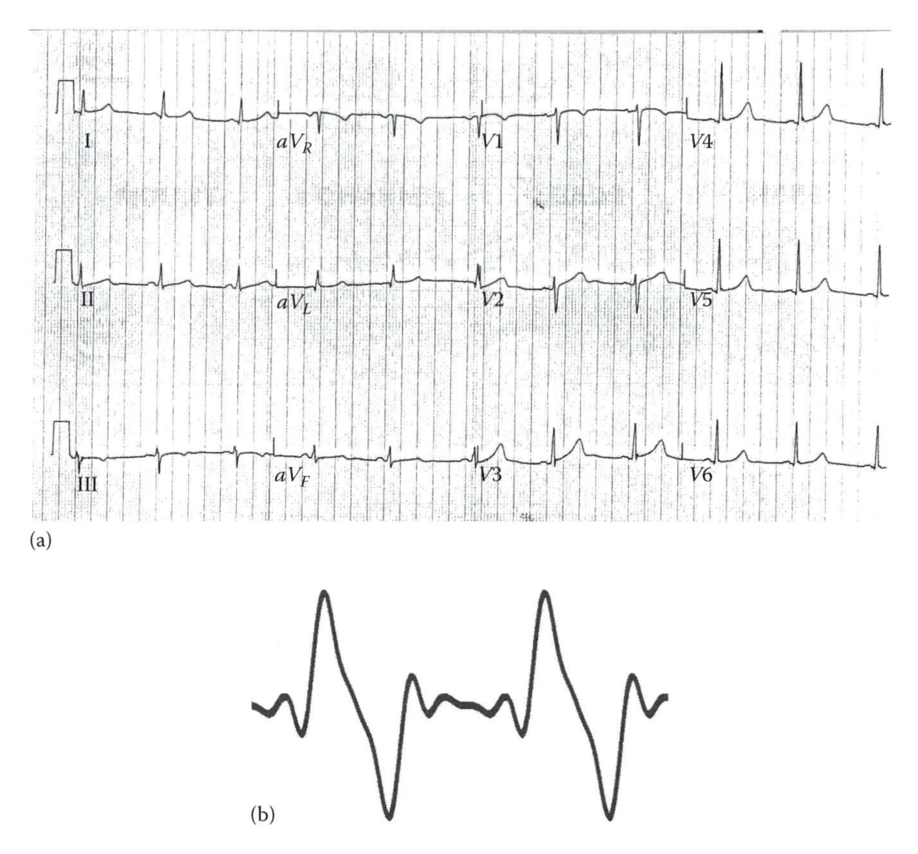

FIGURE 9.18 (a) Normal ECG with a rate of 60 beats per minute or a frequency of 1 Hz, and (b) ECG dissected in the first eight harmonics, added up to give a close match with the original.

more common in teenagers and preteens who may have never considered having a heart disease. One potential origin for the sinus arrhythmia may be the vagus nerve, which regulates respiration as well as heart rhythm. The nerve is active during respiration and through its effect on the sinus node, causes an increase in heart rate during inspiration and a decrease during expiration.

Accurate detection of fetal heart signals during pregnancy is another area where the frequency and wavelet analysis is vital to provide important information on potential fetal cardiac diseases. A different type of standard ECG recordings from the leads placed on the abdomen of the mother is used to monitor the fetal ECG. The observed maternal ECG waveforms are not necessarily noisy but are in fact superimposed on the fetal ECG. The maternal ECG will overpower the fetal signals due to the relatively low-power fetal ECG. Additionally, there will be multiple interference sources. The P and T waves from the maternal ECG can easily be identified in most cases. The fetal heart rate is generally significantly faster than the maternal heart rate, which allows separation of the mother's and the baby's ECG using filters designed in the frequency domain.

Since ECG has a large statistical basis and rarely perfectly reproducible, the direct analytical schemes based merely on sine and cosine transformations are not adequate. As a result, it is often the case that raw ECG recordings, assuming ergodicity, and the correlation function are first estimated and then the power spectrum of the signal is used for the frequency analysis. The details of this process were discussed in Part I of the book.

Several frequency effects measured by the electrodes are not necessarily associated with the true frequency spectrum of the cellular activity. Many have been caused by different sources of noise such as the breathing signals and the electromyography (EMG) of other skeletal muscles. Such noises are often filtered in the frequency domain. For instance, a notch filter at the main power frequency is always applied to filter out equipment and capacitive noise.

As mentioned earlier, one of the obvious skeletal motion artifacts are the breath signals, which have both the chest and diaphragm muscles involved. Both groups of muscles are large muscles, and the EMG resulting from the muscular excitation produces large signal amplitudes. Since the breathing motion is often a regular process and has much slower rate than the heart rate, it may be easily distinguished. However, the electrode motion resulting from the breathing action has a modulation effect on the spectrum content of the measured signal. An effective method of filtering these types of electric interference signals out is by triggering the measurement on the motion that is causing the electric noise. In addition, the inhale and exhale process can be monitored by flow probes and subtracted from the detected ECG signal.

9.5.3 Wavelet-Domain Analysis

Since action potentials are mainly stochastic in nature, wavelet analysis of a single action potential may not provide the reliable data required for accurate diagnosis. However, when observing a repetitive signal (such as ECG) as a resultant of the summation of many action potentials, the wavelet-domain features can identify the relative contributions of the higher frequencies (lower scales).

The wavelet features used in the analysis of ECG often detect the existence of a scaled or shifted version of a typical pattern or wave. Wavelet decomposition using mother wavelet resembles the general shape of the QRS complex, which reveals the location, the amplitude, and the scaling of the QRS pattern quantitatively. Wavelet analysis is also performed using Daubeches and Coiflet wavelets.

A typical application of the wavelet analysis is the separation of the mother's and the baby's ECG. As mentioned earlier, the waveform of the fetal ECG is similar to that of the adult ECG in the wavelet transform (WT) domain, except for the scale of the signal. The wavelet decomposition of the observed signal can effectively separate the mother's ECG from the baby's, simply because the two ECG signals reside on different scales.

9.6 SUMMARY

In this chapter, the function and structure of the heart as well as the origin of the ECG signal are briefly described. This chapter also introduces a number of cardiovascular diseases that can be diagnosed using ECG. The processing methods commonly used for processing of ECG are also covered in this chapter.

PROBLEMS

9.1 Import the data in the file "p_9_1.xls" in MATLAB® and plot the signal.* In order to do so, use File/Import Data... on the main MATLAB menu and follow the steps in loading and naming of the data. The file contains the signals of a two-electrode recording of a normal ECG over a period of 1 min.

a. Determine the PP interval and the RR interval for both signals.
b. Use DFT to describe the signals in the frequency. Determine the heart rate.
c. Isolate one typical period of the signal, i.e., one cycle containing P-QRS-T. Calculate the duration of P, T, and QRS waves.
d. Comment on the differences between the values captured in parts a, b, and c across the two signals.

9.2 Import the data in the file "p_9_2.xls" and plot the signals. The file contains the signals of an eight-electrode recording of an abnormal ECG describing AF. Choose the signal of recording II for your analysis.

a. Repeat the calculations in parts a, b, and c of Problem 9.1 on the recording II.
b. Compare a single period with one period of the signal in Problem 9.1 and comment on the differences.

9.3 Import the data in the file "p_9_3.xls" and plot the signals. This signal is one recording out of 12 recordings of an ECG with bundle-branch block. For this ECG signal, we focus on the signals in the recordings I and II.

a. Repeat the calculations in parts a, b, and c of Problem 9.1 on the recordings I and II.
b. Using "wavemenu" and Daubeches 1 mother wavelet, decompose the signal into five levels. Comment on the contents of each decomposition level. Apply denoising option to filter out the noise.
c. Repeat part b using Daubeches 2 mother wavelet.
d. Compare a single period with one period of the signal in Problem 9.1 and comment on the differences.

9.4 Import the data in the file "p_9_4.xls" and plot the signal. This is a fifteen-channel recording of a myocardial infarction ECG. Use signal II for the following analyses:

a. Repeat the calculations in parts a, b, and c of Problem 9.1 on the recording II.
b. Using "wavemenu" and Daubeches 1 mother wavelet, decompose the signal into five levels. Comment on the contents of each decomposition level. Apply denoising option to filter out the noise.
c. Repeat part b using Daubeches 2 mother wavelet.
d. Compare a single period with one period of the signal in Problem 9.1 and comment on the differences.

---

* All ECG recordings in the problem section of this chapter were taken from PhysioNet, http://www.physionet.org/. The research resource for complex physiologic signals: MIT, Cambridge, MA.

9.5 Import the data in the file "p_9_5.xls" and plot the signal. This file contains the ECG signal of VT with clear AV dissociation.

a. Repeat the calculations in parts a, b, and c of Problem 9.1 on the recording.
b. Using "wavemenu" and Daubeches 1 mother wavelet, decompose the signal into five levels. Comment on the contents of each decomposition level. Apply denoising option to filter out the noise.
c. Compare a single period with one period of the signal in Problem 9.1 and comment on the differences.

9.6 Import the data in the file "p_9_6.xls" and plot the signals. This file contains fifteen-electrode recording of the ECG for a case of myocardial infarction with apparent ST elevation. Use signal II or II for your analysis.

a. Repeat the calculations in parts a, b, and c of Problem 9.1 on the recording.
b. Compare a single period with one period of the signal in Problem 9.1 and comment on the differences.
c. Is the amplitude the only discriminating factor in the diagnosis of this patient's ECG?

10 Electroencephalogram

10.1 INTRODUCTION AND OVERVIEW

The brain acts as the central control and data processing unit for the biological medium. The neural activity of the brain uses action potentials by which the brain activity can be recorded by means of electrodes, as in electroencephalogram (EEG), or by magnetic inductors, which form a signal called magnetoencephalogram (MEG). In this chapter, we focus on the EEG.

Electroencephalogram is the combination of the three words electro, encephalo, and gram. The first term, electro, pertains to electric and the second term, encephalo, which stems from the Greek words *en-kephale*, means "in-head" and stands for the brain. The third term, gram, represents the act of recording. Putting the three words together, electroencephalogram means the recording of the electric activities of the brain.

In 1929, a German psychiatrist named Hans Berger experimented by placing electrodes on the head of his daughter and verified his hypothesis that the brain exhibits electric activity. He measured the brain waves of his daughter when she was doing mental arithmetic. He also discovered that the activity increased when she was trying to perform difficult multiplications. From this evidence, he deduced that the wave patterns observed in the brain recordings reflected the depth of the brain activity.

In this chapter, we focus on the biological roots of EEG as well as the diseases often diagnosed by analysis of EEG. We also discuss the computational techniques typically used to process EEG signal.

10.2 BRAIN AND ITS FUNCTIONS

The brain is an organ that is part of the central nervous system (CNS). The brain monitors and regulates unconscious bodily processes, such as digestion and breathing. The brain also coordinates most voluntary movements of your body. It is also the site of conscious thinking, allowing you to learn and create. A frontal cross section of the brain and brain stem is illustrated in Figure 10.1. As can be seen in Figure 10.1, the gray matter and the white matter form the major part of the brain. The gray matter is the outside shell of the brain and is made up of a body of nerve cells. The nerve cells (also called neurons) perform the actual signal processing inside the brain. The white matter in the core of the brain comprises the nerve axons, linking to the gray matter (cortex), the brain stem, and the peripheral motor and sensory units. Both the gray and the white matter have connective tissue intertwined for support.

As shown in Figure 10.1, the cortex forms the outside layer of the wavy upper structure of the brain, which is called the cerebrum. This is where the nerve cells are located. Below the brain is the cerebellum, which is split into two halves. The cerebral cortex also has two hemispheres. It has been determined that for right-handed

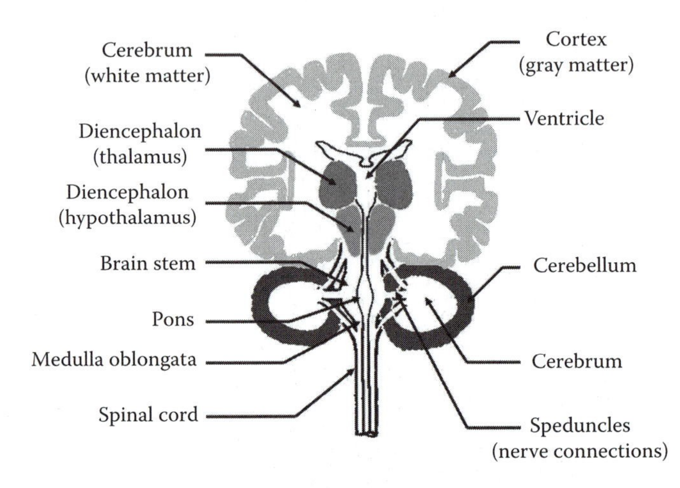

FIGURE 10.1 Schematic anatomy of the brain with the major functional components identified. The main source for EEG signals is from the cortex of the cerebrum.

people the left hemisphere manages speech, reading, writing, logical thinking, and predominantly controls the right side of the body. The right hemisphere, on the other hand, manages artistic and creative ability and movements on the left side of the body and is primarily involved in artistic creativity.

Each part of the brain has been specialized to provide certain functionality. The front section of the cerebrum manages speech, thought, emotion, problem solving, and skilled movements. This part is referred to as the frontal lobe. Moving toward the rear of the head, behind the frontal lobe is the parietal lobe, which identifies and interprets sensations such as touch, temperature, and pain. At the very back of the brain is the occipital lobe, which collects and interprets visual images. On either side of the occipital lobe are the temporal lobes, which process hearing and store memory. The cerebellum coordinates muscle action and is involved with posture and balance maintenance. The cerebellum helps to control and coordinate familiar movements. Initially, when an individual is in the process of learning a new activity, such as riding a bike, the cerebrum directs the muscles to move. At the point where the motion becomes common nature, the cerebellum takes over the muscle controls.

The diencephalon is positioned in the center, directly underneath the cerebrum and on top of the brain stem. It contains the thalamus and the hypothalamus. The thalamus acts as a relay station for incoming sensory nerve impulses. The hypothalamus plays a vital role in regulating body temperature, among other things. The hypothalamus controls the release of hormones from the nearby pituitary gland.

The brain stem is responsible for continually regulating the various life support mechanisms, such as your heart rate, blood pressure, digestion, and breathing, as well as involuntary activities such as swallowing and sneezing.

Other parts of the brain are the diencephalons, the brain stem in the center, and the spinal cord below the brain stem. Nerve impulses carrying different kinds of information travel to and from the brain to and from the spinal cord. The spinal cord will branch the signal to the target areas of the extremities or the designated organs to accomplish the desired result. The spinal cord also conveys the sensed signals from the peripheral nervous system (PNS) to the brain.

Due to the importance of the brain and its delicate nature, the brain is protected by three membranes called the meninges. The space between the meninges is filled with a liquid called the cerebrospinal fluid. Despite these layers of protection, different types of damages to the brain can cause physiological and mental problems for the patients. Specifically, damage to a specific region of the cerebrum results in impaired functions associated with that part. For example, a stroke in the motor area of the right hemisphere will cause paralysis of all or part of the body's left side. Such damages may also affect speech. It was observed that with training and determination, surviving neurons in the neighboring regions can be taught to take over at least a portion of the original functionalities.

Now that we have familiarized ourselves with the physiology and the functions of the brain, next we explore how EEG is created and measured.

10.3 ELECTROENCEPHALOGRAM: SIGNAL OF THE BRAIN

It has been estimated that the number of nerve cells in the brain is in the order of 10^{11} nerve cells. Especially, the neurons in the cortex are strongly interconnected. A cortical axon may be covered with between 1,000 and 100,000 synapses. The steady-state nerve potential is negative and is typically around −70 mV. The peak of the action potential is positive 30 mV and lasts approximately 1 ms. The peak-to-peak amplitude of the nerve impulse is thus approximately 100 mV. Every neuron in the gray matter displays a release of action potentials throughout the course of receiving and processing sensory inputs coming from other neurons or external stimuli. ECG is the spatially weighted summation of all these action potentials measured at the surface of the skull.

Since the initial discovery of the electric activity of the brain, the ability to measure this activity using EEG has been perfected. The EEG technology is very inexpensive and accurately measures brainwave activity in the outer layer of the brain. Sensitive electrodes are attached to the skull, and signals are recorded in either unipolar or bipolar fashion. The depolarization signals from the brain cells are attenuated while passing through the connective tissue, the brain fluid, and the skull and skin, which have complex impedances. In order to collect the relatively small signals from the brain activity, the skull needs to be prepared for quality contact to at least overcome the impedance mismatch created by the hair and dead skin on the skull, which prove to be poor conductors.

The collected signals on the surface of the skull are amplified to give a graph of electric potential versus time. Usually, the electric activity of the brain needs to be compared at different spots on the head simultaneously. The most common recording technique applies 21 electrodes and an equal number of channels for EEG measurement. Other measuring techniques are in use that may record from 64 electrodes to as many as 256 electrodes. The frequency range of the amplifiers used to record the brain waves needs to be from 0.1 to 100 Hz to ensure proper registration of all periodic details.

The most common EEG measurements are made with the electrodes placed in an internationally recognized configuration illustrated in Figure 10.2. This standard

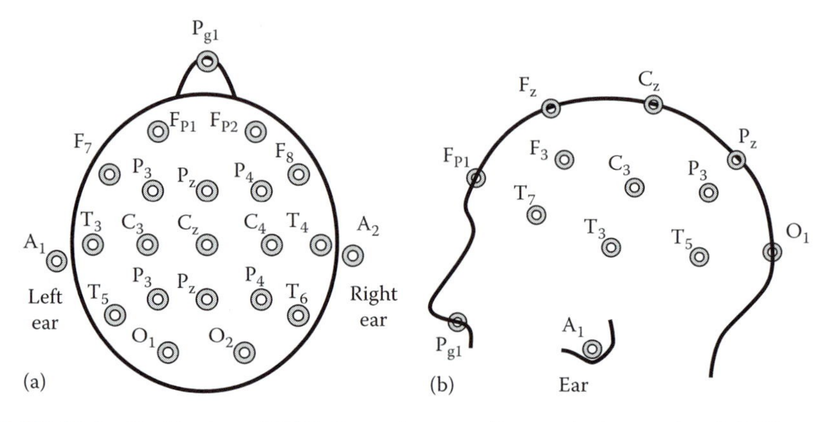

FIGURE 10.2 Positioning of EEG electrodes according to the international 10/20 system. The letters F, T, C, P, and O represent the anatomical sections referred to as frontal, central, parietal, and occipital, respectively. (a) Top view of the head with 21 electrodes, plus one on each ear, and the nose acts as reference point. (b) Left side view of the head with electrodes placed in relation to parts of the brain that have been identified as the main location of particular mental and motor functions.

allows reproducibility and comparison of recorded EEG with the reported EEGs of the recognized cases of physical and/or mental disorders. This standard technique has the electrodes at 20° angles with each other across the middle of the skull in a hemispherical matrix and at approximately 10° above the eyes.

EEG is often used to diagnose seizure disorders, tumors, head injuries, degenerative diseases, and brain death. EEG is also heavily used in research on brain function and activity. The most frequent application of EEG is in the recording and analysis of evoked potentials (EPs) and event-related potentials (ERPs) of the brain. In such applications, the EEG signals respond to specific stimuli such as auditory and visual inputs and are recorded. EPs and ERPs are instrumental in investigating how long it takes for the brain to process different kinds of information in response to the designed stimulation. EPs are also used to monitor the level of attention as well as stress during various experiments. EPs and ERPs will be described later in this chapter when the clinical applications of EEG are explained.

The major drawback of EEG is that it cannot reveal from which structure inside the skull a specific part of the signal has originated. This is due to the fact that, as mentioned earlier, the EEG is a spatial summation of all action potentials coming from billions of neurons at different depths below the cerebral cortex. Hence, in sensitive applications where the functional information from the structures deep within the brain has to be extracted, functional magnetic resonance imaging (*f*MRI) is used. The principles and applications of *f*MRI will be discussed in detail in Chapter 15. The structural as well as functional information provided by the *f*MRI allows brain activity to be determined in relation to specific locations in the brain.

Knowing the general characteristics of EEG, next we start the analysis of typical EEG signals in the frequency domain.

10.3.1 EEG Frequency Spectrum

The EEG signal is often interpreted based on the presence and absence of particular waves with known frequencies. The presence or absence of these waves indicates certain physiological conditions that are extremely useful in diagnostics. The typical waves classified in the EEG signal are alpha (α), beta (β), delta (δ), and theta (Θ) waves. The presence and strength of each of these waves can be easily detected using discrete Fourier transform (DFT) of the EEG signal (in deterministic analysis of the signal) or using the power spectra of the EEG signal (in stochastic processing of EEG). The definition of each wave identifies the formation of band-pass filters needed to extract these waves.

The normal adult, in a physically relaxed state while having the eyes closed, produces a rhythmical brain wave with a frequency of 8–14 Hz, which is called alpha wave. Generally, the alpha wave disappears when the eyes are opened; however, they may still be present if the person is in a state of extreme relaxation. Since these waves were discovered first, they were labeled as alpha waves. From the definition of the alpha wave, it is clear that in order to extract this wave component, one needs to pass the EEG through a band-pass filter with the pass band set to 8–14 Hz.

The frequency band of the beta waves is 14–50 Hz. The beta waves are prevalent in the regions of parietal and frontal lobes. Beta waves are often associated with problem solving and logical thinking. As will be discussed later, beta wave is the major component observed in an important stage of healthy sleep. In order to extract the beta wave, a band-pass filter with the pass band set to 14–50 Hz must be used.

The delta waves have a frequency range of 0.5–4 Hz and are detected in infants and sleeping adults. The band-pass filter needed to extract delta wave has a pass band of 0.5–4 Hz.

The theta waves fall in the frequency range of 4–8 Hz and are measured in resting and sleeping adults and in children while awake. This wave can be separated using a 4–8 Hz band-pass filter.

Representative signals from the four frequency bands of the brain activity are illustrated in Figure 10.3. Additionally, specific spikes associated with epileptic

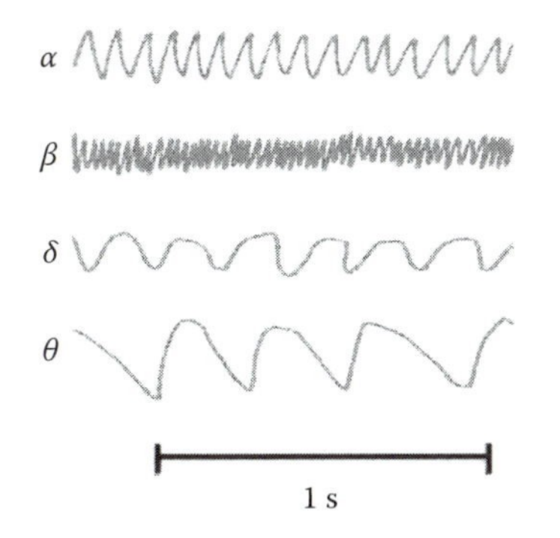

FIGURE 10.3 Representative frequency patterns from the four spectral groups in the EEG. Alpha waves (α) generally cover the spectral range of 8–14 Hz, beta waves (β) span the spectrum between 14 and 50 Hz, while delta waves (δ) range from 4 to 8 Hz and theta waves (θ) are in the frequencies covered by the spectrum from 0.5 to 4 Hz.

episodes with no particular frequency spectrum are also observed in EEG. A newborn's EEG generally has a frequency range between 0.5 and 2 Hz. The frequency spectrum of a baby's EEG increases rapidly by the second year when short episodes of alpha waves can be distinguished. At the age of 14, the EEG is identical to that of a grown adult.

Before discussing the significance of EEG, it is very insightful to explore the physical rules governing the formation of major frequencies in the EEG spectrum. The coherence and formation of the higher frequencies in EEG can be explained as a wave interference phenomenon on purely physical grounds. When a depolarization potential is generated in a cell, it travels over the surface of the cortex in the conducting media. Consider the distance traveled by a neural signal in time t as d. Then, assuming the speed of neural signal propagation as V, we have

$$d = V \cdot t \tag{10.1}$$

On average, the distance from the frontal to the posterior area of the brain spans approximately 0.2 m. In addition, we know the speed of propagation for current in biological media is approximately 5 m/s. This means, according to Equation 10.1, the duration to traverse the distance from front to back of the cortex comes to 0.04 s. In reality, this wave travels back and forth between the front and back of the brain. Modeling this phenomenon as a standing wave (a pattern formed by a forward and a backward moving wave), would generate a primary one-half wavelength standing wave. This means that the entire length of the wave, or the period T of the standing wave, will be 0.08 s. Calculating the frequency of this wave, we have

$$f = \frac{1}{T} = \frac{1}{0.08} = 12.5\,\text{Hz} \tag{10.2}$$

This would be a frequency in the alpha spectrum. Higher frequencies can easily be portrayed as higher harmonics this frequency. Lower frequencies, however, will not fit the standing wave theory. This phenomenon could be one of the possible explanations that higher frequency brain activity often produces synchronized recordings of multiple electrodes; even though the sections of the brain that are sending signals are in unison, they are anatomically and physiologically not connected to the phenomenon producing the EP.

Next, we briefly discuss the significance of EEG in medical diagnostics.

10.3.2 Significance of EEG

EEG is the most commonly used clinical measure in diagnostics of almost all types of neurological disorders. Some of the main applications of EEG are briefly described in the following, and more detailed applications of EEG will be discussed later in this chapter.

During an important stage of sleep called rapid eye movement (REM) sleep, a strong beta wave pattern of 40 Hz was observed in the sleep EEG. During sleep, short burst of frequencies between 12 and 14 Hz also appear in the EEG. These bursts are called spindles. The presence of beta (and to some degree, alpha) during sleep describes why a major application of EEG is the diagnostics of different types of sleep disorders. For instance, a healthy night sleep must contain a rather long REM period that is typically detected by the occurrence of beta waves. The absence or the short duration of beta (and other similar waves) often indicates an abnormal sleep.

Due to the age dependency of the EEG signal, this signal has significant applications in the diagnostics of age-related disorders. It is known that during childhood the dominant EEG frequencies increase with age. A newborn baby has frequencies ranging from 0.5 to 2 Hz. At the end of the second year, the EEG already displays short stretches of alpha waves. At the age of 14, however, the brain wave pattern is virtually undistinguishable from an adult. The presence or absence of certain frequencies in a person belonging to a particular age group is an indication of abnormality of the brain activities.

In general, the measure of conciseness can be derived from the frequency components of the EEG signal, i.e., as higher frequencies are detected, the patient is more alert and mentally occupied. In addition to the increase in frequency with increased activity, the neural activity will show less coherence (i.e., more chaotic behavior) with an increase in the alertness. This is due to the fact that in an alert brain, each neuron acts more and more independent from its neighbors and desynchronization becomes more prevalent. The measurement of general electric activity of the brain is called spontaneous activity, which represents the apparent chaotic brain activity.

There are two internationally accepted methods of testing the brain activity that are commonly applied in clinical measurements. These two methods are EP recordings and ERP recordings. These two methods will be explained next.

10.4 EVOKED POTENTIALS

EPs are the EEG signals generated under external stimuli such as auditory input or visual input. EPs are typically used to diagnose the sensory properties and also the motor pathways within the specialized sections of the CNS. The different types of EP measurements form three classes of measurements: auditory evoked potentials (AEPs), somatosensory evoked potentials (SEPs), and visual evoked potentials (VEPs). These methods of stimuli to perform diagnostic utilities are discussed next.

10.4.1 Auditory-Evoked Potentials

AEPs are used to check for hearing damage and the source of the damage, either mechanical or neurological. During the course of AEP measurement, tones with different frequencies are played on a headphone attached to the patient's ears. While the tones are played, the EEG signals are recorded and marked according to the frequency of the tone. In the processing step, the correlation between the tone signal and the recorded EEG will determine the sensitivity of the CNS to the played tone. More specifically, when the brain is not responding to a tone with a particular frequency, the case can be diagnosed as pathological. The real problem observed in

AEP can be due to damages either in the ear or in the CNS. Further tests will verify the exact source of the abnormality observed in the AEP.

Certain pathological neurological sensory conditions as well as mechanical pathological auditory conditions can be treated by surgical methods. The importance of the AEPs can be further realized knowing that the AEPs serve as the main diagnostic tool to detect these conditions.

10.4.2 Somatosensory-Evoked Potentials

SEPs are accomplished by the application of electric impulses administered to the skin of the arms or legs. The response of the CNS to these stimuli is then measured and analyzed to identify the sensitivity and functionality of the neuromuscular system under study. It is often the case that the stimuli are applied to the arm or leg that is closest to the muscular system under study.

Under normal conditions, these electric impulses delivered through electrodes pass through the skin and result in motor neuron actions. These neuron actions are typically followed by muscle contractions. The muscle contractions are stimulated by delivery of currents in the range of 25–50 mA. The electric impulses are usually delivered in pulse mode to avoid saturation and muscle fatigue. The pulse durations are varied between 100 μs and 1 ms. It is standard procedure to apply the stimulus at various distances from the location where the EPs are recorded.

The measured time delay between the stimulus and EP is often treated as the main indication of pathological characteristics. A long observed delay indicates that the neural pathways involved in the transmission of the stimuli to the brain are somehow damaged. The SEPs are typically used as the main diagnostic tools to identify neuromuscular disorders. They are also utilized to measure the depth of anesthesia in some specialized surgeries.

10.4.3 Visual-Evoked Potentials

VEPs are EEG signals measured when the patient is subjected to the visual stimuli. The applied visual stimuli often contain high-contrast patterns stretching the entire field of view. Such stimuli typically generate sensory potentials that are transmitted to the brain and are reflected in the measured EEG. The main part of the brain that registers VEPs is the primary visual cortex, located on the rear of the head in the occipital lobes of the brain. However, other areas of the brain have been found to show EPs as well.

During the course of measuring VEPs, there cannot be any distractions, especially other visual disturbances, because the brain stimulus needs to be responding only to the applied visual stimulus. A standard visual stimulus is the use of a checkerboard that changes the location of the black and white squares. Other stimuli are flashes of light that turn on and off with a certain frequency and other light-intensity patterns. One aspect of designing useful visual stimuli is calibration and standardization of the stimuli. The aspects of the stimuli that need to follow certain standards include the light color(s), the light intensity, the pupil diameter, and the degree of eye fixation on the stimulus.

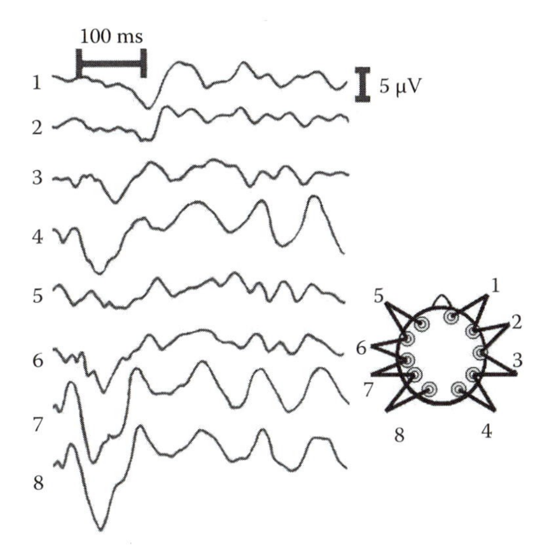

FIGURE 10.4 Representative bipolar EEG of a visual evoked response using the electrode placement from Figure 10.2.

As in other types of EPs, the existence and amplitude of the response to a certain stimulus as well as the latency in the response are often the most informative features of the recorded signals. In the experiments using flashing lights with different frequencies, the frequency spectrum of the response of the visual system is identified and analyzed. As discussed in Chapter 2, the phase of the frequency response indicates the delay (latency) of the response.

The EEG from a VEP is illustrated in Figure 10.4. As can be seen in these bipolar recordings, the signal is strongest near the section of the brain that processes visual input. The visual input is processed in the rear of the head, with the left brain processing the information of the right eye. The signals that are recorded at greater distance from the active brain are displaying lower amplitude potentials and also have a delay with respect to the main evoked response potential.

10.4.4 Event-Related Potentials

ERPs that are closely related to EPs investigate the response of the CNS to psychophysiological events. ERPs detect the EEGs resulting from a combination of various stimuli. The stimuli are designed to emulate the environment of the event to be studied, for example, sensory stimuli such as smell, electric currents, and muscle stimuli in response to the challenge reflecting the event to be studied.

While the most common stimuli for ERPs are light and visual patterns, there is a difference between typical stimuli used in EPs and ERPs. In ERPs, by arranging the stimuli according to specific archetypes, the brain is tested for its response to complicated tasks, and, simultaneously, we study the sensory perception as well as the cognitive processes of the brain. This means that in ERPs, the stimuli are often a combination of the basic stimuli in EPs to better emulate the environment in which the brain needs to be tested.

Since the stimuli are not very specific, the ERPs are extremely small in amplitude. The standard mode of operation in such situations is to perform repetitive measurements and to average the signals. Ideally, all the signals in these repeated experiments must have a similar response (in the strict theoretical sense); often in practical applications, the measured signals are stochastic signals that are in the best condition stationary processes. As discussed in the analysis of stochastic processes, averaging the actual responses would increase the signal-to-noise ratio; however, the unique response of a single stimulus may be lost. In typical analysis of EPs and ERPs, stochastic analysis is often preferred over the deterministic signal processing.

The investigation of EPs and ERPs usually focuses on establishing characteristic changes in typical signal components. These characteristic features usually receive a designation based on the polarity of the initial signal deflection, either positive or negative, in combination with the time lag in milliseconds. For instance, P300 stands for a positive peak after 300 ms. As another example, an auditory stimulus will have a typical response signal with approximately 100 ms latency compared to the applied stimulus. Such a response is typically a negative deflection and is referred to as N100, due to the 100 ms delay and the negative nature.

ERP EEG measurements are often used to investigate neurophysiologic correlation between factual knowledge, awareness, and attention. ERP measurements can also be used to identify specific components or patterns in the electromyogram (EMG) signal, which is the electric activation of muscle tissue. The EMG will be discussed later in a separate chapter.

10.5 DISEASES OF CENTRAL NERVOUS SYSTEM AND EEG

In clinical applications, EEG is commonly used to diagnose diseases in the CNS. While the cerebellum, thalamus, and spinal cord do not offer large enough signal amplitudes to make clinical observations, signals originated at the cortex are heavily used for biomedical diagnostics. A typical use of EEG, as discussed later, is the diagnosis of epilepsy. This is the application that made EEG a routine clinical test of the CNS. Some of the important diagnostic applications of the EEG are described next.

10.5.1 EPILEPSY

Epilepsy is a chronic illness identified by irregular occasions of unconsciousness, sometimes associated with violent convulsions. It is a pathological condition of a group of nerve cells firing harmoniously with a certain frequency. With the default location of the nerve cells in the cortex, this will manifest in a measurable EEG signal. It is estimated that approximately 1 out of 2000 people per year will develop some type of epilepsy. In addition, it is speculated that 1 out of every 20 people will have at least one spontaneous epileptic occurrence in their lifetime.

From the standpoint of diagnostics, it is a definite inconvenience that epileptic attacks are relativelv unpredictable. However, sometimes epilepsy can be induced under laboratory conditions. In general, epilepsy may be induced by periodic events such as flickering lights in a discotheque or while traveling down a road lined with trees, providing an alternating sun-shade sequence. In the clinical environment, a minor event may sometimes be induced by mechanical stimulus such as tapping on the arm. The frequency of epileptic EEG signals usually displays depolarization spikes at 3 Hz intervals.

Epileptic events are characterized in various forms. One method of identifying different stages of epilepsy is the discrimination between the duration of the epileptic events and the intervals between the events. The nomenclature for this designation uses the terms "petit mal" and "grand mal" from French, meaning "small bad" and "severe bad" episodes, respectively. The petit mal frequently occurs in children and is fairly brief in duration, but it may occur very frequently. During the several seconds or minutes of the petit mal attack, the patient will endure minor spasms, mostly in the face, jaw, and hands. There are not too many consequences involved with a petit mal attack. The other classification is grand mall, which results in violent convulsions and the patient will lose consciousness.

Another classification method for the types of epilepsy distinguishes general and partial seizures, nonepileptic seizures, and the most severe: status epilepticus. The general seizures are subdivided in severity as absence, atonic, tonic–clonic, and myoclonic. The absence corresponds mostly to the petit mal of the previous system of classifications and the tonic–clonic is equivalent to the grand mal seizure. Partial seizures are subdivided in simple and complex. The nonepileptic seizures will change the patient's behavior for a brief period of time and resemble the symptoms of the standard minor stages of general epileptic seizures. One main characteristic of nonepileptic seizures is that they are not generated by electric disturbances in the cortex. The status epilepticus involves sustained epileptic attacks associated with nonstop seizures and convulsions. The status epilepticus can result in death when no immediate medical attention is provided. Patients may have only one type of epilepsy or a combination of several classified stages at different times.

The characteristic feature of an epileptic assault is an abrupt onset with perfectly synchronized action potentials across all 20 electrodes. Therefore, the amplitude of high-frequency epileptic EEG is much higher than the normal delta wave. The mechanism driving an epileptic assault is still not completely understood. The EEG of an epileptic attack called a "petit mal" is illustrated in Figure 10.5. The recording uses only four bipolar measurements from the electrode placements in Figure 10.2. As is evident from the recordings of different locations in Figure 10.5, there appears to be an overall chaotic disturbance in the EEG of the entire cortex.

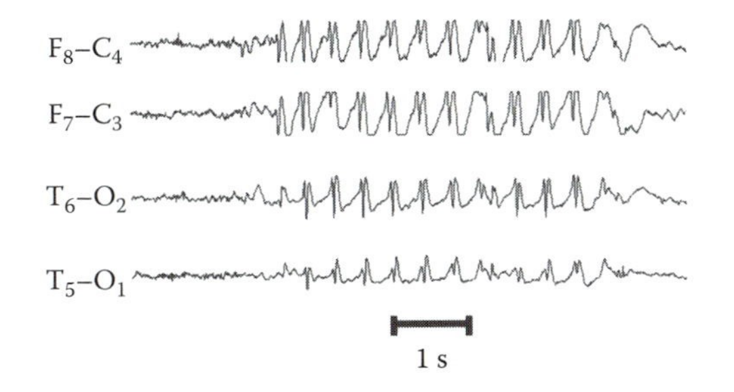

FIGURE 10.5 Epileptic recording of four bipolar measurements of a petit mal epoch from Alpo Vaerri and a research team at the Tampere University of Technology, Tampere, Finland.

The focal location of the origin of the epileptic signal is usually determined by finding the inverse solution to a so-called equivalent dipole source from the EEG recordings. The equivalent dipole source feature was described in Chapter 8. Combining the spatial distribution with the temporal information of the representative features in the EEG signal from many electrodes can usually resolve the source location with relatively high degree of accuracy.

10.5.2 Sleep Disorders

Due to the distinguished differences in frequency content of the awake and sleep EEG, the EEG recordings are heavily used in diagnosing sleep disorders. As mentioned earlier in this chapter, the EEG of a person at rest is in the low-frequency ranges, especially with the eyes closed. However, there are different stages in sleep that can be identified using EEG. The various sleep stages with the associated EEG signals are illustrated in Figure 10.6 in comparison with the EEG of a person that is solving a complex problem and thus exhibits beta waves.

Several criteria have been adopted to identify the different sleep stages. As mentioned previously, the most important stage of sleep, at least in terms of clinical use, is characterized by REM. The eye movement is controlled by muscles and the activation of the muscles in turn gives an electric depolarization signal that is stronger than the EEG. While the muscle activation signals in the EEG recordings due to the eye movement may not be perfectly filtered out, these signals will need to be identified and categorized. The electric activity associated with the muscle movement is monitored under an algorithm called the EMG. EMG is covered in Chapter 11. The combined EMG and EEG recordings can be used to score sleep stages. This is typically done by analyzing the data to obtain representative features describing the muscular and neural activities. Since the frequency range and the signal patterns of the expected eye movements are typically known beforehand, EMG and EEG can be separated on the signal processing level using typical signal processing procedures such as DFT and wavelet transform (WT).

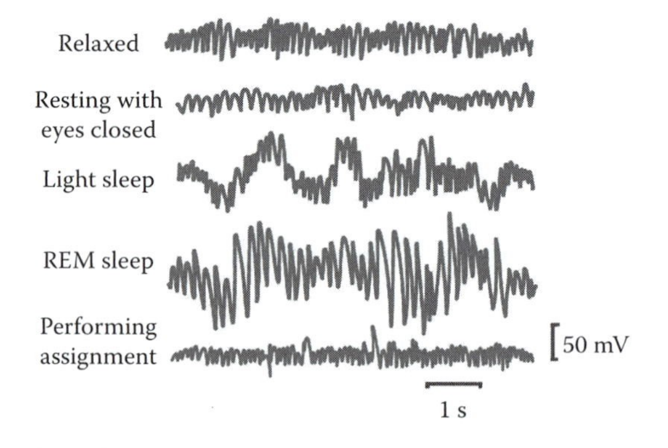

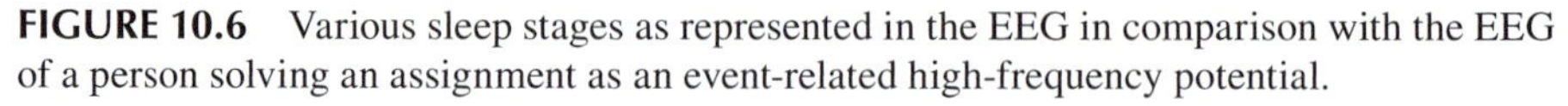

FIGURE 10.6 Various sleep stages as represented in the EEG in comparison with the EEG of a person solving an assignment as an event-related high-frequency potential.

In a typical use of the EEG for diagnostics of sleep disorder, the features captured from several hours of sleep EEG are compared to the features of standardized cases of normal and abnormal cases. The standardized data file is often called a score file. The comparison of patient feature matrices to the standard score file provides a platform for automated sleep pattern recognition. Ideally, the score system provides the tool needed for automated identification of sleep disorders.

10.5.3 Brain Tumor

The EEG can also indicate the presence of brain tumors. Both malignant and benign masses in the brain can be the cause of epileptic episodes. In most cases, the presence of a tumor will reveal a focal source in the spatial EEG recordings. The tumor can be regarded as an intermittent dipole, which can be located by reverse solution to the spatial EEG recordings. The tumor will cause the greatest disturbances closest to the tumor and will thus be identified by the electrode placement. Due to the relatively inexpensive nature of EEG recording, they are used as the initial examination of patients suspected of having a brain tumor. The next step in the detection of the brain tumor will be an MRI or a positron emission tomography (PET) session; both techniques will be covered in Chapters 15 and 17, respectively.

10.5.4 Other Diseases

Another common use of EEG is the diagnosis of meningitis. Meningitis is an infection of the membranes that surround the brain, which may sometime cause inflammation of the brain itself. Meningitis will typically result in capricious bursts of electric potentials at high frequency from randomized locations in the cortex that are reflected in the EEG. With an infection of the meninges, which surrounds the cortex, a disturbance of the depolarization of the gray matter neurons can be expected. The result is usually wave trains of 1–1.5 Hz. The meningitis provokes the cortex, but not in one place only. The infection-excited wave trains may also randomly shift in the spatial recordings.

Parkinson's disease is the process of diminishing neural activity due to the fact that nerve cells are consistently dying. This is an irreversible process in most cases, but when diagnosed in an early stage, there is medication that can slow the process down. The EEG of a Parkinson's disease patient resembles that of a toddler or a young child.

10.6 EEG FOR ASSESSMENT OF ANESTHESIA

During anesthesia, drugs are administered that are specifically aimed to depress nerve cell activity. The effects of anesthetic and analgesic drugs result in specific unusual patterns that can be observed in the EEG. Another cause for the slowing of EEG is a lowered oxygen content of the blood (hypoxia) or a lowered carbon dioxide concentration (hypocapnia). A severe increase in carbon dioxide concentration (hypercapnia) will cause a decrease in the EEG spectrum as well, while a small increase in the carbon dioxide content can result in an increase in the spectral content of the EEG.

When the normal brain pattern with standard frequency content is alternated by periods of EEG signal that have an extremely low frequency content (flat EEG), this is identified as burst suppression. Burst suppression has been linked to a diminished metabolic function of the cortical neurons. This is usually an indication of deprived oxygen supply to the brain. Additionally, in anesthesia monitoring, this burst suppression is often seen in relation to the dosage changes of various anesthetic drugs.

EEG monitoring to determine the consciousness of a patient predominantly focuses on the spectral content of the EEG. This monitoring can take place either in the operating room (OR) during or after surgery, or in the intensive care unit (ICU) for a patient that may appear to be in a coma. The existence of more significant higher frequency contents in an EEG signal generally indicates a more alert state of consciousness.

10.7 PROCESSING AND FEATURE EXTRACTION OF EEG

In order to maximize the information extracted from the EEG signal, the signals need to be analyzed and characteristic features must be revealed. Some typical methods used for processing and featuring extractions of an EEG are described next. We start this section with the description of typical noise sources for EEG signal.

10.7.1 Sources of Noise on EEG

Several features will provide signals that are much more powerful than the EEG signals, such as muscle contractions and eye movement. The eye is a large dipole and as such produces a large signal under ordinary conditions. The eyes move left to right at approximately 10 times per second to prevent saturation of the rods and cones in the retina. Both eyes move, by definition, in unison and will provide both left and right eye signals in both left and right brain. This phenomenon can be eliminated by placing the reference electrode on the nose, thus providing a signal cancellation through electronic processing. Using differential amplification, the eye movement will be expressed in all electrodes and will be rejected by the common mode rejection factor of the amplifier.

Another potential source of noise is electrode motion. Each electrode forms an electrochemical equilibrium with the skin of the head, and when the electrode is moved, the equilibrium will need to be reestablished. This type of noise is easily identified because of the magnitude of the motion artifacts but, at the same time, will require considerable time to reestablish equilibrium. This motion artifact caused by the electrodes can also be compensated for using signal processing if the range of frequency for the motion artifact is different from the measured EEG signal. For instance, since this motion often has a frequency less than a few Hz, a low-pass filter can eliminate most of the noise without affecting the high-frequency waves in the EEG.

Another frequency artifact observed in the EEG is due to the temperature-dependent nature of this signal. Generally, a slowing of the EEG activity is observed during hypothermia, when the body temperature drops below 35°C. This does not necessarily mean the patient has suffered any brain damage. This is why it is often recommended that EEG signals are taken in a room with a fixed temperature and illumination settings.

Other sources of error can be introduced by the leads acting as antennas picking up ambient alternating signals through induction. Sources include the socket power, switching of equipment, and motion by the technicians in the earth's magnetic field. An often overlooked but significant source of error is the saline drip from the intravenous line. The salt solution may cause spikes in the recordings when dripping.

The muscle contractions of the face caused by blinking, the chest motion due to respiration, and the ECG are all significant sources of fluctuating electric potential that cannot be simply ruled out and need to be filtered during the measurement of the EEG. The muscle signal artifacts are generally characterized as relatively high frequency variations.

Filtering specific frequency bands from the EEG can be used to reduce the influence of muscle activities as well as other sources of noise listed earlier. This is explained in more detail next.

10.7.2 Frequency-Domain Analysis

The use of a low-pass filter with a cutoff frequency around 12.5 Hz is necessary to ensure that the residual muscle activities do not interfere with EEGs beta activity. However, this is not desirable in most recordings, since the true beta activity and spike-type activity will also be attenuated or even obscured. In case the interference from the external source noise is persistent, some form of filtering will have to be incorporated. An adaptive digital notch filter, which allows all frequencies to pass through except for the frequencies in the narrow band of the interfering noise, is often preferred over a simple low-pass filter.

Conversely, when only a specific frequency range of the EEG requires particular interest, a band-pass filter can be applied to filter out low-frequency muscle activity and high-frequency interference from instrumentation to extract the pure EEG signal. The high-frequency components to be filter out include the power supply's frequency (50 or 60 Hz) and the high-frequency muscle activity.

A main method of EEG feature extraction in the Fourier domain is evaluation of the power of specific frequencies in the power spectra of the signal. A full frequency spectrum recorded from all over the head with 64 electrode placements during a 1 s segment is shown in Figure 10.7. As mentioned before, due to the noisy nature of the EEG, it is often preferred to treat EEG as a stochastic process, and as a result, the frequency analysis of the signal is performed using the power spectra of EEG. The frequency spectrum of the EEG signal can be easily computed by taking the DFT of the EEG correlation function. While an equipment artifact that operates in a specific frequency range may not reveal itself clearly in unprocessed EEG traces, a spectral analysis will quickly reveal any irregular pattern of higher harmonics in the frequency spectrum.

The EEG spectrum is often analyzed only over consecutive short-time segment. The short-time interval of frequency analysis is called an "epoch." The longer the selected epochs targeted for frequency transformation, the better the frequency resolution. However, there is a trade-off in taking longer time segments since they will result in a lower time resolution. The time resolution can be improved by shifting epochs forward over the chosen time segment. The best accuracy in time resolution

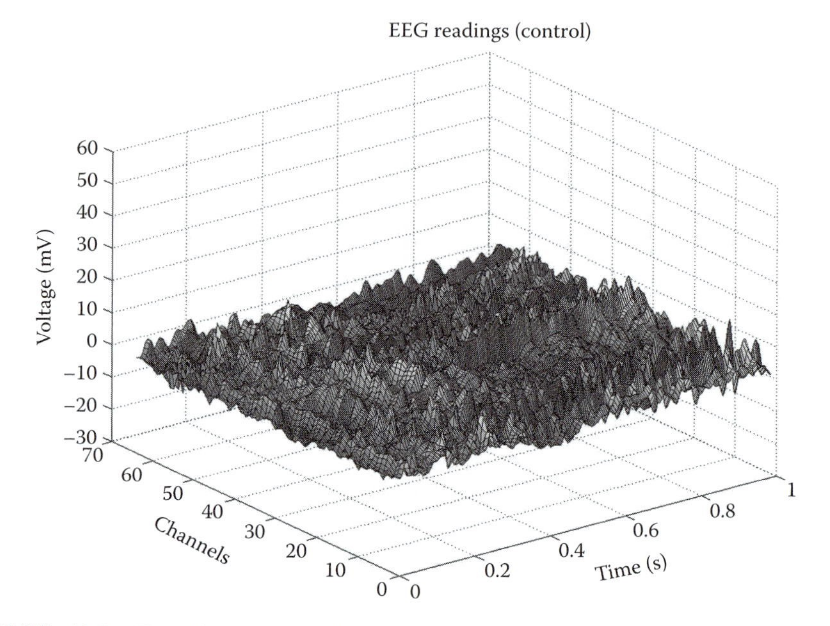

FIGURE 10.7 Two-dimensional display of a normal frequency spectrum recorded with a 64-electrode placement for an awake resting person in a 1 s interval. (Courtesy of Dr. Henri Begleiter, Neurodynamics Laboratory, State University of New York Health Center, Brooklyn, NY.)

can be obtained by using short-time shifts, in the order of 10 ms. Most benefits will be in the recognition of fast-changing signals such as epileptic seizure analysis.

The main frequency components of a typical EEG, alpha, beta, delta, and theta waves, are informative frequency components that are easily extracted from the power spectra and are heavily used in the diagnostics of EEG.

Another useful frequency measure applied in the analysis of EEG is called spectral edge frequency (SEF). This measure is of particular importance in the analysis of the depth of anesthesia. The SEF quantifies the influence of the highest frequency range in the power spectrum of EEG. The SEF identifies the relative strength of the high-frequency components in the signal and is therefore an indication of the power distribution over the frequency spectrum. The depth of anesthesia is often identified as a reduced influence of the high frequencies in EEG. This means that a reduction in SEF corresponds with a deeper level of anesthesia.

Similarly, another frequency measure is defined as the median peak frequency (MPF), which is the frequency located at 50% of the energy level. This MPF indicates the general shift in frequencies, in contrast to the SEF, which gives the overall high-frequency share. The MPF is also used in the analysis and quantification of anesthesia depth.

10.7.3 Time-Domain Analysis

Artifact detection in time domain is usually based on the empirically determined amplitude thresholds. An artifact is usually defined as the instantaneous EEG amplitude exceeding a threshold that is at least six times the average amplitude of the recording over the preceding 10 s. This criterion needs to be combined with boundary conditions of the algorithm that ensure the capture of the entire artifact.

Electric signals originating from muscles usually have a steeper slope than the average EEG signal. The use of slope threshold or steepness threshold can be used to minimize the influence of these types of muscle artifacts. The slope of a curve is found by estimating the first derivative of the signal. The first- and second-order derivatives of the slope are also used to form a complexity measure from the EEG signal. These measures are highly similar to signal complexity and signal mobility measures introduced in Part I of the book.

Other complexity measures such as fractal dimension and entropy are also heavily used as features of the EEG signal. A very important rule regarding the fractal dimension of the EEG signal indicates that the fractal dimension of EEG falls by age. This means that older people often have much smaller fractal dimensions compared to younger people. An intuitive justification of this phenomenon is based on the internal complexity of the brain. From the definition of fractal dimension, it is evident that systems with complex modular structure will provide a higher fractal dimension. More specifically, a system, where many active subsystems generate signals, will produce an overall signal that reflects the intrinsic hierarchical or modular structure in the form of a highly fractal signal. In a young brain where all parts of the brain are active, the hierarchical and modular structure is more significant. But, as the person grows older, some parts of the brain become considerably less active, which in turn reduces the complexity of the EEG signal. The same decreases in other complexity measures are recorded in EEGs of older people.

It is also reported that all complexity measures of the EEG signal and, in particular, the fractal dimension decrease in diseases such as epilepsy and Alzheimer's. This is again due to complexity reduction of the brain due to the reduction in modularity of brain activities. The reduction of almost 30% fractal dimension of EEG in epilepsy is used as a diagnostic criterion to detect epilepsy.

An efficient method of EEG analysis is designed based on the coherence of the recorded signals, as described in the following.

10.7.3.1 Coherence Analysis

Another type of EEG characterization is based on the synchronicity of any pairs of signals in the 20 channels. The measure of coherence between channels can reveal details on the efficiency of the brain functions. One common method of EEG synchronicity analysis is achieved by comparing the recordings of the electrodes in the left brain to the corresponding electrodes in the right brain. A powerful tool for this type of comparison is averaging, gated by specific stimuli such as the ERP methods, which will be covered in the following subsections.

Coherence analysis is also performed between the specific waves (frequency bands) of the EEG signals. In the description of the alpha wave spectrum, it was indicated this spectrum represents a significant level of consciousness. Since the patient is alert during both alpha and beta rhythms, especially during the beta rhythm, these wave patterns will display a certain level of coherence. In contrast, since the theta waves are generated under relaxation with little or no sensory input. These waves do not display any significant amount of coherence, as there is no common denominator driving this activity. One possible explanation of the fact that the coherence analysis of neither delta nor theta spectra reveal any useful task-related information is the fact that the wavelength of these waves is too long to be recognized with a high enough accuracy to produce the benefits of coincidental detection.

10.7.4 Wavelet-Domain Analysis

As shown in Chapter 5, wavelet techniques are typically used for the detection of known waveform patterns against a noisy background signal.

A major application of wavelet analysis is processing of EEG by detecting spike-like epileptic patterns. The detection of epileptic pattern is of particular concern because, in most suspected epileptic cases, these patterns appear at random and only for brief periods of time. Due to infrequent occurrence of these patterns, Fourier analysis can miss these patterns. In addition, since the patterns of these spikes are often known beforehand, one can design a wavelet method to not only detect the existence of such pattern but also identify the exact time of the occurrence of these abnormal patterns.

An important issue in wavelet analysis of EEG is the choice of epoch length. When analyzing a single epoch, the total number of sequences available is of direct influence on the standardized time period testing. This influence is due to the unreliable intercorrelation between adjacent sequences. Epoch lengths of 1–2 s duration are recommended for EEG processing. This duration guarantees a widespread stability in the data features. This is even more important when using low sample frequencies.

The wavelet analysis is particularly important in analysis of EPs. Wavelet analysis of EP finds the typical shape of the EP pattern by finding the largest coefficients identifying the highest correlation of decomposed signals with the pattern of applied stimuli. In other words, when a decomposed version of the signal at a certain level shows a high correlation with the stimuli pattern, the resulting waves in the decomposed signal identify a good estimation of the EP pattern.

Wavelet is also helpful in the determination of synchrony at the scalp. Specifically, the determination of the exact delay between two patterns can quantitatively identify the level of synchrony of the two waves. This decomposition is used in a number of measures of harmonization, where the measures are based on both amplitude and phase information.

Wavelet analysis can also be used for denoising and filtering of the EEG signal. Often the very low scales, i.e., high frequencies, identify the additive noise, and, by removing the low-scale components, the signal can be filtered. This was demonstrated in the chapter dedicated to wavelet analysis.

10.8 SUMMARY

In this chapter, we described the recording of nerve cell electric activity in the brain by means of a signal called EEG. EEG can be characterized by four specific frequency ranges that roughly differentiate different mental activities. Alpha waves are associated with sensory input and data processing. Higher frequencies in the beta spectrum are characteristic of problem solving and complex tasks. Lower frequencies such as delta and theta waves are prevalent in children and during rest. There are several standard ways of providing calibrated tests on the functioning of the brain. Many tests involve sensory stimuli and specific restrictive assignments to generate EPs. Typical diagnostic applications of EEG analysis are as follows: diagnosis of epilepsy, monitoring of brain activity of patients under anesthesia, analyzing sleep disorders, and initial tests for identifying suspected brain tumor.

PROBLEMS

10.1 Import the EEG signal in the file "p_10_1.xls" and plot the 10 channels.* The sampling rate was 256 samples per second with 3.9 ms period.
  a. Determine the dominant frequency of channel 0 and compare this to the dominant frequency of channel 8.
  b. In channel 0, using the power spectra of the signal, locate the motion artifacts that are characterized by a gradual change in the trend (DC offset) of the signal. This artifact is resulting from either electrode movement or muscle action.

10.2 Use the MATLAB® to read the file "p_10_2.xls" and plot the four graphs. The sampling rate of this data file is 100 Hz, and the file spans 10 s worth of data. The data are of a suspected petit mal assault in a 13-year-old patient.†
  a. Detect the spike-and-sharp-wave complexes with wavelet analysis and determine the duration of these events.
  b. Using the duration of these events, and by considering the typical frequency or duration of petit mal patterns, verify that these assaults fall in the petit mal category.

10.3 Import the data in file "p_10_3.xls" and plot the EEGs. The sampling rate of the data was 173.61 Hz. The EEG pattern of "p_10_3.xls" represents a grand mal assault.‡
  a. Determine the normal EEG frequency spectrum.
  b. Determine the onset of the epileptic EEG pattern.
  c. Plot the power spectrum of the signal.
  d. Calculate the fractal dimension, signal complexity, and signal mobility of this signal and compare it with the same values for the signal in Problem 10.4.

10.4 Import the data in file "p_10_4.xls" and plot the single EEG. This file shows tonic–clonic or grand mal assault seizures. The data were recorded with a C4 electrode on the right central portion of the scalp with the earlobe as reference.

---

* The data file "p_10_1.xls" is a portion of 64 recordings of a study by Dr. Henri Begleiter at the Neurodynamics Laboratory at the State University of New York Health Center at Brooklyn in the effects of alcoholism on the brain activity and on the EEG.

† The data file is from Alpo Vaerri and a research team at the Tampere University of Technology, Tampere, Finland.

‡ Courtesy of Ralph G. Andrzejak, Department while at the Department of Epileptology of the University of Bonn, Bonn, Germany.

The file contains a 1 min episode-free segment followed by the epileptic attack.* The total file duration spans 3 min with post-seizure activity. The sampling rate is 102.4 Hz.

a. Detect the spike-and-sharp-wave complexes with wavelet analysis and determine the duration of these events.
b. Verify that these assaults fall in the grand mal category since the duration is longer than a few seconds.
c. Locate the post-seizure activity, and determine the dominant frequency(ies) in the spectrum of the epileptic attack and the post-seizure epochs.

10.5 Import the data in file "p_10_5.xls." Each event spans 512 data points (256 prestimulation and 256 poststimulation) stored with a sampling frequency of 250 Hz. This file represents 16 trials of VEP.† All 16 trials are stored consecutively in a single column.

a. Plot the EEGs of 16 visual stimuli in 16 different graphs.
b. Identify the start of the VEP.
c. Determine the duration of each of the 16 events.

* These data were supplied by Rodri Quian Quiroga of The University of Leicester, Great Britain while at California Institute of Technology in Pasadena California.

† The data were acquired by Martin Schuermann at California Institute of Technology.

11 Electromyogram

11.1 INTRODUCTION AND OVERVIEW

Electromyogram stems from three terms: electro, which means pertaining to electric activity; myo, which has a Greek root meaning muscle; and gram, which stands for recording. Electromyography, or EMG, refers to recording of muscle's electric activities.

As mentioned in the previous chapters, every cell creates some electric activity as part of its normal functioning. This rule is also applicable to the muscle cells. Having this rule in mind, EMG can be defined as a signal that records the electric activities generated by the depolarization of muscle cells during muscle contraction, and the nerve impulses that initiate the depolarization of the muscle.

The first action potentials generated by human muscle contraction were recorded by Hans Piper in 1907, and ever since EMG has emerged as vital signal in medicine. Specifically, in today's medicine, a number of neuromuscular disorders are diagnosed using EMG. In this section, the nature of this signal, as well as the computational methods to process this signal for different medical applications, is discussed. We start this section with a brief review of muscle, its structure, and electric activities. The anatomy and physiology of the muscle provides a better insight to the origin of the EMG signal itself.

11.2 MUSCLE

Muscles provide motion in response to nerve impulses. From the system theory standpoint, the roles of muscles can be better understood when focusing on a typical neuromuscular activity such as a "reflex." The reflex loop is described as follows. An assortment of external stimuli, for example, the touch of a hot object, is received by the receptors in the body. The nervous system processes this information, either consciously or involuntarily, and issues a response to respond and react to the situation perceived. This response is transmitted to the muscles through the network of nerves. As the muscles execute the command, a mechanical motion is created to react to the stimuli. For instance, in the previous example of touching a hot object, as a result of the muscle activations, the head retracted. As can be seen from the earlier example, muscles are at the end of a reflex loop and often respond by forming a muscle contraction.

There are two main categories of muscle that can be distinguished based on their anatomy and on the particular functions they perform. The largest group of muscles is the group of skeletal muscles, which control posture, generate heat, and provide motion control. The skeletal muscles are mostly influenced by the brain in a conscious act.

The second group of muscles is the group of smooth muscles. Smooth muscles provide rhythmic motion outside the control of the brain (involuntary). The heart is entirely made of smooth muscles of different size and function. As mentioned in the previous chapter, the smooth muscle of the heart is called cardiac muscle and plays a central role in synchronization of cardiovascular activities. Smooth muscle tissue is generally found in the abdomen and in arteries. Even though smooth muscles are not controlled voluntarily, they are controlled by the autonomic nervous system. Unlike in the skeletal muscles, the depolarization wave front is not delivered to the entire smooth muscle system at once. Rather, the smooth muscle cells transmit the depolarization signal from cell to cell, to produce a wavelike contraction mechanism. The transmission between the individual cells takes place through intercalated disks, which are incorporated in the smooth muscle cell itself. This process was previously described in Chapter 10 with more details for the smooth muscles of the heart.

Regardless of the exact type of the muscle, every muscle has the following four characteristics: excitability, contractility, extensibility, and elasticity. The excitability represents the phenomenon of the effect of an external stimulus to contract. The contractility means that the muscles have the ability to contract or shorten themselves. The extensibility represents the ability of the muscles to stretch by external force and to extend their length. Finally, the elasticity signifies the fact that muscles have the ability to return to the original shape after contraction or extension.

In principle, a nerve cell provides a train of impulses delivered to a muscle or a group of muscles. These impulses depolarize muscle cell(s) and cause the muscles to contract. The frequency of the nerve impulses determines the process of muscle depolarization and muscle contraction. Due to the central role of this nervous excitation process and in order to better describe the nature of the EMG, next we will focus on the concept of a "motor unit" as part of the driving mechanism in the operation of the muscle contraction.

11.2.1 Motor Unit

Several muscle fibers are innervated by only one single motor neuron or motoneuron. The structure containing the motor neuron and its connected muscle fibers is known as the motor unit. In other words, a motor unit is composed of a single nerve fiber (neuron) and all of the muscle fibers it innervates. All the motor neurons innervated by the same nerve cell fire in concert whenever an action potential is conducted along the neuron. Each muscle is composed of a number of motor units, and each motor unit, as mentioned earlier, is driven by a neuron. Depending on the collective effects of the information coded in the nerves deriving a muscle, a particular action (e.g., contraction or relaxation) is performed by the muscle. Absence of any electric impulses will make the muscle relax.

The chemical process under which the neuron stimulates the fibers in a motor unit, illustrated in Figure 11.1, can be briefly described as follows. As can be seen in Figure 11.1, under the influence of an external action potential transmitted by a nerve cell, the axon of the nerve cell ending in a synapse releases a chemical substance called a neurotransmitter (acetylcholine: ACh) that travels the distance between the nerve cell and the muscle cell. The ACh attaches to ACh receptors

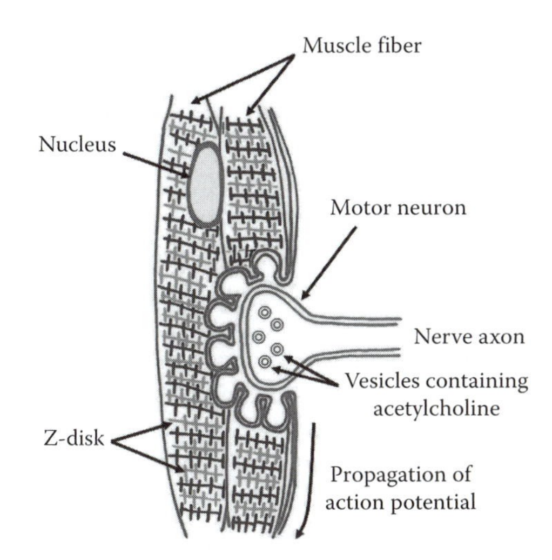

FIGURE 11.1 Motor units are composed of a nerve fiber, and the muscle fibers are innervated by this nerve fiber at the motor plate. The motor plate is a synapse junction that releases ACh in between the muscle fibers.

located on the postsynaptic membrane of the muscle cell. The area on the muscle cell that receives the neurotransmitter is called the motor end plate, a specialized section of the muscle sensitive to this ACh. The binding of the ACh to the motor end plate of the sarcolemma (the cell membrane of the muscle cell) initiates a release of sodium anions across the sarcolemma, causing the muscle cell to depolarize. The contraction mechanism will be further described later under a section dedicated to muscle contraction.

During neural activation of the muscle, each complete motor unit is either on or off, as the entire unit is driven by only one nerve cell. In this way, all muscle cells grouped together in one muscle contract together to perform work. The motor units of one muscle group may originate from different nerve cells. Motor units are interwoven with the muscle, so that various motor units will control one entire muscle made up of many muscle cells. This principle is known as redundant circuits. When one circuit fails, there is always a backup circuit to complete the task. Because the alpha neurons that innervate the motor units have their origin in the spinal cord, spinal cord injury may result in loss of motor function.

Depending on the size and level of control of the muscle, only a single motor unit may affect the area where the muscle is placed. The number of muscle fibers in a motor unit ranges from only a few to many thousands of muscle fibers. For more intricate muscle groups, such as those operating the fingers, several motor units will control one muscle group, and less information about that particular muscle function can be derived. As a rule of thumb, if a muscle is expected to perform very delicate and versatile activities, then each motor unit of the muscle is expected to initiate only a fine motion. For such muscles, the number of motor units consists of only a few muscle fibers. As example of such a muscle, we can name extraocular muscles where each motor unit consists of only five or six muscle fibers. On the other extreme, there are rather larger muscles in charge of relatively coarse motions. In these large muscles, which include the large muscle of the lower limb such as gluteus maximus, each motor unit engages approximately 2000 muscle fibers.

In order to see how contraction is performed by a muscle, we need to focus on the internal structure of a typical muscle and describe the interaction among the molecules involved in the process of contraction.

11.2.2 Muscle Contraction

A muscle is made up of several muscle cells, and every muscle cell has a larger number of muscle fibers. Each muscle fiber is made of strands of tissues, called fibrils composed of smaller strands, called filaments. As shown in Figure 11.2, the muscle structure has two types of filaments: actin and myosin. Both actin and myosin are large proteins that can be polarized. The actin and the myosin are arranged in interspaced configuration in which each actin and myosin has generally three neighbors of the opposite kind, as shown in Figure 11.2. The disk formed by an actin and its neighboring myosin is called a Z-disk.

In contrast to the nerve cells (neurons), the muscle cells depolarize by the release of calcium ions into the muscle fiber. The neural impulse transferred across the synaptic junction between the nerve and the muscle by ACh initiates a chemical mechanism that depolarizes the muscle cell. The muscle cell releases calcium ions stored in cisternae throughout the muscle cell under the influence of the depolarization. As a result, the calcium ions flow in between the fibrils. The myosin and actin filaments have macromolecular chains that are attached to the filaments on one side. These large molecules normally lay along the length of the filament, but when the filament is depolarized by the calcium ions, these molecules are repelled. When repelled, these molecules form an angle with the filaments. The heads of the actin and the myosin are of opposite polarity and attract each other, thus pulling the actin into the myosin structure.

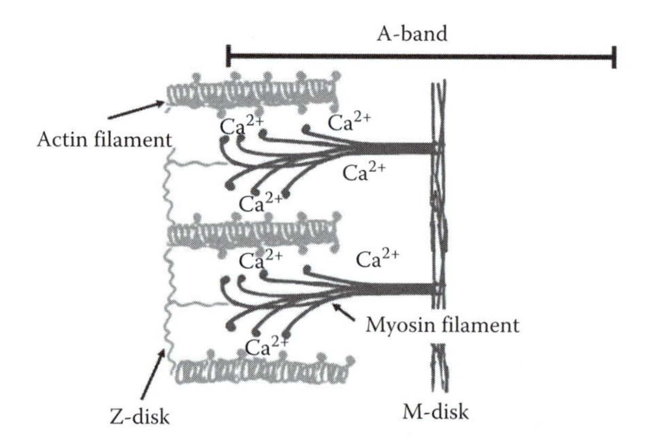

FIGURE 11.2 Actin–myosin unit used for muscle contraction.

The result of this repulsion is that the filaments come in closer proximity to each other, i.e., the chains on the actin filament attract the chains on the myosin filament, pulling the actin filaments closer to the myosin filaments, resulting in a shortening of the myofibril and therefore the entire muscle cell. After this stage, the muscle cell subsequently goes through a repolarization phase, releasing the calcium ions. The calcium release process takes only several milliseconds, after which the process can start over. This depolarization and calcium release process repeats itself many times over all sections of myofibrils within one single muscle cell, resulting in a significant shortening of the muscle cell.

The frequency of the muscle depolarization is a function of the frequency of the impulse trains in the stimulating nerve. The neuromuscular depolarization process can be described as a binary mechanism, and the higher the frequency of pulses, the stronger the contraction will be. A single muscle depolarization effect will last between 5 and 8 ms.

There are two methods of muscle contraction: isometric and isotonic. Under isometric contraction, the muscle is not allowed to shorten, while under isotonic contraction, a constant force is applied by the muscle.

In general, not all muscle cells contract simultaneously; some remain idle and take over when the contracting muscle cells relax. This operation is controlled by distribution of the firing sequence of various motor units to provide a desirable action by the muscle.

11.2.3 Muscle Force

The tension exerted by the muscle fibers is a function of the length of the overlap between the actin and myosin. The collection of two neighboring Z-disks, as shown in Figure 11.3a, is called a sarcomere. The length of the sarcomere determines the maximum force that can be applied. The force diagram illustrated in Figure 11.3b illustrates the fact that there is a maximum force that can be applied before the force start decaying with increased contraction. In point A of this diagram, the actin and myosin are virtually separated, and the muscle is completely extended. The force increases linearly with contraction to point B. At this point, the actin filaments are in close proximity to each other. In point C, the actin filaments are touching and will start repelling each other. When point D is reached, the actin filaments will overlap, and the repulsion will reduce the muscle force dramatically. Beyond point A, the molecular chains will start forming permanent chemical links.

The total force that a muscle can apply is a direct function of the number of muscle fibers. The force is approximately 30–40 N per cross-sectional area in square centimeter of muscle tissue. The amount of force is a function of the frequency of the pulse trains as well as the total duration in which the pulses appear in the stimulating neuron. This phenomenon is shown in Figure 11.4. As can be seen, after a certain period of pulse activation, the force plateaus and exhibits a saturation effect.

Knowing how muscle contracts, extends, and produces force, we are ready to discuss the formation and measurement of EMG.

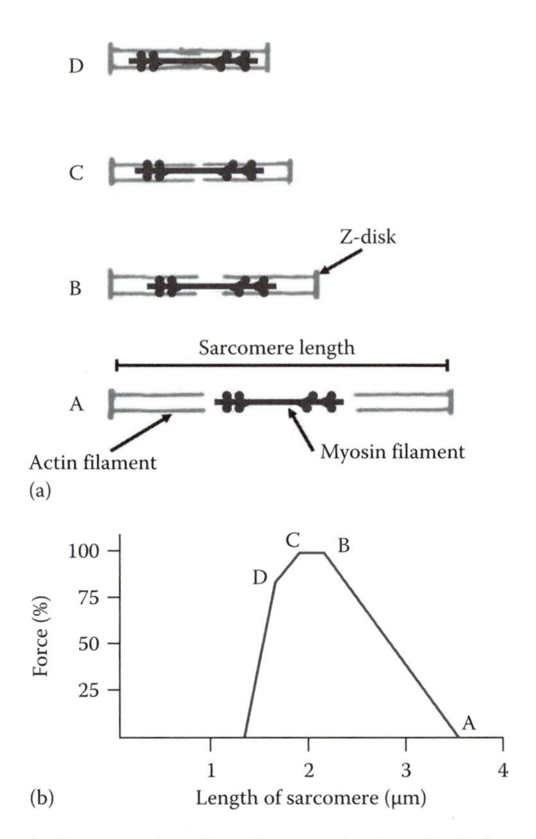

FIGURE 11.3 Muscle force as a function of contraction length. (a) State of each action; and (b) position in force-length curve.

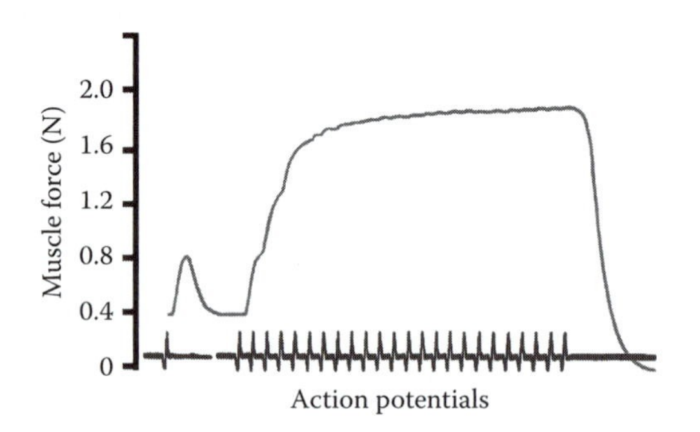

FIGURE 11.4 Diagram of contraction EMG under continuous stimulus by action potentials.

11.3 EMG: SIGNAL OF MUSCLES

There are two general methods of recording the electric activities of muscle tissue. One method applies electrodes on the skin and records a surface EMG. The second method actually inserts needles with electrodes into the muscle itself.

In most applications, what we measure as EMG is the spatially weighted sum of the electric activities of a number of motor units that are collected on the surface of the skin. In other words, a typical EMG signal is the resultant of the electric activities of many motor units that are weighted according to the amount of the fat and skin between each motor unit and the electrode as well as the distance of each motor unit from the location of the electrode. Electrodes placed on the skin surface can be used to monitor the coordination of entire muscle groups; however, not much will be known about the individual muscle cells from this. In general, this technique is used to identify which muscle groups are involved in a particular motion or action. A representative unfiltered surface EMG of the gluteus maximus is shown in Figure 11.5.

If the electric activities of a specific motor unit (or only a few motor units) are to be measured, subcutaneous concentric EMG needle electrodes are used for measurement.

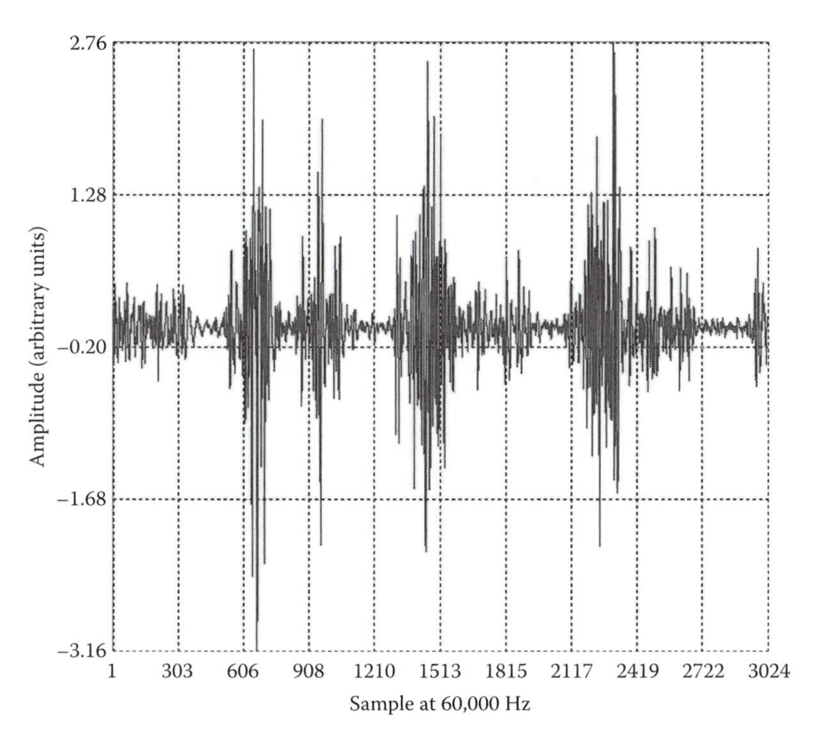

FIGURE 11.5 Raw EMG signal of the gluteus maximus. (Courtesy of Motion Lab Systems, Inc., Baton Rouge, LA; Courtesy of Edmund Cramp.)

In such EMG recordings, electrodes incorporated in very fine needles can be inserted in the muscle itself. These electrodes record the electric potential generated by the depolarization of the muscle cells directly surrounding the needle electrode. More specifically, in such neuromuscular measurements, the electric activity of a single motor unit is directly measured. When a needle has more than one electrode, bipolar measurements can be made to derive potential gradients within the muscle. Figure 11.6 illustrates the different phases of electrode placement. During needle insertion, illustrated in Figure 11.6a, there is a short burst of activity. When an axon of a nerve is touched, there may be several repetitions of bursts of activity. The transition from rest to various stages of activity shown in Figure 11.6b is characterized by the frequency of the measured potentials.

Regardless of the type of electrode used for measurement of EMG, it is important to note that the muscle potential spikes observed during muscle contraction are not true action potentials of individual cells. As described earlier, the potential of muscle excitation is mostly due to calcium ions instead of the regular sodium, potassium, and chlorine ions in a neural action potential. The measured potential on the skin or inside a muscle using needle electrodes is a triphasic potential phenomenon.

The measured amplitude of the excitation potential will be an indication of the distance between the muscle fibril and the electrode. Amplitude will diminish with the square of the distance to the source since the equipotential surface forms a

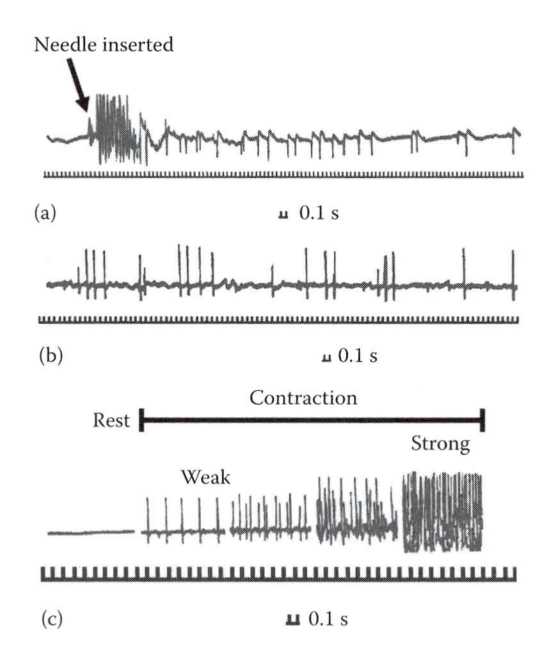

FIGURE 11.6 Illustration of the different phases of electrode placement: (a) During insertion, there is a short burst of activity; (b) when an axon of a nerve is touched, there may be several repetitions of bursts of activity; and (c) transition from rest to active in different magnitudes.

spherical geometry as it moves away from the source. Muscle potentials usually range from 2 to 6 mV and last for 5 to 8 ms.

The raw EMG (before filtering) is often considered as the most noise-like signal among almost all biomedical signals. This noise-like form makes the processing of EMG relatively different from ECG and EEG, which are described in other chapters. The specific processing methods suitable for analysis of EMG will be described later in this chapter.

11.3.1 Significance of EMG

In this section, we focus on the characteristics of muscle that can be determined by EMG. In general, two major characteristics of muscle are evaluated using EMG. These characteristics are conductivity and excitability.

In the first type of EMG analysis, the conductivity of the muscle is assessed by spatially mapping the pattern and speed of muscle conductivity. In this type of analysis, specific stimuli (e.g., weak electric or nonelectric shocks) are applied to a particular position on the muscle while the EMG at several points along the muscle is measured and analyzed. The spatial spread and timing of the spikes observed on the EMG is expected to reveal any damage to the muscle fibers.

Another typical experiment based on EMG measures the excitability of a muscle. In such experiments, typically, electric or nonelectric (e.g., mechanical) stimuli with different amplitudes are applied to a point on the muscle, and the EMG of neighboring positions is measured. The relative response of different points to different levels of stimulation is then used to analyze the excitability of the muscle at different points.

Other types of EMG experiments include identification of the muscle strength. The total force of a muscular contraction and the number of motor units activated in a muscle activity are directly reflected in the amplitude of EMG. As a result, EMG is sometimes used to measure the force exerted by a muscle. In doing so, one would need to consider factors such as the size of the muscle, the position of the muscle (i.e., distance between muscle and electrode), and the thickness of the subcutaneous fat (i.e., electric insulation between muscle and electrode).

In every one of the aforementioned EMG-based experiments, certain technical and practical issues must be considered. These issues that can affect the EMG readings include skin preparation, orientation of the electrodes with respect to the muscle fiber direction, and the exact type of electrodes used for measurements.

One particularly significant application of the EMG signal is the opportunity to operate artificial prostheses with the electric signal of other muscles still functional. This means that when a person loses an extremity and starts using an artificial prosthesis, there is a need to allow the person to initiate the commands for certain types of motion in the artificial limb. In such cases, often the EMG of some other still functional muscles is used to create the command. This is done by measuring the EMG of the healthy muscles, and based on the type of motion of the healthy muscle and therefore the shape of the EMG signal, the desirable command is detected and sent to the prosthetic limb.

Most often in prosthesis, the EMG-based command drives servomotors that are battery operated. These servomotors, for instance, control the motion of prosthetic limbs.

Using other muscles to drive prosthetic systems needs a significant period of training for the person using the system.

Knowing the overall needs to EMG signals, next we focus on the diagnostic applications of EMG.

11.4 NEUROMUSCULAR DISEASES AND EMG

The majority of muscular diseases have a neurological basis. Several neuromuscular diseases are diagnosed by processing of the EMG signal and detecting particular deviations from the normal EMG. In diagnostics using EMG, the exact deviations identify the source of the disorder. Many examples of EMG abnormalities root in factors such as disorder in the cell body of the nerve cell, disturbance in the axon of the nerve delivering the excitation, failing of the neuromuscular transmission within the motor unit, defects in the muscle cell membrane, and finally general imperfections in the entire muscle.

The partial or complete loss of EMG signal is often due to the loss of nervous excitation. The nerve cell attached to the motor unit may degrade at various locations between the spinal cord and the motor unit, thus depriving the muscle of the action potential. This in turn results in significant reduction in EMG strength or even the complete loss of this signal.

Muscular disorders will require different types of clinical attention than nervous disorders. The EMG will most likely not reveal the neurological cause of the visually observed abnormalities in the muscle function. This importance of this statement can be further realized knowing that the neurological degeneration can be as far away as the spinal cord.

Several examples of diseases related to either the neural mediation or the muscular dysfunctions are Parkinson's disease, radiculopathy, plexopathy, polyneuropathy, myopathy, and anterior horn cell disease or amyotrophic lateral sclerosis (ALS). A brief description of some of these diseases will be given when we focus on the use of EMG in diagnostics of motor neurons and motor unit–related diseases. In all aforementioned diseases, the EMG signal is frequently used to discover the different types of nerve damage and other physiological disorders involved. Next, we explore the EMG changes in such abnormalities.

11.4.1 Abnormal Enervation

When the nerve cell has effectively been destroyed, there will be no more action potentials delivered to the motor unit that enervates the muscle fibrils. Damage to the motor neuron can result from several illnesses, among which polio is an example.

When the continuity of the axon of an enervating neuron has been compromised by mechanical or physiological means, the motor unit will be denervated. The muscle is thus partially paralyzed, and, with increasing damage, more severe paralysis will occur. A denervated muscle fibril shows a particular pattern in the EMG when it starts producing spontaneous depolarizations several days after the onset of denervations. These spontaneous random depolarizations are called fibrillations, which are short fluctuations with small amplitude. Mechanically these muscle fibrils will show contraction twitches with minimal contractibility; however, the entire muscle may not be noticeably affected.

In case of muscle denervation, generally the composition of the EMG recording gets even more complicated. In the normal cases, one axon of a single neuron innervates only a single motor unit. However, when neurons leading to a motor unit die, the affected muscle fibers can be innervated by branches from adjacent stimulating neurons. The adjacent neurons form extensions on the abnormal motor unit that can typically control several dozen muscle fibers. This process is referred to as collateral enervation.

In collateral enervation, the measured EMG might be composed of the signals from several neighboring motor units. Specifically, collateral enervation affects the EMG recording in such as way that an increase in amplitude and duration of the waveform is observed. In addition the configuration of the EMG becomes more complex because one neuron is innervating more muscle fibers and the motor unit is spread out over a larger area.

11.4.2 Pathological Motor Units

Knowledge of the functions of individual motor units makes it possible to develop an understanding of some of the major pathological conditions that affect predominantly the skeletal movement.

The relatively well-known condition of muscular dystrophy includes muscle fiber degeneration and a direct interference with the contractile ability of the muscle fibers. The EMG characteristics of muscular dystrophy are recurring sequences of myotonic episodes.

One of the main disorders in peripheral motor neurons is anterior horn cell disease, or ALS. This is a disease in which the motor units are affected as a result of nerve degeneration. This affliction is also known as Lou Gehrig's disease. The ALS is known to affect about 1 in every 100,000 people. The symptoms are severe muscular atrophy associated with extreme weakness. The disease can result in death often as a result of failure in the respiratory muscles. In this case, the EMG shows spontaneous activity, aberrant discharges, abnormal recruitment, reduced interference pattern.

In a disease called radiculopathy, the nerve cells leading to the motor units are ischemic and are subjected to an inflammatory process. In this disease, the EMG reveals the signs of focal demyelination of the nerve cell (i.e., the damage or lack of myelin cover around the axon). Radiculopathy is also characterized by the excitation frequency that suddenly drops followed by an immediate increase in the depolarization frequency. Under acute severe compression of the axon of the nerve cell, the EMG shows fibrillations with 10–21 days following the injury to the nerve cell.

Plexopathy, another disease associated with the damage on the stimulating nerve, involves either the brachial or lumbosacral plexus. The visible results are decreased movement capabilities and a diminished sensation. This type of neural disease can be caused by inflammation or compression of the nerve. The EMG signals are similar to those observed in radiculopathy, combined with a different pattern in the central nervous system observed in EEG signals. This is the major difference between radiculopathy in which central nervous system is unaffected and plexopathy in which the brain waves too show some irregular patterns.

Polyneuropathy is a disorder of the peripheral nerves. The distal nerve axons are more likely to be affected than the proximal fibers. The EMG of the patients suffering from polyneuropathy shows signs of denervation of the muscle. Myopathy is a purely muscular disorder. The pathological symptoms are related to ion channel dysfunction in the motor units. One chronic disorder that may be associated with neuromuscular causes is cerebral palsy. Cerebral palsy is actually a brain disorder in the motor areas of the cerebrum.

11.4.3 Abnormal Neuromuscular Transmission in Motor Units

Certain diseases are known to cause abnormal transmission within motor units. The most known case of such abnormality is myasthenia gravis.

The pathological condition of myasthenia gravis involves a blockage of the nicotinic ACh receptors on muscle fibers, leading to paralysis. This is a chronic illness classified by abnormal rapidly occurring fatigue in the skeletal muscles. The first contraction will proceed normally, while the subsequent contractions become increasingly weaker. The EMG in this situation is characterized by omission of depolarization spikes and decreasing amplitude over time, as shown in Figure 11.7.

In Alzheimer's disease, the neurotransmitter ACh is selectively destroyed, and, thus, muscle function is impaired. Another well-known muscle-related disease is anterior poliomyelitis, which affected hundreds of thousands of children before a vaccine was developed, specifically attacking and killing motoneurons in the anterior (ventral) spinal cord. Multiple sclerosis is another relatively common disease that involves demyelination of the motor axons in the ventral roots and somatic nerves.

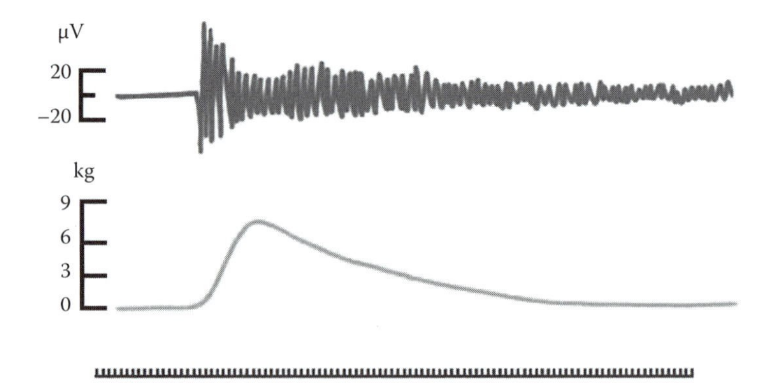

FIGURE 11.7 EMG of myasthenic muscle.

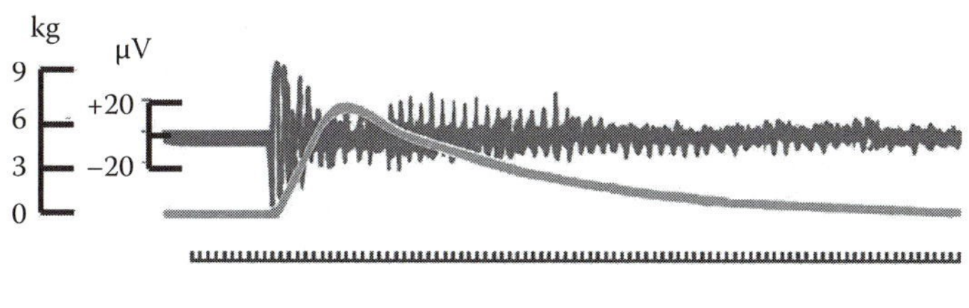

FIGURE 11.8 Rapid decay of a single depolarization excitation seen in the EMG of myotony.

Parkinson's disease may be the most well-known type of neuromuscular disease. Parkinson's disease is a disease of the motor unit in which the regulation of an important neurotransmitter, called dopamine, is severely disturbed. Parkinson's disease is often identified by the muscle tremors, especially visible continuous shaking of the hands. Other symptoms include the loss of the ability to move fast, the rigidity of muscles, and the loss of muscular reflexes that maintain posture.

11.4.4 Defects in Muscle Cell Membrane

Defects in the muscle cell membrane are the result of genetic influences. This type of muscle damage is called myotony. The contraindications are that the muscle cannot relax and the contraction lasts substantially longer than for a healthy muscle. An example of an EMG of a myotone muscle is presented in Figure 11.8. The deeper laying cause of the malfunction may be related to a malfunctioning ACh metabolism in the cell membrane.

General imperfections of the muscle tissue are classified as muscular dystrophy. In such diseases, the muscle fibers themselves degenerate over time, resulting in a total lack of EMG signal. These diseases often show gradual decrease of the EMG strengths through a few weeks or even a few months.

11.5 OTHER APPLICATIONS OF EMG

We discussed some of the main applications of EMG in medical diagnostics. This signal is used in several other applications. Some of other applications of EMG are discussed later.

Muscles undergoing fatigue portray visible changes in their EMG. These changes include reduction in EMG amplitude, reduction in EMG power, and reduction in the power of high-frequency contents of EMG derived. Generally muscle fatigue is expressed as a reduction in the higher-frequency content with a shift in power to the lower frequencies. Trials on muscle fatigue are usually performed under isometric muscle action for reproducibility purposes. All these changes can be accurately measured with signal processing techniques. For instance, a high-pass filter captures the fast variations, and the power of these components is used to evaluate muscle fatigue.

The timing of the depolarization spikes in EMG signal in reference to the neural impulses is used to identify the conduction and time response of muscles, as discussed earlier. Signal processing can be used to detect these peaks and measure the time distance among these peaks. The information obtained from event timing studies will identify muscle conduction and general muscle health issues.

The force generated by a muscle directly affects the amplitude and frequency of the EMG signal. Just like in measuring fatigue, different signal processing measures, especially the root-mean-square (RMS) value, can be used to quantitatively measure the muscle activity for such studies.

The ratio between muscle force and muscle contraction is an important measure in evaluating the muscle condition and is often referred to as muscle's mechanical resistance. In calculating resistance, while muscle contraction is often measured by direct measurement of the length of the muscle, muscle force is sometimes replaced by the power of EMG as a more quantitative measure of force.

In surgery, where local anesthesia has to be performed, the anesthesiologist needs to have a measure of how deep the local anesthesia is. The muscular response to electric stimuli can help determine the level and depth of anesthesia and identify the need to administer additional anesthetic drugs. In many cases, anesthesiologists use the power of EEG (windowed over a period of at least several minutes) as the indicator of anesthetic efficacy.

Under certain conditions, the EMG of the contractions during childbirth is used as a feedback mechanism to help the mother concentrate on the contractions. In this case, the EMG is converted into an audible signal to make the onset of the contraction more noticeable.

11.6 PROCESSING AND FEATURE EXTRACTION OF EMG

After discussing the origin of the EMG signal and its applications in biomedical diagnostics, next we focus on the typical processing methods applied for filtering and analysis of EMG.

11.6.1 Sources of Noise on EMG

In order to achieve two-way motion, for example, extending and flexing an arm, a minimum of two muscle groups will be needed. Every skeletal muscle has an antagonist to stretch the contracted muscle after relaxation. Since each muscle can only perform a one-way motion, it receives and generates only a binary signal, which can be either on (i.e., contraction) or off (i.e., no contraction).

This agonist–antagonist principle is essentially the main source of cross talk and noise in EMG, as it is almost always difficult to record the surface EMG of the agonist muscle without recording some of the electric activities of the antagonist muscle. More specifically, due to the low resistance of the body around muscle cells, the surface electrodes will detect action potentials of several muscle groups including the antagonist muscles simultaneously.

This cross-talk effect can be avoided, at least to some extent, by filtering the recorded signals and applying threshold detection to eliminate the signals from distant muscle groups. Other sources of noise on the surface EMG are ECG and breathing signals. These noise sources can be rather successfully filtered using band-pass filters centered around the main frequency spectrum of the EMG signal.

A major source of noise in EMG is the motion artifact. This noise is caused by unwanted motion of electrodes, wires, and muscles. However, since the frequency range of the motion artifact is between 0 and 20 Hz, this source of noise can be easily filtered using a low-pass filter, as discussed next. Before explaining the filtering methods, however, it is insightful to note a significant difference between EMG and other signals that affects the acquisition and therefore the noise susceptibility of EMG. A major difference between EMG and other biomedical signals such as the EEG and ECG is the fact that EMG does not use a single reference electrode while the other two do. The single reference electrode is not a feasible option since each muscle that is investigated can be in any part of the body of the subject under investigation. For the heart and the brain, this is not a serious concern since the ECG and EEG are recorded in the same anatomical location every single time. The differential nature of EMG acquisition helps reducing the noise during the acquisition step and therefore simplifying the filtering step in the signal processing level, discussed next.

11.6.2 Time-Domain Analysis

For the signal processing, as with other signals mentioned in the previous chapters, there is a standard set of features that can be used to investigate and compare the clinical significance of the image. The features of interest in 1-D muscle signal image processing are the power distribution of signal in specified frequency ranges, wavelet coefficients at different scales, complexity, and mobility, and additionally fractal dimensions are always informative features for any kind of biomedical signal. However, some specific features are more frequently used for the analysis of EMG signals than for other signals. These tools are RMS analysis and average rectified (AVR), as introduced next.

Since EMG is the signal for several muscle cells combined, averaging can reveal commonalities that will get lost in the collective signals. The energy of the EMG signal, as a common denominator, can provide the clinical relevance of the muscle group as a whole. Assuming that the EMG signal is expressed as the discrete signal x, the RMS measure is defined as

$$\text{RMS} = \sqrt{\frac{\sum_{i=0}^{N-1} x^2(i)}{N}} \quad (11.1)$$

The RMS value, which describes the average level of second-order variations in the signal, is often used to express the power of the EMG signal. The power of the signal can define muscle fatigue, evaluate the strength the force generated by the muscle contraction, and assess the ability of a muscle to handle mechanical resistance.

While the second-order power, which constitutes the core idea of RMS, is a useful measure in energy evaluation, first-order deviations of EMG are also used to assess this signal. Representing the EMG signal as x, another important feature called the AVR value measure is defined as

$$\mathrm{AVR} = \frac{\sum_{i=0}^{N-1} |x(i)|}{N} \tag{11.2}$$

AVR describes the average of absolute variations in the signal and is often used to express the smoothness, or respectively the nonsmoothness, of the signal.

11.6.3 Frequency- and Wavelet-Domain Analysis

A typical frequency spectrum of EMG is shown in Figure 11.9. As can be seen, the typical frequency range of the EMG signal is between 50 and 500 Hz. Analyzing the frequency spectrum shows that the maximum energy of the EMG is between 70 and 300 Hz.

The frequency range shown in Figure 11.9 also tells us that the best type of filter to separate typical EMG from the noise is a band-pass filter with the passband of 20–500 Hz. Even though the frequency range of most EMG signals is limited on the upper side by 500 Hz, some EMG tests with muscles under loads connected to them can register frequencies much higher than the range seen in the typical EMG signal.

One fundamental concept of EMG analysis is the acquisition of the frequency features from the power spectrum. During the initial contraction, the frequency spectrum

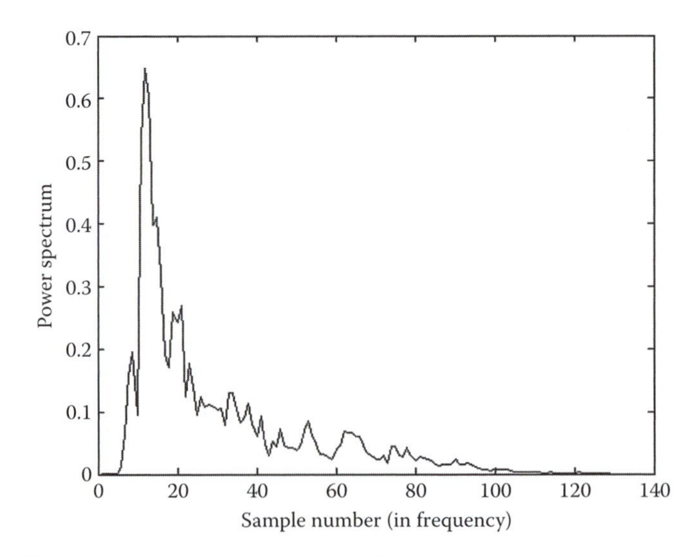

FIGURE 11.9 Typical frequency spectrum of EMG of muscle applying stress. (Courtesy of Motion Lab Systems, Inc., Baton Rouge, LA; Courtesy of Edmund Cramp.)

is mostly in the higher frequencies, while, after fatigue, the power spectrum shifts toward lower frequencies. The shift in the dominant frequencies in each of the states, rest and contraction, is an indication of the muscle status.

The use of wavelet analysis of EMG signals shows advantages in the detection of changes in the wave patterns during stimulated recordings. For instance, isometric contraction is controlled by the patient and can be performed in various modes. Rapid contraction will have a different EMG pattern than slow initiation of the contraction.

Wavelet analysis is also applied to detect the presence or absence of some expected patterns in healthy and abnormal cases. Wavelet analysis is also used to decompose the signal and detect the delays in response to the stimulations. Specifically, detection of the delays in the response times of motor units using wavelet and STFT can help identify the state, size, and of the density of the motor units involved in the neuromuscular task. Large motor units are generally faster in response compared to the smaller motor units. Daubechies wavelets have been shown useful; however, other wavelets can reveal details in different aspects of the signal structure and elaborate on the muscle recruitment process.

11.7 SUMMARY

In this chapter, we first described the origin of electromyogram (EMG) and the way this signal is formed and measured. Then we briefly reviewed the applications of EMG in diagnostics of several neuromuscular diseases. Finally, we reviewed the main time-, frequency-, and wavelet-domain methods for filtering, feature extraction, and analysis of EMG.

ACKNOWLEDGMENT

The source of all EMG signals used in this chapter is Motion Lab Systems, Inc., Baton Rouge, LA; Courtesy: Edmund Cramp.

PROBLEMS*

11.1 Import the data in the file "p_11_1.txt" in MATLAB® and plot the signal. In order to do so, use File/Import Data ... on the main MATLAB menu and follow the steps in loading and naming of the data. The file contains one single muscle signal from a 40 month old patient; the first column is the time, and the second column is the data.

a. Determine the frequency spectrum or power spectrum.
b. Using "wavemenu" and Daubechies 1 mother wavelet, denoise the signal and locate significant features of the EMG signal.
c. Calculate the AVR value of the EMG signal.

* Problems 11.1 through 11.5 use data obtained from http://www.physionet.org/physiobank/database/gait-maturation-db/

11.2 Import the data in the file "p_11_2.mat" in MATLAB and plot the signal. In order to do so, use File/Import Data ... on the main MATLAB menu and follow the steps in loading and naming of the data. The file contains one single muscle signal from a 61 month old patient; the first column is the time, and the second column is the data.

   a. Repeat the calculations in parts a, b, and c of Problem 11.1.
   b. Compare a single period with one period of the signal in Problem 11.1 and comment on the differences.
   c. Analyze the shift in the frequency spectrum to lower frequencies compared to Problem 11.1.

11.3 Import the data in the file "p_11_3.txt" in MATLAB and plot the signal. In order to do so, use File/Import Data ... on the main MATLAB menu and follow the steps in loading and naming of the data. The file contains one single muscle signal from an 80 month old patient; the first column is the time, and the second column is the data.*

   a. Repeat the calculations in parts a, b, and c of Problem 11.1 on the EMG recordings.
   b. Using "wavemenu" and Daubechies 1 mother wavelet, decompose the signal into five levels. Comment on the contents of each decomposition level.
   c. Repeat part b using Daubechies 2 mother wavelet.
   d. Compare a single period from the EMG data file from this problem with one period of the EMG signal in Problem 11.1 and comment on the differences.

11.4 Import the data in the file "p_11_4.mat" in MATLAB and plot the signal. In order to do so, use File/Import Data ... on the main MATLAB menu and follow the steps in loading and naming of the data. The file contains one single muscle signal from a 130 month old patient; the first column is the time, and the second column is the data.

   a. Repeat the calculations in parts a, b, and c of Problem 11.1 on the EMG recordings.
   b. Using "wavemenu" and Daubechies 1 mother wavelet, decompose the signal into five levels. Comment on the contents of each decomposition level.
   c. Compare a single period with one period of the signal in Problem 11.3 and comment on the differences.

11.5 Import the data in the file "p_11_5.txt" in MATLAB and plot the signal. In order to do so, use File/Import Data ... on the main MATLAB menu and follow the steps in loading and naming of the data. The file contains one single muscle signal from a 163 month old patient; the first column is the time, and the second column is the data.

   a. Repeat the calculations in parts a, b, and c of Problem 11.1.
   b. Using "wavemenu" and Daubechies 1 mother wavelet, decompose the signal into five levels. Comment on the contents of each decomposition level.
   c. Repeat part b using Daubechies 2 mother wavelet.
   d. Identify the onset of contraction in EMG.

---

* Courtesy of http://www.physionet.org/physiobank/database/gait-maturation-db/

e. Compare the frequency content of before and during contraction.

11.6 Import the data in the file “p_11_6.csv” and plot the signal.* In order to do so, use File/Import Data … on the main MATLAB menu and follow the steps in loading and naming of the data. The file contains the signals of a two-electrode EMG recording of 10 different muscle groups of a person standing erect and at rest. The scanning rate was 60,000 Hz.

a. Repeat the calculations in parts a, b, and c of Problem 11.1 on the recording EMG1, the adductor: EMG6, and the tibia anterior: EMG7.
b. Using “wavemenu” and Daubechies 1 mother wavelet, decompose the signal into five levels. Comment on the contents of each decomposition level.
c. Repeat part b using Daubechies 2 mother wavelet.
d. Identify the onset of contraction in EMG6 and EMG7.
e. Compare the frequency content of both EMG6 and EMG7 before and during contraction.

11.7 Import the data in the file “p_11_6.csv” and plot the signal.* In order to do so, use File/Import Data … on the main MATLAB menu and follow the steps in loading and naming of the data. The file contains the signals of a two-electrode EMG recording of the gluteus maximus. The scanning rate was 60,000 Hz.

a. Repeat the calculations in parts a, b, and c of Problem 11.1 on the recording EMG2, EMG3, and EMG4.
b. Using “wavemenu” and Daubechies 1 mother wavelet, decompose the signal into five levels. Comment on the contents of each decomposition level.
c. Repeat part b using Daubechies 2 mother wavelet.
d. Identify the onset of contraction in EMG3 and EMG4.
e. Compare the frequency content of both EMG3 and EMG4 before and during contraction.

* Courtesy of Edmund Cramp, Motion Lab Systems, Inc., Baton Rouge, LA. http://www.motion-labs.com

12 Other Biomedical Signals

12.1 INTRODUCTION AND OVERVIEW

Besides the main biomedical signals introduced in the previous chapter, there are some other signals captured from other biomedical system that are used for medical diagnostics. In this chapter, we briefly introduce some of these signals and discuss their applications in medicine.

12.2 BLOOD PRESSURE AND BLOOD FLOW

In our description of an electrocardiogram (ECG), we reviewed the functions of the cardiovascular system. Blood pressure is one of the vital signals used to detect a wide range of abnormalities. In typical measurements of the blood pressure, many clinical processes are limited to measurement of only systolic and diastolic pressures (as opposed to the entire signal). However, when the entire blood pressure signal is collected, much more information can be extracted from the data.

Typical measurements of blood pressure signal can be categorized as extravascular and intravascular measurements. The typical measurement of blood pressure, which is often limited to measurement of systolic and diastolic pressure, is the popular sphygmomanometer and stethoscope system, which is considered as the gold standard of extravascular blood pressure measurement systems. On the other hand, the intravascular measurement of blood pressure signal is often conducted using arterial catheter placement. The catheter placement is often used to measure the entire blood pressure signal as opposed to recording only the high and low peaks in the sphygmomanometer and stethoscope system.

A typical blood pressure signal over two pulses is shown in Figure 12.1. As can be seen in the figure, this stochastic but periodic signal can be readily analyzed using Fourier techniques. In practical applications, after decomposition using Fourier transform or FT (or more precisely discrete Fourier transform or DFT), the amplitude of the FT (or the poser spectrum in stochastic analysis of the signal) in six frequencies are calculated and analyzed. These six frequencies are the pulse rate, f_0; its second harmonic, $2f_0$; the third harmonic, $3f_0$; the forth harmonic, $4f_0$; the fifth harmonic, $5f_0$; and finally the sixth harmonic, $6f_0$. The reason for the popularity of these frequencies is the fact that most of the energy of the blood pressure signal is contained in these harmonics. Moreover, the relative strength or weakness of these harmonics is often associated with certain abnormalities. The preceding discussion explains why Fourier analysis is often used for processing and analysis of blood pressure signal.

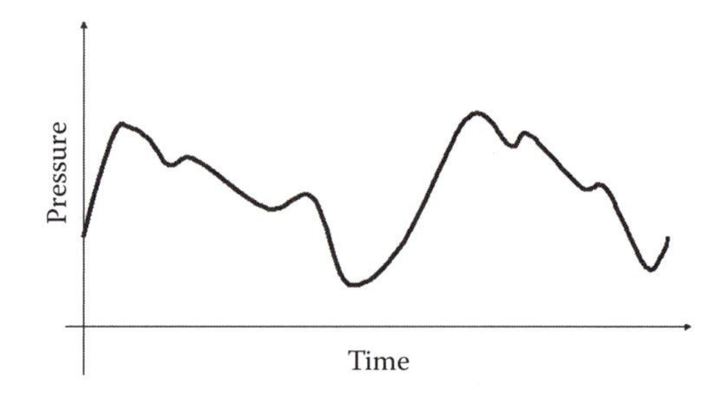

FIGURE 12.1 Typical blood pressure signal.

Blood pressure is so commonly used in clinical diagnostics that it is difficult to point out to the main applications. However, it is widely believed that almost all cardiovascular diseases somehow alter the blood pressure signals, and, therefore, the blood pressure signal can be used for detection of such abnormalities. In addition, most of the other diseases not directly related to the heart are also detected or diagnosed at least partially using the blood pressure. For instance, a number of chronic headaches are often associated with high blood pressure. Moreover, blood pressure signal is one of the best signals to detect some less severe types of internal bleedings.

Blood flow signal is greatly related to blood pressure. In the measurement of the blood flow, one needs to know the speed of the blood at a certain point. There are many techniques to detect this quantity. Indicator dilution method is one of these methods in which an agent is injected into the blood, and then the concentration of the agent is measured in time. The faster the dilution of the agent occurs, the more the blood flow is. In other words, the dilution of the agent is measured, and based on that the blood flow is estimated. The recording of dilution constitutes a signal that can be processed using signal processing techniques. Another similar method for the measurement of the blood flow is based on the measurement of thermal dilution. In this method, the temperature of an added agent (often saline) through time is monitored to estimate the blood flow. There are other methods of measuring the blood flow including the ultrasonic method, electromagnetic flow, and the Fick technique. The changes in the blood flow in a tissue through time have been used to analyze the condition of the tissue.

12.3 ELECTROOCULOGRAM

Electrooculogram, or EOG, is a signal that is measured on the skin around the eyes. EOG is often used to measure the gaze angle and assess the dynamics of the eye motion. The electrodes are placed on the sides of the eyes for measuring the horizontal motions of the eyes (Figure 12.2) and above and below the eyes when the vertical elements of the motion and gazing are studied and assessed (Figure 12.3). In each case, differential amplifiers are used to detect any potential difference between each pair of electrodes caused by the motion of the eye. More specifically, this potential difference is the result of a dipole (i.e., eye ball) changing the potential balance

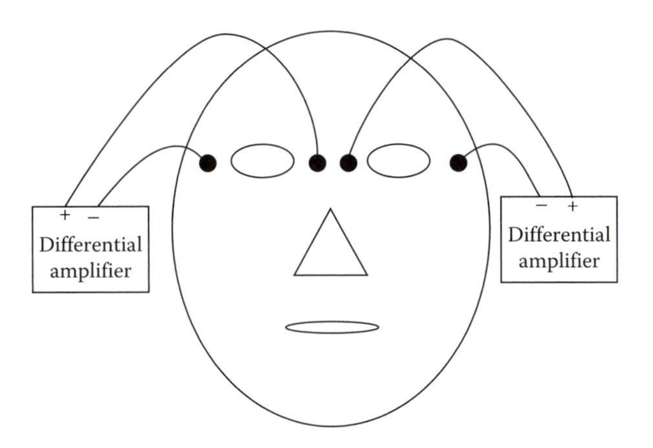

FIGURE 12.2 Detecting horizontal motion of the eyes using EOG.

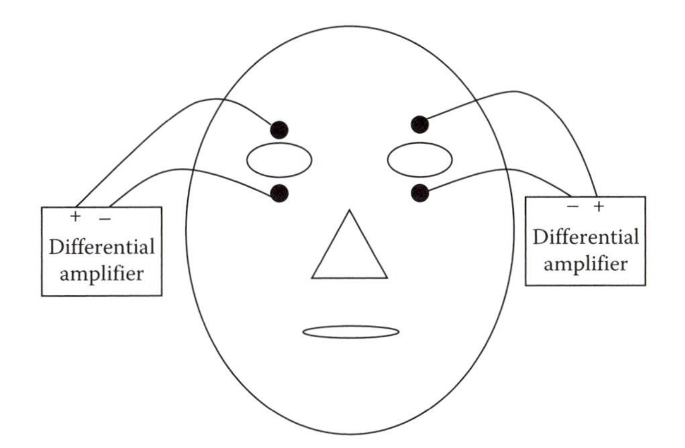

FIGURE 12.3 Detecting vertical motion of the eyes using EOG.

between the two points where measurements are taken. This potential is primarily generated between cornea and retina (i.e., corneoretinal potential) and is often between 0.4 and 1.0 mV. EOG is, as previously mentioned, a weaker version of this potential measured on the surface of skin and often has the amplitude of a few microvolts up to tens of microvolts.

There are more complete measurements of EOG that simply use more electrodes and capture both horizontal and vertical motion and gazing for both eyes.

The EOG signal, being the result of the eye motion, is often in the frequency interval 0–100 Hz. The frequency range of EOG is identified by the mechanical limitations of the eye motion. It is often required that the 60 Hz noise (due to power supply) be removed to have a more reliable EOG reading.

The main clinical application of EOG is detection and assessment of degenerative muscular disorders. Laziness of the eyes in tracking moving objects, detected by analysis of EOG, is an efficient way of assessing such disorders. In a typical experiment, the moving object on a monitor is shown to the patient and as the patient tracks the object with his or her eyes, the EOG is captured and analyzed. The lag between the moves of the cursor and the electric activities captured by EOG provides the metric needed for diagnostics.

Another major application of EOG is helping severely paralyzed patients. It is estimated that number of patients in the United States whose spinal injuries have paralyzed them from neck down is about 150,000. EOG provides these patients the means to communicate with their caretakers and computers. In order to do so, a large board is placed in front of the patient that is divided to an array of command. For instance, a place on the board is marked as "copy" and another part as "paste." By analyzing the EOG, a computer identifies the gaze angle and based on that identifies the command the patient is trying to execute. Similar systems have been successfully used for navigation of aircrafts and boats.

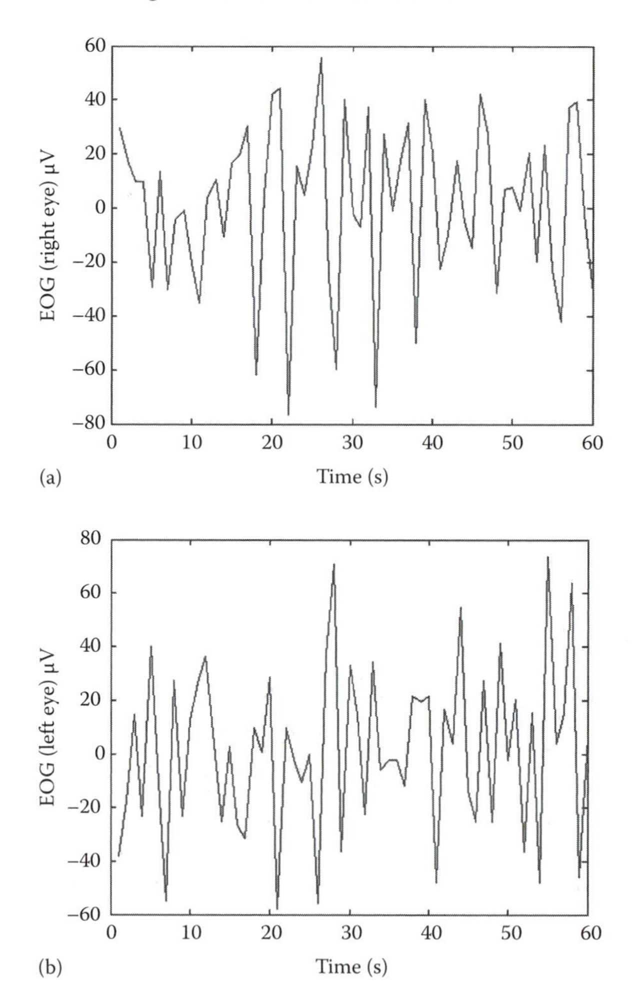

FIGURE 12.4 (a) Right and (b) left EOGs sampled at 50 Hz. (From Goldberger, A.L. et al., *Circulation*, 101, 23, e215, June 13, 2000, Circulation Electronic Pages; http://circ.ahajournals.org/cgi/content/full/101/23/e215).

The main processing techniques applicable to EOG are FT and wavelet transform (WT). Certain domain-related features are also calculated from EOG. For example, the difference between the timing of the cursor move and the eye response can be calculated simply based on the direct measurement of the time difference between the rising edges of the two signals.

The long recordings of EOG are also used for the study of sleep. Figure 12.4 shows the recordings of the right and left EOGs, sampled at 50 Hz during a sleep study in which a number of physiological signals during sleep are recorded and correlated.

A very closely related signal called "electroretinogram" or ERG has been used for very similar applications. This signal that is the potential difference among the retina and the surface of the eyeball is known to be highly correlated with EOG, and, as a result, EOG is often used in many applications to represent ERG.

12.4 MAGNETOENCEPHALOGRAM

The signal known as "magnetoencephalogram," or MEG, is essentially the magnetic equivalent of EEG. In other words, while EEG captures the activities of the brain neurons through detection of the changes in the electric activities on the surface of the head, MEG measures the changes in the magnetic field caused by the activities of the brain neurons. From electromagnetics, we know that any changing electric field causes a magnetic field that is proportionally related to the electric field. As a result, the changes in the electric charges of the neurons create a magnetic field that can be measured to detect the activities of the brain. MEG measures the extracranial magnetic fields produced by intraneuronal ionic current flow within appropriately oriented cortical pyramidal cells.

At this point, we need to address the following question: "If MEG captures almost the same information as EOG, why do we need MEG at all?" The question becomes more relevant if we consider the fact that the instrumentation needed to measure MEG is significantly more complex and expensive than that of EEG. It seems that since we can capture the same information using much less expensive EEG machines, there would be no need for MEG. The answer to this question is twofold. First, EEG is captures on the surface of the skull and therefore is suitable to many sources of noise such as the electric activities of the muscles close to electrodes. The lack of skin contact facilitates using MEG to record DC and very-high-frequency (>600 Hz) brain activity.

In addition, the MEG is capable of detecting the electric activities of the neurons deeper in the brain, as opposed to the EEG signals that are often due to the neurons closer to the surface of the brain. More specifically, MEG has selective sensitivity to tangential currents (from fissural cortex) and less distorted signals compared with EEG. This allows MEG to provide much better spatial and temporal accuracy. A major advantage of MEG is determining the location and timing of cortical generators for event-related responses and spontaneous brain oscillations. MEG provides a spatial accuracy of a few millimeters under optimal conditions, combined with an accurate submillisecond temporal resolution, which together enable spatiotemporal tracking of distributed neural activities, for example, during cognitive tasks or epileptic discharges.

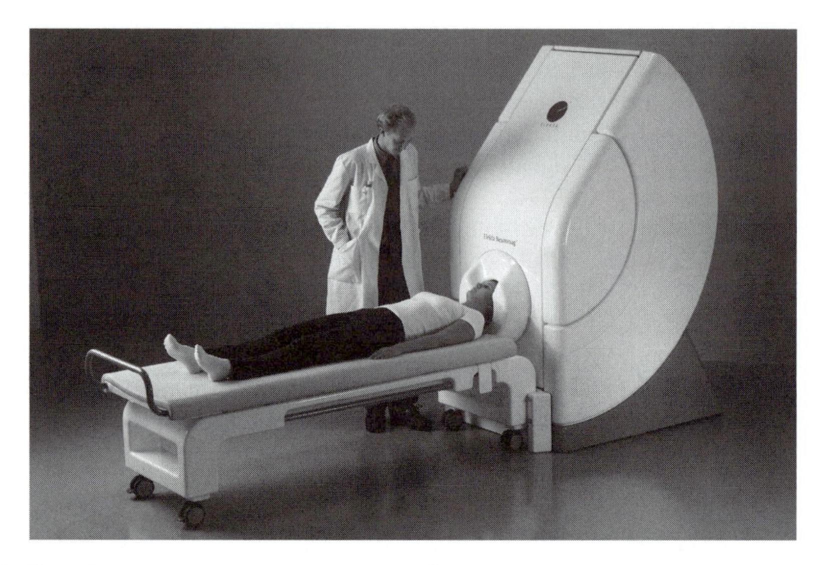

FIGURE 12.5 MEG machine with large SQUID. (Image courtesy of Elekta.)

A typical MEG machine is shown in Figure 12.5. As can be seen, the machine utilizes large superconducting quantum interference devices (SQUIDs) as a sensor of weak magnetic fields. MEG signals have a typical strength of a few pT (picotesla) and SQUID sensors can capture both natural and evoked physiological responses observed in MEG.

The main source of interference in MEG measurements is the magnetic field of the Earth. This source of noise is systematically filtered in the MEG machines. Due to the resemblance of MEG and EEG, the same processing techniques used for EEG are also applied for analysis of MEG.

MEG studies in psychiatric disorders have contributed materially to improved understanding of anomalous brain lateralization in the psychoses, have suggested that P50 abnormalities may reflect altered gamma band activity, and have provided evidence of hemisphere-specific abnormalities of short-term auditory memory function. The clinical utility of MEG includes presurgical mapping of sensory cortical areas, localization of epileptiform abnormalities, and localization of areas of brain hypoperfusion in stroke patients. In pediatric applications, MEG is used for planning of epilepsy surgery and also provides unlimited possibilities to study the brain functions of healthy and developmentally deviant children.

12.5 RESPIRATORY SIGNALS

A group of respiratory signals are commonly applied for clinical assessment of the respirator systems. A group of such signals capture both the timing and breadth of the respiration. For instance, motion sensors placed on the chest can capture the respiration timing and volume. It is also common to measure thoracic and abdominal excursions for the diagnostics of respiratory system. A sample of typical recordings of thoracic and abdominal excursions measured by inductive plethysmography bands is shown in Figure 12.6.

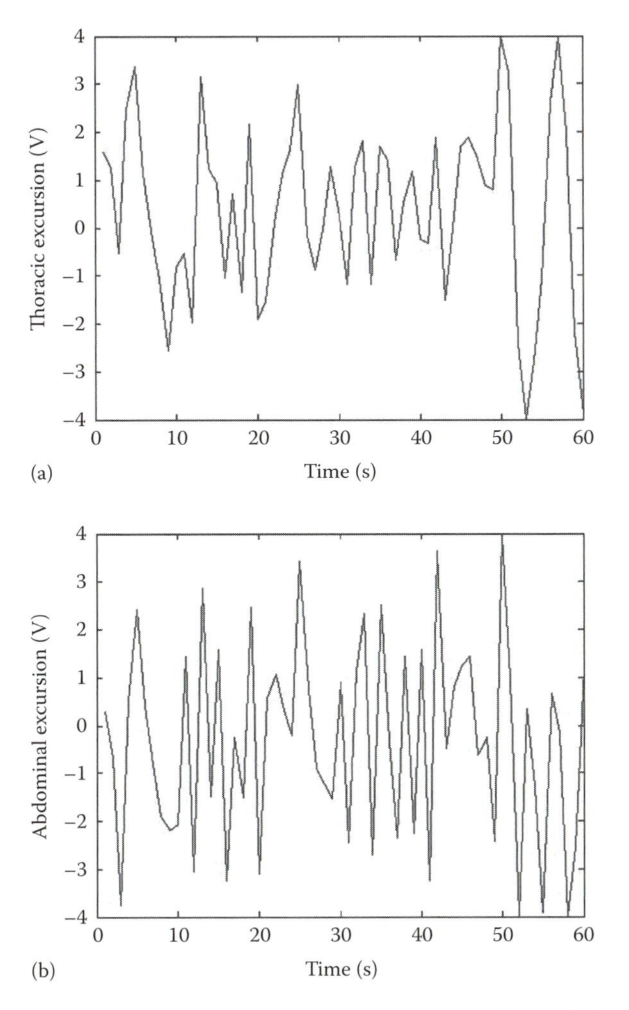

FIGURE 12.6 (a) Thoracic and (b) abdominal excursion signals sampled at 50 Hz. (From Goldberger, A.L. et al., *Circulation*, 101, 23, e215, June 13, 2000, Circulation Electronic Pages; http://circ.ahajournals.org/cgi/content/full/101/23/e215).

There are also other signals that detect the gas flow and strength of the exhaled gas to detect the depth of breathing. A popular signal measured during many clinical monitoring is the airflow signal detected by a nasal–oral thermocouple. This signal is an indication of the mechanical strength of the respiratory system. The signal is sometimes used to monitor the patient's respiration during sleep. A typical airflow signal measured during sleep is shown in Figure 12.7.

Another category of respiratory signals expresses the chemical contents of the exhaled gas. The most important signal in this category is the partial pressure of CO_2 in the exhaled gas. This signal is measured using a specialized light emitting diode whose illumination depends on the CO_2 contents of a volume of gas. This signal is applied to assess the quality of gas exchange in alveoli.

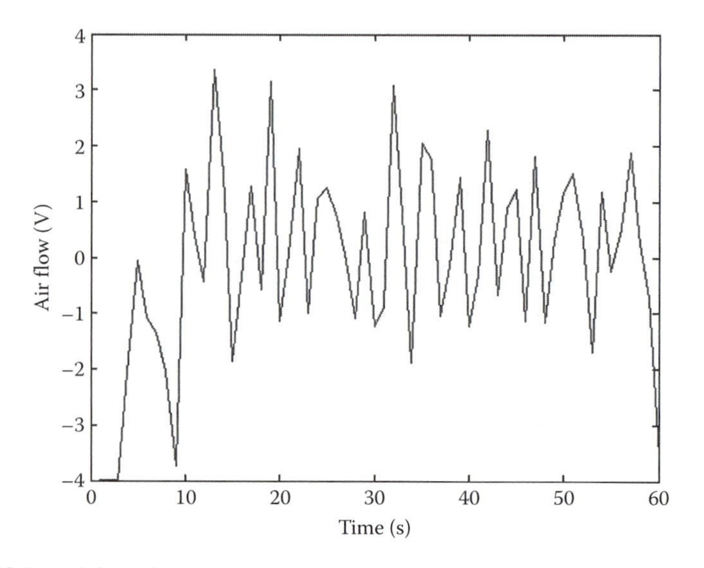

FIGURE 12.7 Airflow signal sampled at 50 Hz. (From Goldberger, A.L. et al., *Circulation*, 101, 23, e215, June 13, 2000, Circulation Electronic Pages; http://circ.ahajournals.org/cgi/content/full/101/23/e215).

12.6 MORE BIOMEDICAL SIGNALS

There are many more biomedical signals that are used for so many clinical and research applications. In this section, we describe some of these signals very briefly.

A signal used for diagnostics of the heart is the heart sound. The heart sounds are the sounds made by the flow of the blood in and out of the heart compartments. In order to measure the heart sounds, often mechanical stethoscopes are used to amplify the sounds. However, since these devices are known to have an uneven frequency response, they somehow distort the sounds. From the signal processing point of view, these changes in the heart sounds made by the mechanical stethoscopes are direct filtering of the actual sounds (i.e., inputs) based on the internal structure of the stethoscope (i.e., mechanical filter), which provides an altered perceived sound (output). While electronic stethoscopes overcome these problems and provide much less distorted version of the actual sounds, physicians have not generally accepted these electronic devices.

The typical changes in the frequency of the heart sounds result in murmurs that are often associated with the imperfections in the heart valves or the heart walls. In infants, the existence of the heart murmurs is often caused by the flow of blood from one side of the heart to another, through the hole between the two sides. This hole is often filled a few weeks after the birth, which in turn stops the heart murmur.

Audiometric measurements and assessments are perfect examples of using FT to evaluate linear systems. In audiometric studies, tones (sinusoidal beeps) of different frequencies are played for the patient through a headphone and the auditory system's response to these tones are measured (often via electrodes measuring the electric activities of the brain). The strength or weakness of the response to each frequency is used to evaluate the performance of the auditory system in those frequencies. This is simply forming the system function $H(f)$ using impulses of different frequencies. The bell shape for the response, i.e., $H(f)$, is often considered a healthy shape, and any irregularity in the response function is measured as the deviation of the curve from a healthy normal bell-shape curve.

12.7 SUMMARY

In this chapter, we reviewed a number of biomedical signals that are used in clinical and research applications. These signals include respiratory signals, cardiovascular signals such as blood pressure and heart sounds, and MEG. Similarities of these signals to other signals discussed in more detail in the previous chapters allow us to process these less widely used signals using the same methods discussed in the previous chapters.

PROBLEMS

12.1 An airflow signal, $g(t)$, is given in file "p_12_1.mat." Load this file from the CD and write MATLAB® codes to perform the following:

a. Plot the signal in time. Also, plot the magnitude of the DFT of the signal.

b. What is the dominant frequency of this signal? What does this frequency (or equivalently, its corresponding period) represent?

12.2 An airflow signal, $g_1(t)$; an abdominal excursion signal, $g_2(t)$; and a thoracic excursion signal, $g_3(t)$, are given in file "p_12_2.mat".* These signals are captured from the same person during sleep. Load this file from the CD and write MATLAB codes to perform the following:

a. Plot the signals in time and frequency and comment on the dominant frequencies of the signals.

b. Find the correlation function among the three signals and comment on the identified correlations.

REFERENCE

Goldberger, A.L., Amaral, L.A.N., Glass, L., Hausdorff, J.M., Ivanov, P.Ch., Mark, R.G., Mietus, J.E., Moody, G.B., Peng, C.K., and Stanley, H.E. (2000, June 13). PhysioBank, PhysioToolkit, and PhysioNet: Components of a new research resource for complex physiologic signals. *Circulation* 101(23):e215–e220.

* From Goldberger et al. (2000).

Part III

Processing of Biomedical Images

13 Principles of Computed Tomography

13.1 INTRODUCTION AND OVERVIEW

Before applying any image processing technique described in the previous chapters to analyze a biomedical image, one needs to create an image. This is often done using computational techniques specialized to exploit the physical laws governing the imaging system as well as the tissue to be imaged. Despite the differences in the physical laws and principles of imaging modalities such as MRI, x-ray CT, ultrasound, and PET, surprisingly, the core computational techniques used to create an image in all these modalities are more or less the same. These computational techniques are often referred to as "computed tomography" or CT. We start this section with the description of the main concepts of CT and its importance in biomedical image processing.

While mathematical representation of CT (as will be discussed in detail) is rather complex, the concept of CT is very much simple and intuitional. Simply put, CT is a process in which the contents of a black box are estimated and visualized based on the reading and measurements made on the surface or around the box. In other words, in CT, one needs to know the contents of a box without opening it. This simple definition explains the importance of CT in biomedical sciences. In medical diagnosis, physicians need to "see" the inside of a body as a two-dimensional (2-D) or three-dimensional (3-D) image noninvasively, i.e., without having to cut the skin, organ, or tissue. The popularity and widespread use of all the existing imaging systems in the recent decades witness to the importance of CT.

From the simple definition of CT given earlier, one might think that this is not a feasible task and no math can handle it. In order to see if this task might be possible even without any math, let us make a quick journey to our younger age. Piggy banks are not only popular play objects among children but also the best examples to witness to the feasibility of CT. Children are often curious to know how full or empty their piggy banks are, i.e., they try to estimate the contents of their black box (piggy bank) at least roughly. In order to do so, they shake (i.e., "stimulate") their piggy bank and get two types of feedback: tactile and audio information. Based on the way the shacked piggy bank "touch" and "sound," children decide not only whether it is full or not but also whether the contents are mainly notes or coins. This CT process happens in the brain apparently without any math as most of these children do not even know how to add numbers!

The reader might think that the examples of CT are limited to early medical imaging, but CT problems are encountered in many areas of science such as nondestructive tests (e.g., estimating the internal structure of a crystal without breaking it), remote sensing (e.g., using satellite image to estimate the shape and distribution of weather fronts), and mining (e.g., discovering the existence of a particular mineral inside a mountain or deep under the ground).

Returning to our discussion of CT for biomedical imaging, from the standpoint of how the system is stimulated and how the measurements are made, CT systems can be categorized into three most commonly used types: attenuation tomography, reflection tomography, and refraction tomography. A brief and high-level description of these three approaches that avoids any mathematical formulations is given in the following.

13.1.1 Attenuation Tomography

In this technique, as shown in Figure 13.1, the system is stimulated by an energy source on one side of the tissue, and the power (or amplitude) of the energy reaching to the other side of the tissue is detected on the other side and is measured. The energy beams such as x-ray are known to travel mainly through straight lines through biological tissues with little or no reflection or refraction (i.e., bending the path and deviation from a straight line). As a result, for such energy beams, assuming a straight pass between the source (transmitter of the beam) and the receiver (detector of the energy beam) is reasonable.

While we are not planning to cover electromagnetic laws to determine when significant reflections or refractions are produced, a simple rule of thumb based on the relative size of the smallest objects in the tissue (e.g., blood vessels, tumors, and so on) to the wavelength of the energy beam can be given here. This rule of thumb states that no significant reflected echoes or refraction is produced if the wavelength of the energy beam is much smaller than the size of the smallest objects in the tissue to be irradiated. In simple words, if the wavelength is small, then the beam can be assumed to pass through the tissue without much reflections or refractions. Knowing that x-ray has a very small wavelength (less than 10 nm), when the objects to be identified are bones or medium- to large-size blood vessels (even to some degree small blood vessels), one can safely assume that x-ray attenuation tomography can be performed without concerns regarding significant

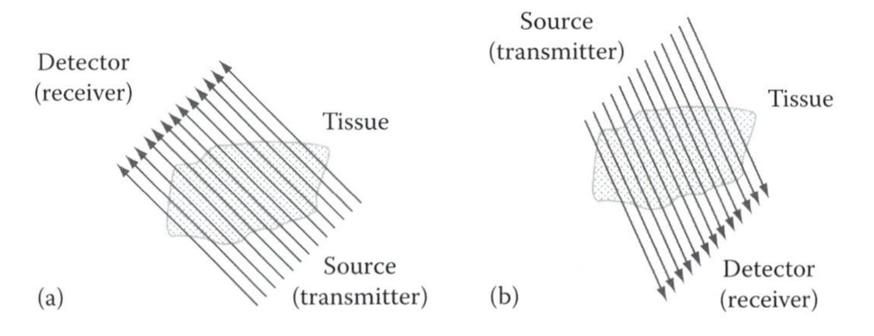

FIGURE 13.1 Attenuation tomography (a) parallel measurements along the same direction and (b) along several directions.

amount of reflection or refraction. On the other hand, for medical ultrasonic waves, the typical wavelength is in the order of a few millimeters and therefore will produce significant echoes and diffraction.

Returning to the mechanism of attenuation tomography, often, the process of irradiation on one side and measurement on the other side is repeated on several points along the same direction (i.e., parallel lines in Figure 13.1a) and along many directions (Figure 13.1b), and the resulting attenuation values are used to create an image of the internal structure of the tissue.

13.1.2 Time-of-Flight Tomography

In the description of attenuation tomography, we did not use the concept of the time needed for beams to pass through different tissues as a means of tomography. This is due to the fact that in some image modalities such as x-ray, due to very high speed of the beam (speed of light for x-ray), it is extremely difficult to measure the very short time periods often encountered. In many such cases, designing hardware to measure such short time intervals is practically impossible. However, in some image modalities, such as ultrasonic imaging, the speed of the propagation of the energy is rather low, and we have the means (e.g., hardware) to measure the resulting time intervals. For such technologies, a different type of tomography is often used that creates an image of the tissue based on the differences in the speed of the energy beam in different objects inside the tissue or, equivalently, the time it takes for the beam to "fly" through different objects. Time-of-flight or TOF tomography is a popular technology that is described here.

In order to better describe the physical concepts involved in this type of tomography, we postpone describing this technique until the chapter on ultrasonic imaging. However, the principle techniques are applicable to all types of image modality.

13.1.3 Reflection Tomography

In some types of imaging modalities, the transmitted beam is reflected on the surface of the objects inside the tissue. In reflection tomography, as shown in Figure 13.2, the tissue is stimulated (i.e., irradiated) by an energy source on one side of the tissue and the power of the reflected beams is measured on the same side of the tissue (often using the same measurement device as both transmitter and detector). In other words,

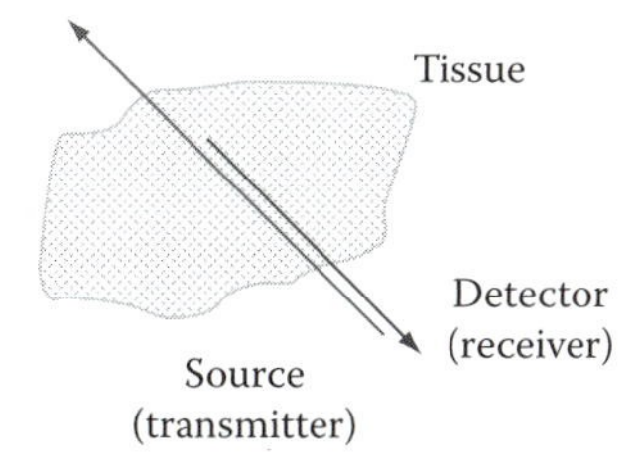

FIGURE 13.2 Schematic diagram of reflection tomography.

the reflected signals are received by the detectors (located on the same side as the transmitters) as the "echoes" of the transmitted signals. The energy beams such as ultrasonic waves create more significant reflection echoes when traveling within biological tissues that can be detected with rather simple piezoelectric probes. As a result, for such energy beams, assuming a straight pass between the source (transmitter of the beam) and the receiver (detector of the energy beam) is reasonable. Just like in attenuation tomography, the measurement process is repeated on several points, and the resulting reflections are used to create an image of the internal structure of the tissue.

For more clarity of the physical description of the system, we again focus on ultrasonic reflection tomography and again have to delay describing the technical and mathematical description of the reflection tomography until the basic concepts of ultrasonic imaging are explained.

13.1.4 Diffraction Tomography

For many energy sources, the irradiate beam bends as it hits the objects in the tissue. This is the basis for diffraction tomography. In such topographic measurements, as shown in Figure 13.3, the tissue is stimulated by an energy source one side of the tissue and the power of the diffracted beams is measured on theoretically all around the tissue. This type of tomography constitutes the most difficult and challenging task in terms of creating mathematical techniques to produce an image of the irradiated tissue. Just like in other types of tomographic systems, the measurement process is repeated on several points along the same direction and along many directions, and the resulting reflections are used to create an image of the internal structure of the tissue.

In terms of the computational techniques used to conduct this type of tomography, one needs to include all wave equations and apply computational techniques that are beyond the focus of the this book and are not discussed here.

As mentioned earlier, the formulation and structure of most of the computational methods used for CT are the same or similar for all modalities. As a result, we formulate the major part of the problem based on the most intuitive one, i.e., x-ray attenuation tomography, and then when dealing with other types of tomographic tasks, the differences and extensions are further described.

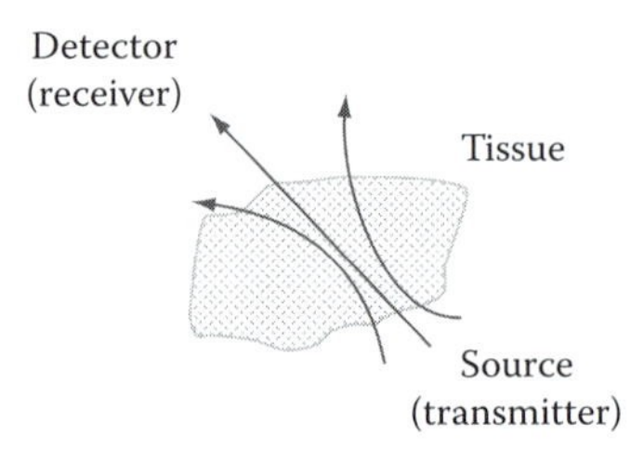

FIGURE 13.3 Schematic diagram of diffraction tomography.

13.2 FORMULATION OF ATTENUATION COMPUTED TOMOGRAPHY

In this section, a mathematical formulation of tomography is presented. In any tomographic system, a particular physical property of the tissue is used to generate an image. For example, in attenuation tomography, the characteristics used to distinguish the points from each other, and therefore create an image based on these differences, is absorption index. In other words, if the absorption index of a point (x, y) is shown by a 2-D function $f(x, y)$, the tomographic image created will represent the tissue based on the differences among the absorption index of each point inside the tissue.

The main difficulty of almost all imaging systems is the fact that the value of the function $f(x, y)$ cannot be measured directly; rather, what is often measured is an integral in which $f(x, y)$ acts as an integrand. In order to see this more clearly, let us examine attenuation tomography more carefully. As can be seen in Figure 13.4, the beam "i," generated by the transmitter, undergoes attenuation at every point (x, y) proportional to $f(x, y)$. Showing the length of a small path around the point (x, y) as "ds," the amount of dP_i, attenuation from one side of the path ds to the other side of it, can be written as follows:

$$dP_i = f(x,y)ds \tag{13.1}$$

Since the detector is located on the other side of the tissue, the attenuation sensed at the detector reflects the total amount of attenuation all through the path as opposed to a particular point. In other words, the total attenuation on the other side of the tissue is

$$P_i = \int_{Path\text{``}i\text{''}} f(x,y)ds \tag{13.2}$$

The integrals of Equation 13.2 are called line integrals. As can be seen, our measurement gives the result of the line integrals, i.e., the integration of $f(x, y)$ over the entire linear path as opposed to the value of $f(x, y)$ at every point. Now, the task of CT is to use these integral equations and solve for $f(x, y)$. In mathematics literature, such a task is normally referred to as the inverse problem. Intuitively, one can see

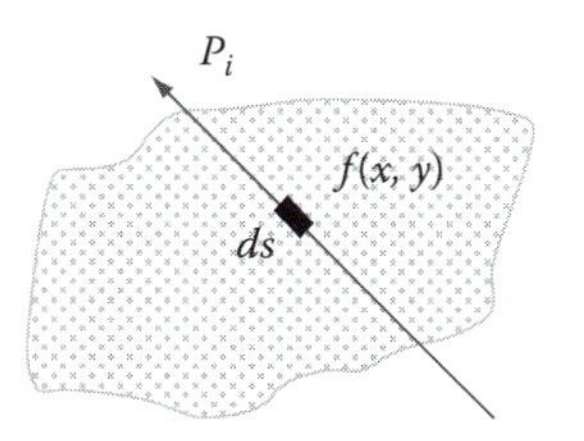

FIGURE 13.4 Attenuation across a differential element of path ds.

that it is theoretically impossible to solve for $f(x, y)$ from only one integral equation such as Equation 13.2. A simple justification of such a claim is as follows: Someone has two numbers in mind and wants you to guess these numbers. As a hint, he or she provides you with the summation of these numbers. Is this hint sufficient to guess every one of those two numbers? Obviously, the answer is no. Getting back to our problem and knowing that integration is nothing but the summation over the differential elements, one cannot find a function $f(x, y)$ from the result of its integral. Then, the question is “how can we solve this problem?” The beauty of CT lies within the simple idea that one can estimate $f(x, y)$ if she or he repeats measurements at different positions and different angles. This is loosely similar to asking the person who has the two numbers in mind to provide you with some other algebraic fact about his or her numbers, for example, to tell you what is two times one number plus the other one. With having another set of algebraic equation, you can solve a system of two equations with two variables to come up with the numbers. In tomography, many measurements at many positions and many directions (as shown in Figure 13.5) are used to create a set of equations that can be solved for $f(x, y)$.

In medical tomography, two types of beam system are used. In the first type, called “parallel beam,” all beams for a given angle are in parallel (Figure 13.5), while in the second type, often referred to as “fan beam,” the beams for a particular angle fan out from the source (Figure 13.6). In this book, we focus on parallel beam formulation, but the extension of the formulation to the fan-beam system is rather more complicated and is not covered in this book.

Despite the differences in physical properties, solving inverse problems in path integrals based on several measurements constitutes the principle of tomography. As a result, in the following section, a detailed description of the techniques to solve the integral equation in attenuation tomography is given.

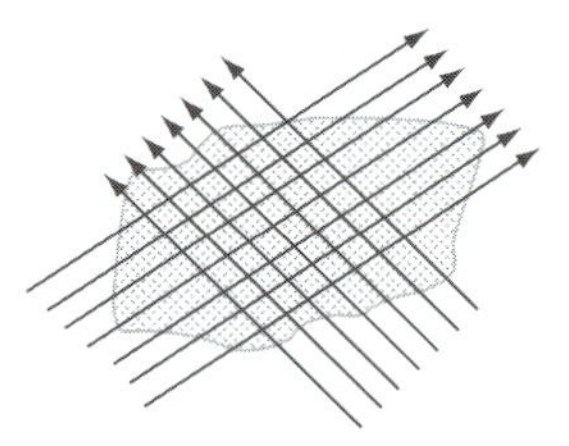

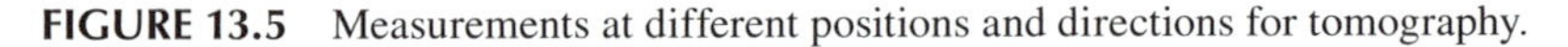

FIGURE 13.5 Measurements at different positions and directions for tomography.

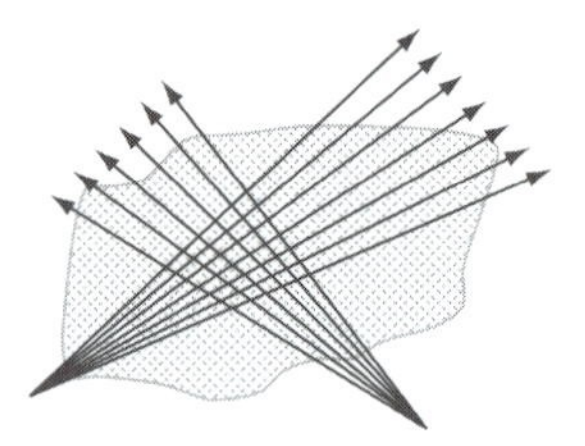

FIGURE 13.6 Fan-beam system.

13.2.1 Attenuation Tomography

In this section, while focusing on attenuation tomography, the main principles of tomography are described. The first step is to device a suitable formulation of "line equation" that matches the ideas of tomography more intuitively. In Figure 13.7, consider the line that forms angle θ with the x-axis and distance t from a parallel line passing through the origin. Such a line can be represented with the following insightful equation:

$$x\cos(\theta) + y\sin(\theta) = t \tag{13.3}$$

The popularity of this formulation of a line lies in the fact that just by looking at the equation, one can know the direction (through θ) and the rectangular distance from the origin (through t).

In addition, such a formulation has more attractive features for tomography. For example, in tomography, often we need to model a number of parallel lines (as in Figure 13.8). In the aforementioned formulation, since the angle θ is the same for all parallel lines, the only thing that changes from one line to another is t.

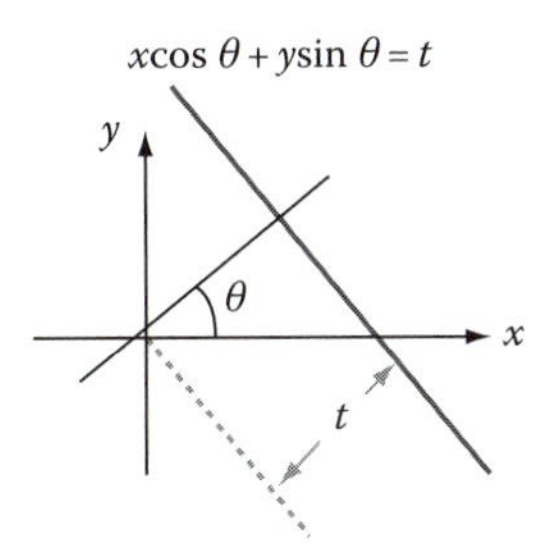

FIGURE 13.7 Line formulation using θ and t.

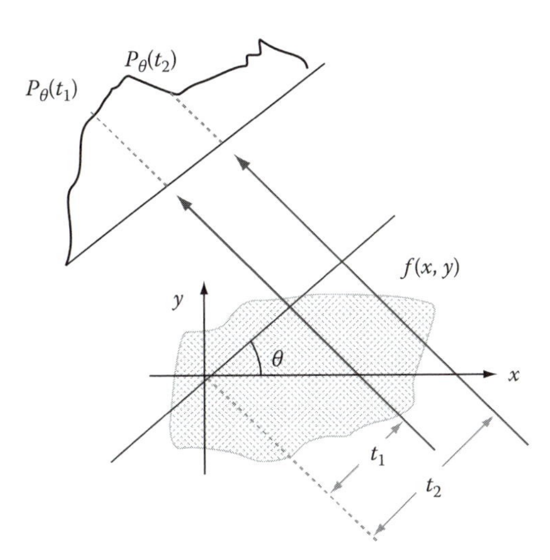

FIGURE 13.8 Forming projection function using parallel beams with angle θ.

Now, assume that at angle θ, we send a number of parallel beams with different t's (as in Figure 13.8) and detect the amount of attenuation (hereafter "projection") at the other side of the tissue. Since for each t we obtain a projection, the resulting projection values can be thought of as a function of t, i.e., the projection function obtained at angle θ can be represented as $P_\theta(t)$. One might argue that since the amount of shift t is often discrete, the function $P_\theta(t)$ should also be a discrete function. While this argument is true and, in reality, both t and $P_\theta(t)$ are discrete, at this point, we restrict ourselves to continuous variables and functions and get back to this issue later on. A typical $P_\theta(t)$ is shown in Figure 13.8, where more attenuation is obtained in the middle. This is due to the fact that the beam has to travel more through the tissue in middle points and therefore gets attenuated more.

Next, we try to see if we can estimate the tissue structure from the projection function, i.e., estimate $f(x, y)$ using $P_\theta(t)$. Let us first explore the integral relation between these two functions again:

$$P_\theta(t) = \int_{(\theta,t)\ line} f(x,y)ds \tag{13.4}$$

As can be seen in Equation 13.4, in order to estimate $f(x, y)$ from $P_\theta(t)$, one needs to solve an integral equation. Before doing so, we first explore special cases of Equation 13.4 that give us more insight to the nature of this equation. These special cases are when $\theta = 0$ (beams parallel with x-axis) and $\theta = \pi/2$ (beams parallel with y-axis). For $\theta = 0$, we have $ds = dy$, and, therefore,

$$P_{\theta=0}(t) = \int_{(\theta=0\,j)\,lines} f(x,y)ds = \int_{-\infty}^{+\infty} f(x,y)dy = P_{\theta=0}(x) \tag{13.5}$$

Equation 13.5 is a single variable integral over y, and the resulting projection function has only one variable x. For $\theta = \pi/2$, $ds = dx$, and, as a result,

$$P_{\theta=\pi/2}(t) = \int_{(\theta=\pi/2\,j)\,lines} f(x,y)ds = \int_{-\infty}^{+\infty} f(x,y)dx = P_{\theta=\pi/2}(y) \tag{13.6}$$

Equation 13.6 is also a single variable integral but this time over x and the resulting projection function has only one variable y. These two special cases will help in our attempt to solve the equations for $f(x, y)$.

The main method to solve the preceding inverse problems applies the Fourier transform (FT). This rather simple strategy has two steps: (1) Use $P_\theta(t)$ to find or estimate $F(u, v)$, i.e., FT of $f(x, y)$ in (u, v) domain and (2) calculate inverse Fourier transform (IFT) of $F(u, v)$ (or its estimation) to obtain $f(x, y)$. As can be seen, the second step is a simple standard routine, and, as a result, conducting the first step, i.e., finding $F(u, v)$ using measurement of $P_\theta(t)$, is the main part of tomography.

In order to see how FT is used for this purpose, first consider FT of the projection function along a particular line for a fixed θ, i.e.,

$$S_\theta(w) = \int_{-\infty}^{+\infty} P_\theta(t)e^{-j2\pi wt}dt \tag{13.7}$$

Also, consider the 2-D FT of the object function $f(x, y)$:

$$F(u,v) = \int_{-\infty}^{+\infty}\int_{-\infty}^{+\infty} f(x,y)e^{-j2\pi(ux+vy)}dxdy \tag{13.8}$$

Now, for $v = 0$, FT along the horizontal frequency coordinate becomes

$$F(u,0) = \int_{-\infty}^{+\infty}\int_{-\infty}^{+\infty} f(x,y)e^{-j2\pi ux}dxdy = \int_{-\infty}^{+\infty}\left(\int_{-\infty}^{+\infty} f(x,y)dy\right)e^{-j2\pi ux}dx \tag{13.9}$$

But from Equation 13.5, remember that $P_{\theta=0}(x) = \int_{-\infty}^{+\infty} f(x,y)dy$, which means Equation 13.9 can be rewritten as follows:

$$F(u,0) = \int_{-\infty}^{+\infty} P_{\theta=0}(x)e^{-j2\pi ux}dx \tag{13.10}$$

Now, from Equation 13.7, we know that $S_{\theta=0}(u) = \int_{-\infty}^{+\infty} P_{\theta=0}(x)e^{-j2\pi ux}dx$, which means

$$F(u,0) = S_{\theta=0}(u) = FT\{P_{\theta=0}(x)\} \tag{13.11}$$

Equation 13.11 finally looks like what we wanted for the first step of our tomography technique, i.e., calculating at least some part of $F(u, v)$ from some part of $P_\theta(t)$. To see what we have obtained more intuitively, consider the visual representation of Equation 13.11 shown in Figure 13.9.

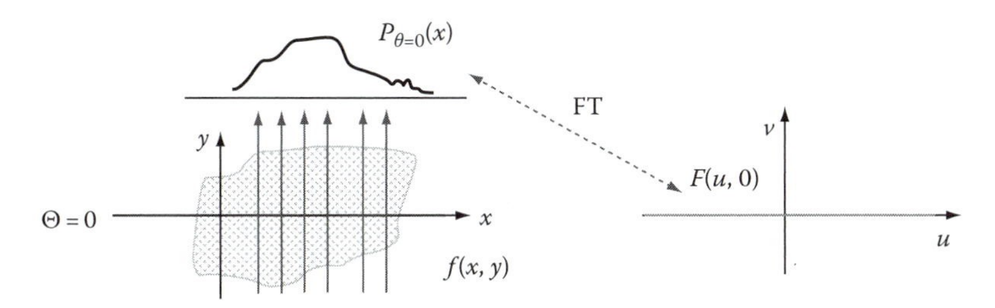

FIGURE 13.9 Visual interpretation of Equation 13.11.

As can be seen in Figure 13.9, one-dimensional (1-D) FT of the projection function for beams $\theta = 0$ (with x-axis in space domain) gives the 2-D FT of $f(x, y)$ on $v = 0$ axis. In other words, one can simply conduct one set of parallel scans along the x-axis and calculate the values of the FT of the resulting projection function to obtain the values of $F(u, v)$ along the u-axis. This is a big step toward our goal of estimating $F(u, v)$, but having $F(u, v)$ only along one axis is not sufficient to form $f(x, y)$, i.e., we need $F(u, v)$ all over the 2-D frequency domain to create a better estimation of $F(u, v)$. Repeating measurement at different angles will produce the values of $F(u, v)$ on different lines in the (u, v) plane. This phenomenon is often referred to as Fourier slice theorem.

13.3 FOURIER SLICE THEOREM

As can be seen in Figure 13.10, Fourier slice theorem simply says that every set of parallel scans at angle θ will produce the values of $F(u, v)$ along one line in the frequency plane (u, v).

Using Figure 13.10, the Fourier slice theorem can be described in the following two steps:

Step 1: Create a set of parallel scans at angle θ and produce the projection function $P_\theta(t)$.

Step 2: Calculate the 1-D FT of the projection function $P_\theta(t)$ to produce the magnitude of $F(u, v)$ along a line passing through the origin with angle θ with u-axis.

It can be seen that if one repeats these measurements on many different angles, the values of the magnitude of $F(u, v)$ can be known along so many lines and that in limit these lines will theoretically cover the entire (u, v) plane (Figure 13.11). After performing scans in many angles, and therefore having many lines in the (u, v) plane, one can calculate the IFT of $F(u, v)$ and produce an estimation of $f(x, y)$.

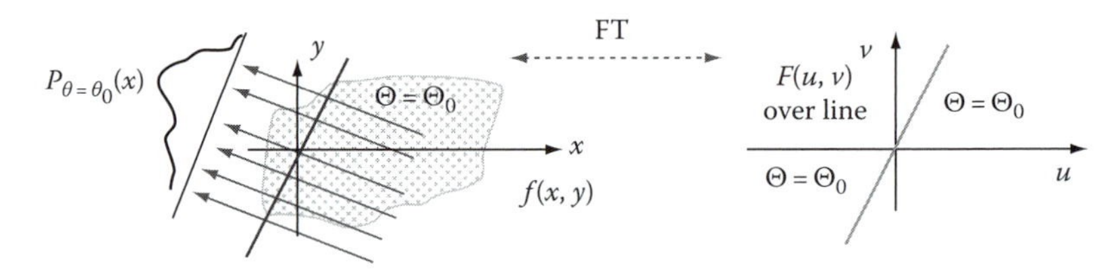

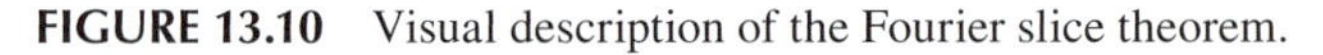
FIGURE 13.10 Visual description of the Fourier slice theorem.

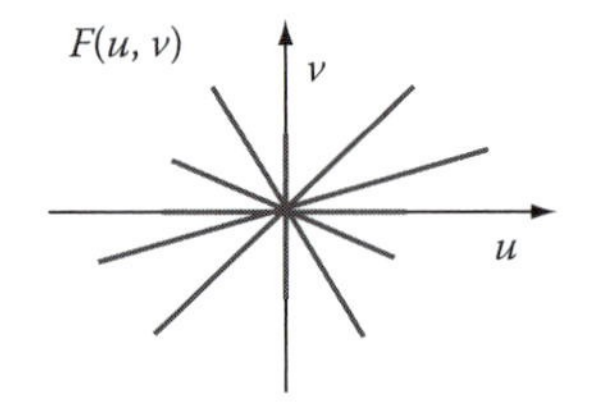

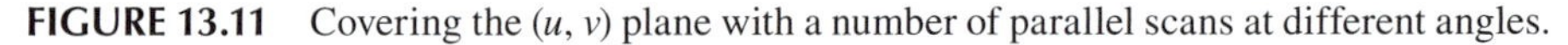
FIGURE 13.11 Covering the (u, v) plane with a number of parallel scans at different angles.

While the principle idea of tomography is as simple and straightforward as what we covered earlier, there are a number of practical considerations that need to be addressed separately. The first issue is the fact that in practical systems, the projection function is a discrete function. In order to see why this is true, let us explore a simplified version of the procedure under which a set of parallel scans are conducted. In practical systems, a number of transmitters with certain physical dimensions are arranged beside each other, along a straight or curved line. The same type of arrangement of receivers (detectors) is made for detectors on the other side of the tissue or object. During scanning, each transmitter sends one scan that is received by the corresponding receiver (detector) on the other side of the object. This describes why you have only a discrete number of scans; the projection function is calculated for a number of points equal to the number of detectors. Obviously, one can make the transmitters and receivers smaller and smaller and, therefore, for the same scanning area, increase the number of points at which the projection function is calculated but can never reduce the size of the transducers ultimately small and form a continuous scan.

Now, knowing that the projection function is a discrete function, instead of performing FT, one needs to perform DFT or fast Fourier transform (FFT). This means that, in reality, instead of knowing the magnitude of $F(u, v)$ on every point along a line, we know this function only on some discrete set of points along the line. In other words, after performing a number of scans, instead of getting Figure 13.11, we will end up with Figure 13.12.

Based on the previous discussion, in order to calculate $f(x, y)$ from $F(u, v)$ known along the discrete lines covering the (u, v) plane, one needs to use 2-D IDFT or IFFT as opposed to the continuous IFT.

Another issue to be addressed about the Fourier slice theorem method is the performance of image reconstruction in the high frequencies. As can be seen in Figure 13.12, the function $F(u, v)$ is known on many points in the vicinity of the origin. This means that since the points on the lines are very close to each other around the origin, we have a lot of information about the low-frequency contents of the image. However, since the lines converge from each other as we move away from the origin, the distance between the points on the lines becomes larger and larger. This means that we know less about higher frequencies of the signal, because the points in which $F(u, v)$ is known are far apart from each other. Let us try to use our knowledge of image processing to visualize how this issue affects the quality of the resulting image. Remember that high frequencies correspond to the edges and textures of the image. This means that if these frequencies are not well known, the edges and texture become vague and fuzzy.

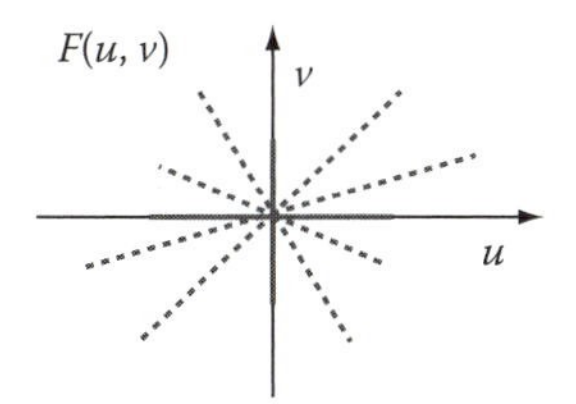

FIGURE 13.12 Covering the (u, v) plane with a number of discrete parallel scans at different angles.

A simple solution for this problem is to make more scans, i.e., make more lines that are closer to each other and therefore create a better representation of the high frequencies. Even though simple in idea, this approach is often limited by the restrictions imposed by the instrumentation and technical issues. Another solution (which is heavily used by the industry) is to design mathematical techniques to interpolate the known points in high frequencies to find more points in high frequency and calculate IFFT of $F(u, v)$ on many more points to create a better representation of $f(x, y)$. There are very many techniques to perform this interpolation, but, in principle, they all share the idea of using the known points to estimate the values of the points in between them. We do not discuss these techniques here, and interested readers can use the list of books and papers provided in this book for further study of these methods.

13.4 SUMMARY

In this chapter, the principle ideas of CT were presented. Knowing that the basic mathematical methods behind all tomographic modalities such as CT, MRI, PET, and some ultrasound imaging systems are the same, covering these techniques in this chapter covers almost all mathematical foundations of medical imaging. In the chapters dedicated to each particular modality, we will describe how the physical principles of each imaging modality provide tomographic equations to be solved by the methods described in this chapter. As described in this chapter, the major mathematical methods for solving the tomographic equations are based on a theorem called Fourier slice theorem that translated the tomographic measurement into a computationally simpler problem in the frequency domain.

PROBLEMS

13.1 During an attenuation tomographic measurement, assume that the two projections at $\theta = 0$ and $\theta = \pi/2$ have resulted in the following projection functions:

$$P_{\theta=0} = \begin{cases} 0 & |t| < a \\ 1 & |t| \geq a \end{cases} \tag{13.12}$$

and

$$P_{\theta=\pi/2} = \begin{cases} 0 & |t| < b \\ 1 & |t| \geq b \end{cases} \tag{13.13}$$

Without using any mathematical calculations and only using heuristics, try to visualize the object being imaged.

13.2 Study the formulation of the 2-D FT in the polar coordinates and explain how this formulation helps with the implementation and usage of the Fourier slice theorem for CT.

14 X-Ray Imaging and Computed Tomography

14.1 INTRODUCTION AND OVERVIEW

Medical x-ray imaging is an imaging modality operating in the x-ray electromagnetic spectrum. The difference with other parts of the electromagnetic spectrum lies in the fact that x-ray operates in very short wavelengths, much shorter than the ultraviolet light of the visible spectrum. The x-ray photon energies range from 10 keV (1.6×10^{-15} J) to 100 keV (1.6×10^{-14} J) or, equivalently, the x-ray wavelengths ranging from 0.124 to 0.0124 nm.

The x-ray energy electromagnetic radiation was discovered by the German scientist Wilhelm Conrad Röntgen (1845–1923) in 1895 while testing a gas discharge tube. The name x-ray was chosen at the time because it was an unknown type of radiation, i.e., at the time it was not known that the x-ray was indeed some type of electromagnetic radiation such as light, only with much shorter wavelengths.

Röntgen's discovery was made when accelerated electrons traveling through vacuum in a glass tube were hitting both the anode and the glass wall. The interaction of the accelerated electrons with the anode or the glass wall apparently produced some form of radiation that made certain materials light up. In the case of Röntgen's experiment, the material that started glowing was barium platinocyanide. The principle of x-ray radiation relies on the deceleration of the electrons during the interaction with the atomic nuclei of the heavy metal anode and the heavy metals in the glass wall where the electron energy is converted into another form of energy, electric and magnetic fields.

The potential for imaging the inside of the human body was almost immediately recognized as the main usage of the piercing new form of radiation and is still one of the most used means of medical imaging with continuously increasing capabilities. In this chapter, we first describe the physics of x-ray and then discuss some of the major imaging methods based on x-ray, including regular x-ray imaging and x-ray computed tomography (CT).

14.2 PHYSICS OF X-RAY

We start this section by introducing some of the main concepts that are heavily used in x-ray imaging. Two of the concepts in x-ray radiography are radiopaque and radiolucent. Radiopaque refers to characteristics of an object that is impenetrable to x-ray. Irradiating such an object with x-ray results in low radiation exposure of the detector on the opposite side of the medium. On the other hand, radiolucent means transparent to x-ray radiation, i.e., high exposure of the detector on the opposite side. The reference material used in x-ray imaging is water that is used as a point of reference or comparison to assess the transparency of other materials. Roughly speaking, water's transparency to x-ray falls in the middle of the range of x-ray absorption.

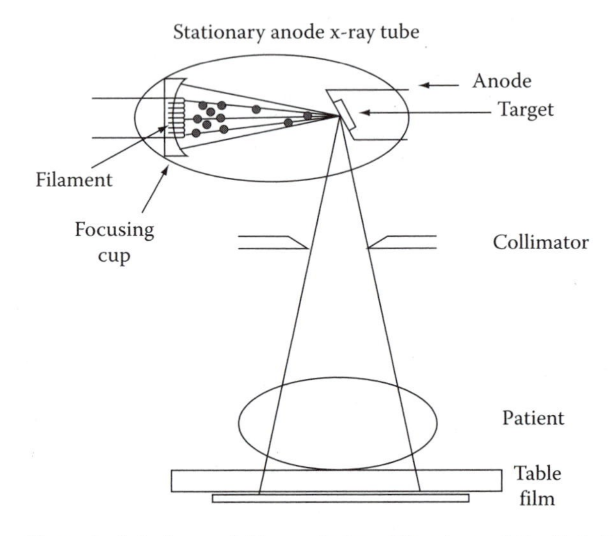

FIGURE 14.1 Characteristic beam delivery design. (Courtesy of Dr. Bob Jones, Lancaster University, Lancaster, United Kingdom. http://www.lancs.ac.uk/depts/physics/physics.htm)

Currently, the method of x-ray generation has not deviated from the original accidental discovery. Figure 14.1 illustrates the generation of x-ray sources used in typical medical imaging applications. A tube with a glow cathode releases electrons, which are accelerated toward a metal anode. The anode is usually made of tungsten. The energy of the x-ray radiation is in direct correlation with the initial acceleration of the electrons measured in the voltage applied between the cathode and the anode. The work, W, performed on the electron during the acceleration is the charge, q, times the electric potential, U. This means that

$$W = qU \tag{14.1}$$

Work and Energy are related by the fact that work equals the change in potential energy PE plus kinetic energy KE:

$$E = PE + KE = W \tag{14.2}$$

In quantum theory, the energy of the photon is all kinetic energy, which is defined as follows:

$$E = KE = \frac{hC}{\lambda} = hf \tag{14.3}$$

where

h equals the Planck's constant
C is the speed of light in vacuum
E is the energy of the photon
λ is the wavelength of the electromagnetic radiation
f denotes the frequency

As can be seen from Equation 14.3, frequency of an electromagnetic wave is related to its wavelength as follows:

$$f = \frac{C}{\lambda} \quad (14.4)$$

Since all the energy of the photon is only kinetic energy, work equals the kinetic energy, i.e.,

$$E = W = qU = hf = \frac{hC}{\lambda} \quad (14.5)$$

Equation 14.5 states that the x-ray's wavelength is primarily identified by the voltage (potential difference) used to create accelerate electrons. However, Equation 14.5 paints the ideal picture of 100% conversion efficiency from the kinetic energy of the electron to the photon, which is highly improbable. In most cases, not all energy from the accelerated electron is released during deceleration when the electron hits the anode. A large portion of energy is converted into heat. In practical systems, even with the highest efficiency, only approximately 1% of the electron energy is converted into electromagnetic radiation; the remaining energy needs to be disposed off as heat. This makes cooling an important concern in x-ray imaging.

As shown in Figure 14.1, the produced x-ray beams are then formed using a collimator. The biological tissues are irradiated with the collimated beams, and the attenuated beams after passing through the biological tissues are then detected by an array of detectors or simply by a sensitive film. This typical setup of biomedical x-ray imaging systems will be discussed later in this chapter.

Based on the choice of the anode material, certain electrons carrying a particular quota of energy are preferably absorbed more than others. This results in an x-ray photon spectrum that is characteristic for the anode material, and it is hence called characteristic radiation. Peaks in the spectrum relate to significantly higher deceleration probability and resonance energy levels of the anode material based on atomic configuration and lattice structure. A representative x-ray spectrum is illustrated in Figure 14.2.

The spectrum emitted by the anode material will range from short wavelengths at the higher energy levels to long wavelengths at the lower energy levels as is clear from Figure 14.2. The shorter wavelengths are most desirable for their ability to make a high level of discrimination capability, which translates to a better image resolution. Conversely, the longer wavelengths are undesirable because of the low resolution and shallow penetration. Therefore, longer wavelengths will need to be eliminated as much as possible since they provide no additional image detail but do add to the damage created by x-ray radiation on biological tissues. Tissue damage takes place at the genetic level, since the wavelengths of x-ray radiation are of the order of the size of the molecular bounds in DNA.

Filtering of electromagnetic radiation at these energy levels can be accomplished by metal plates of various thicknesses in the path of the photon beam. For instance,

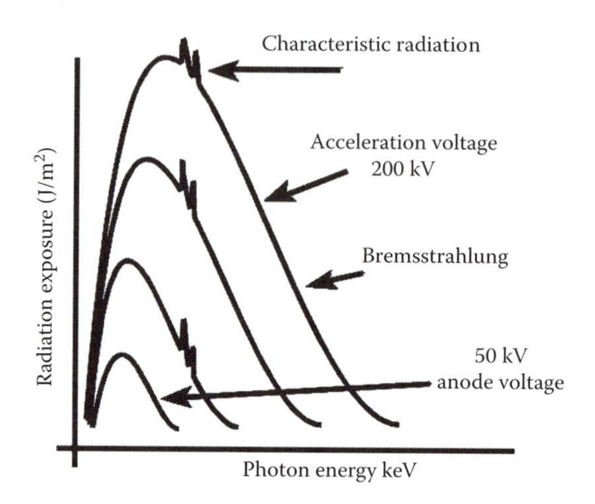

FIGURE 14.2 Example of relative characteristic radiation spectrum resulting from an acceleration energy ranging from 50 to 200 kV. (Courtesy of Dr. Bob Jones, Lancaster University, Lancaster, United Kingdom. http://www.lancs.ac.uk/depts/physics/physics.htm)

aluminum will absorb the majority of the low-energy photons, while the short wavelengths experience minimal adverse effects.

Next, we apply our knowledge of the physics of x-ray to discuss the use of x-ray for imaging and in particular the practical considerations in using x-ray for medical imaging.

14.2.1 Imaging with X-Ray

X-ray radiation produced with <60 kV of acceleration potential is classified as soft x-ray and has electrons with 60 keV (9.6×10^{-15} J) kinetic energy hitting the metal target. This type of radiation is predominantly used for soft tissue imaging, for example, imaging of breast tumors called mammography. When an electric potential of more than 100 kV is used for acceleration, the radiation is categorized as hard x-ray. This type of short-wavelength radiation serves best to image hard tissues like bone or artificial contrast agents. The electromagnetic radiation will pass through either soft or hard tissue based on the photon energy, but the relative amount of absorbed radiation will be proportional to the type and size of tissue.

For imaging purposes, the x-ray energy needs to be converted in a display medium that places the radiation transmitted through the biological medium in the range of human perception. In order to obtain the best quality of an x-ray image, the exposure, the anatomical penetration, and the contrast and resolution on the film or detector array need to be optimized to get the best resolution and contrast for the anatomy of interest while minimizing the radiation hazard to the patient. As will be discussed in detail, the exposure depends on tube operating settings, geometry of the imaging arrangement, and the exposure time. The penetration through the anatomy depends on the characteristics of the respective tissues the beam passes through as well as the anatomical structure of the tissues. The contrast on the x-ray film between anatomical features of interest is of crucial importance in the determination of details. The resulting contract largely depends on the characteristics of the film or other detectors

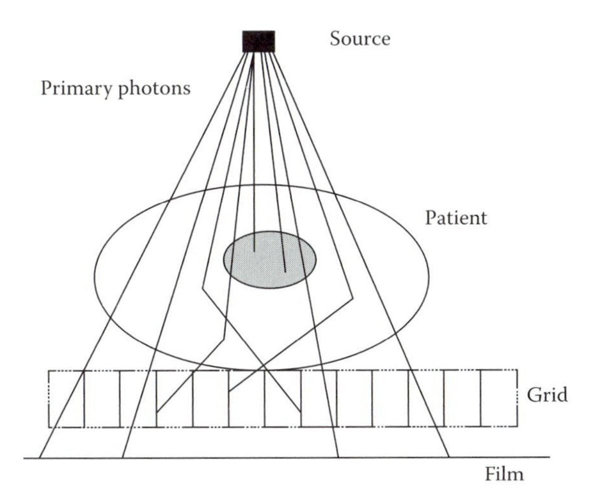

FIGURE 14.3 Illustration of typical uniform x-ray exposure and beam detection geometry to enhance contrast by removing scattered x-ray photons from the detection beam by means of the Bucky roster. (Courtesy of Dr. Bob Jones, Lancaster University, Lancaster, United Kingdom. http://www.lancs.ac.uk/depts/physics/physics.htm)

used for sensing the x-ray. The resolution is determined to a great extent by the geometry of the imaging setup (relative distance between source, patient, and film, and so on). Figure 14.3 illustrates a simplified geometric representation of a typical medical radiography setup. In this diagram, the effects of diffracted photons, which can cause distortion in the resulting images, have been graphically presented.

The next sections will focus on the main practical factors and considerations in using x-ray for medical imaging.

14.2.2 Radiation Dose

The amount of radiation needed to result in accurate images is referred to as the radiation dose. The x-ray radiation exposure is determined by several measures. The exposure is often measured in absorbed radiation dose. The concept of radiation dose plays an important role in all medical x-ray imaging systems and is further described in the following text.

The x-ray exposure, X, is the time exposure to intensity and is the culmination of the intensity exposure over an extended period of time defined as follows:

$$X \propto ZiU^2t \tag{14.6}$$

where

- Z is the atomic number of the target material
- i (mA) is the cathode ray current
- U (kV) is the potential difference between the cathode
- t (s) is the exposure duration

The exposure X is expressed as an energy density (J/m^2).

One can argue that since not all tissues absorb the same percentage of the incident radiation, the exposure X does not give an optimal measure of the radiation absorbed by the tissue. In other words, in order to obtain an accurate reading of the dose, the respective tissues irradiated need to be taken into account. This is why another quantity, the radiation absorbed dose (RAD), is sometimes used an actual indication of the energy absorbed by the medium (biological tissue) per unit mass. However, in dosage assessment procedures, it is often observed that the absorption of the x-ray source is relatively uniform across the entire field of exposure, giving all tissues relatively the same dosage. This observation means that RAD can be often well represented by X.

14.3 ATTENUATION-BASED X-RAY IMAGING

With the knowledge of the operating mechanism of x-ray imaging, we can proceed with the description of the actual image formation. Since almost all commercial x-ray imaging systems, i.e., conventional x-ray machines as well as CT or computed axial tomography (CAT) scan systems, are using attenuation as the major physical quantity to form images, next we focus on the concept using attenuation for image formation.

As mentioned in Chapter 13, in x-ray attenuation tomography, the difference in the attenuation between various tissues forms the basis of the formation of an attenuation contrast image.

The attenuation coefficient, also known as the absorption coefficient, α, plays the central role in x-ray attenuation imaging. This quantity is defined as the proportionality factor for the change in x-ray radiation intensity. In order to formally define this quantity, consider the change in intensity, dI, across a differential element of thickness, dx. This intensity change is proportional to the incident intensity, I_0, and the distance traversed, i.e.,

$$dI = -\alpha I dx \tag{14.7}$$

Integration of Equation 14.14 gives the following expression of exponential decay as a function of distance migrated through the biological medium:

$$I = I_0 e^{-\alpha x} \tag{14.8}$$

or

$$\ln\left(\frac{I_0}{I}\right) = -\alpha x \tag{14.9}$$

where I is the transmitted intensity used for image formation.

As can be seen from the aforementioned formulation, the attenuation coefficient, α, is the reciprocal distance where the intensity decays to e^{-1} or 36% of the initial value.

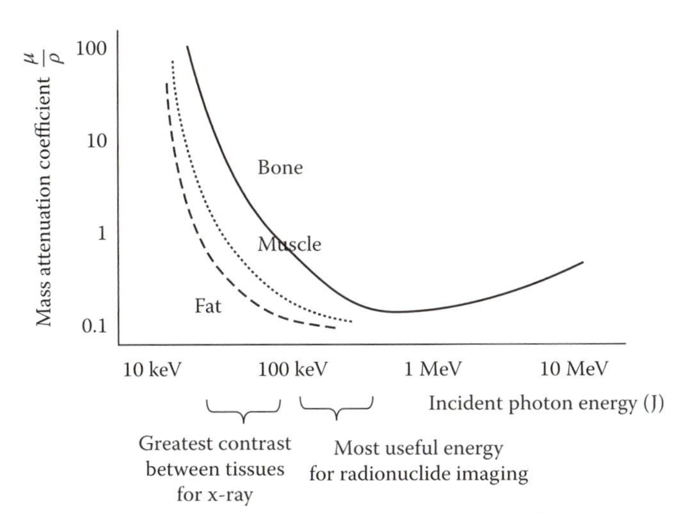

FIGURE 14.4 Energy dependence of the mass attenuation coefficient for three main tissues. (Courtesy of Dr. Bob Jones, Lancaster University, Lancaster, United Kingdom. http://www.lancs.ac.uk/depts/physics/physics.htm)

Accelerated electrons hit anode, producing photons with different levels of energy. Different types of biological tissues have different values of attenuation coefficient. This dependency of the attenuation on the photon energy is illustrated in Figure 14.4. These differences describe why attenuation coefficient can be used to produce an image of the biological systems.

In general, for optimal image formation, the x-ray energy is chosen for maximum contrast, depending on the tissues of interest. As may be concluded from Figure 14.4, the largest gradient in mass attenuation coefficient is in the energy range between 10 and 100 keV. Higher tissue density and associated higher atomic number of the components give greater contrast opportunities; however, soft tissues require greater attention to reveal any contrast.

In order to calculate the amount of attenuation, one needs to detect and expose the amount of the received x-ray energy on the other side of the irradiated tissue. The difference between the transmitted and received energy constitutes a measure of attenuation. Due to the importance of x-ray detection, next, we briefly review the commercially used methods of x-ray detection.

14.4 X-RAY DETECTION

The main methods to obtain an anatomically representative image of a biological medium are discussed in the following.

The most primitive method of measuring x-ray energy is film imaging. In conventional x-ray image formation, the x-ray photons are used to oxidize a sensitive layer made of a silver/bromide/iodine mixture. The amount of radiation exposure determines the degree of oxidation, similar to photographic film imaging. After exposure, the film is developed and a high contrast grayscale image is produced. In general,

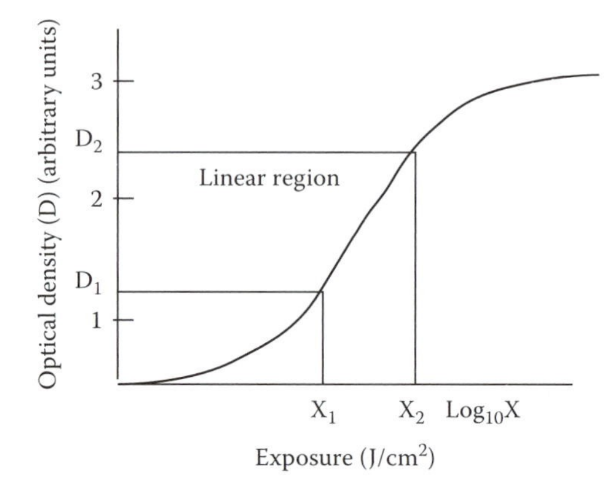

FIGURE 14.5 Illustration of a typical response curve of photographic film plate. (Courtesy of Dr. Bob Jones, Lancaster University, Lancaster, United Kingdom. http://www.lancs.ac.uk/depts/physics/physics.htm)

the film is nonlinear in its response with only a relatively narrow range of energy exposure that is in fact linear. This linear region of sensitivity will need to be utilized to optimally reveal image details. The film sensitivity is expressed in optical density (OD), which is the darkening observed under x-ray exposure. Conventional x-ray is accepted to provide the best discrimination for distinguishing between bone, soft tissue, and lung. In such systems, it is often desired to keep the x-ray exposure amount to the range where the relation between the OD and the exposure is linear, as shown in Figure 14.5. This range allows better control of the exposure while maintaining a proportionally acceptable optical quality of the resulting image. Figure 14.6 shows a typical conventional x-ray machine that applies sensitive films to detect the x-ray attenuation across the irradiated tissues.

Another popular means of image formation is the use of fluorescence induced by x-ray. Fluorescent material emits visible light when receiving the x-ray radiation. This fluorescence can be seen by a charged coupled device (CCD) camera for continuous viewing or still-picture generation. In fluoroscopy, a constant stream of x-ray is delivered and collected in real time. The x-ray radiation is detected by a CCD camera that images fluorescence produced by x-ray photon excitation. Fluoroscopy enables the radiologist to view a changing image continuously, as in an interventional procedure. This technology normally delivers a lower dose of radiation than the previous analog system whilst providing high-definition, high-resolution images. The fluorescence can also be imaged using on regular photographic film. In this case, a fluorescent screen is usually placed on both the front and the backside of the photographic plate to increase efficiency. Each CCD element forms a pixel of the image, or each photosensitive crystal forms a pixel.

Fluoroscopy is very popular in interventional radiology. Interventional radiology encompasses any procedure that is invasive. A representative illustration of an x-ray fluoroscopy imaging device is shown in Figure 14.7. Some examples of invasive procedures involve the insertion of a needle, a cannula (tube), or a catheter, or wire into the patient for diagnosis and/or treatment. Procedures that frequently rely on

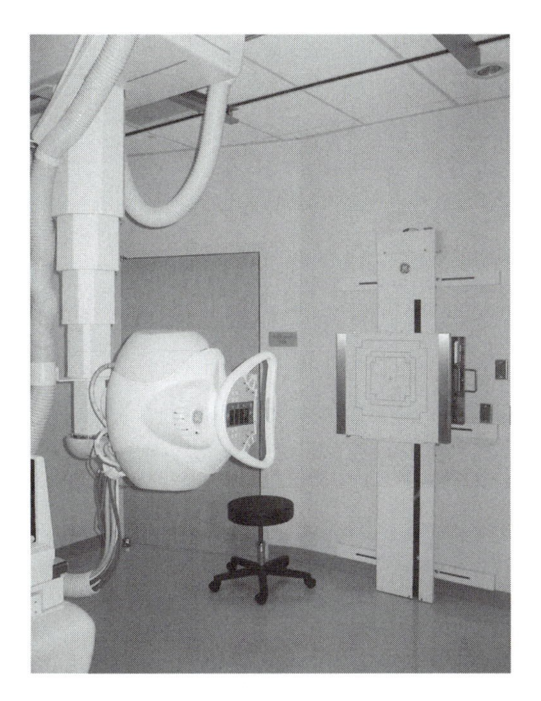

FIGURE 14.6 Illustration of a typical conventional plate photography x-ray machine.

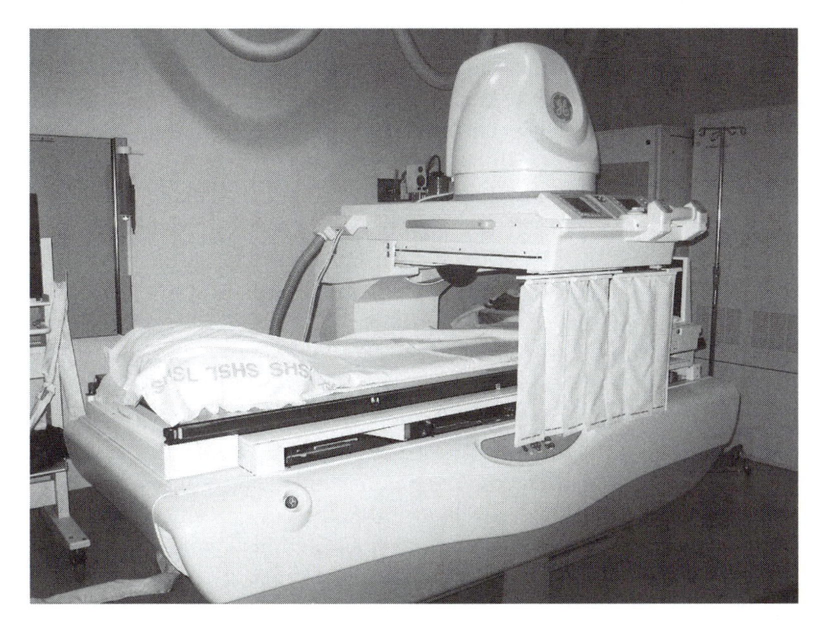

FIGURE 14.7 Illustration of a typical fluoroscopy x-ray imaging device.

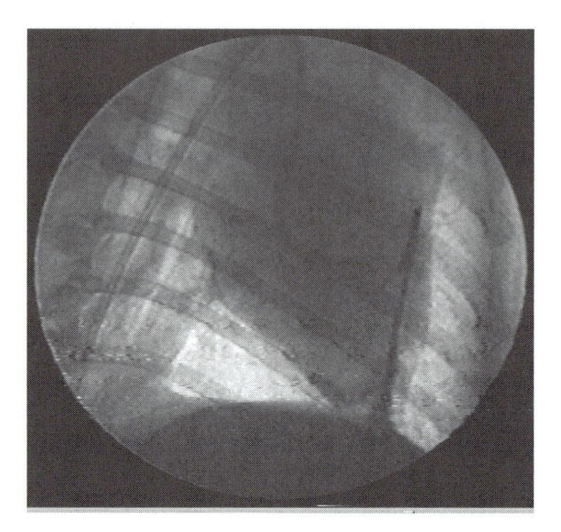

FIGURE 14.8 Fluoroscopic image of electrode placement during heart catheterization. One catheter with four electrodes is placed in a coronary vessel while a second catheter is positioned on the opposite side inside the left ventricle.

fluoroscopy include angioplasty, which is the insertion of a balloon into a vein or artery to widen it and improve circulation. Another application, also in cardiology, is called stenting, which involves the insertion of a tube or wire mash that is expanded by inflating a balloon to keep an artery or a vein open. Other procedures are the monitoring of specific biopsies, for example, lung, breast, renal, liver, and bone. Figure 14.8 illustrates the positioning of electrophysiology catheters in the heart to examine deviations in the ECG locally in relation to suspected conduction problems in the heart under fluoroscopy.

A less popular but substantially higher resolution than the fluorescent plate imaging technique uses a capacitive plate read by a laser beam. A capacitive insulator plate locally loses its charge under irradiation by x-ray radiation. A laser beam sweeps the plate in a line-scan fashion from left to right and from up to down, and the laser reflection changes with the amount of the charge. When using a semiconductor material, this detection scenario becomes a reusable process. This type of image formation can provide very high resolution (approximately 5 μm) due to the small laser spot size. The pixel size here is determined by the data-acquisition rate and the line width of the sweeping laser beam.

The method for x-ray detection used in CT is often based on using scintillation counters. These photomultiplier-type detectors register a current under irradiance by x-ray radiation; the current is directly proportional to the amount of x-ray quanta hitting the scintillator. The image is formed by mapping out the current as a function of location. The current is often converted into a voltage by a high input impedance amplifier in order to reduce the current drain on the device, which negatively influences the detection sensitivity. This method is fast and instantaneously renewable.

Regardless of the specific method used for detection, it is sometimes desirable to increase or enhance detection capabilities using contract agents. One method of detection enhancement is the use of contrast agents that are injected or ingested prior to or during the imaging procedure. The use of contrast agents is fairly common in x-ray imaging. Contrast agents are often radiopaque or radiolucent media introduced to enhance contrast. Several examples of contrast agents are as follows: Barium sulfate for use in the gastrointestinal tract. Not all of the methods to introduce artificial contrast are without hazard. A barium meal is used to explore the digestive system. Iodine compounds are used in blood vessels, which is a nontoxic radiopaque substance. The iodine is injected to visualize blood vessels in angiography, which attempts to visualize the constriction of coronary vessels in particular. Carbon dioxide is used in CT of the colon or in angiography if the patient is allergic to other contrasting agents. Carbon dioxide is radiolucent and will appear as dark spots in images.

Knowing the technologies to create and detect x-ray, next, we focus on the physical factors affecting the quality and resolution of x-ray imaging.

14.5 IMAGE QUALITY

While resolution of the resulting x-ray images can be improved with the image processing methods introduced in the previous chapters, all existing technologies attempt to improve the quality of the image in the acquisition stage to have a much higher quality image.

The four issues that affect the resolution of the details in x-ray imaging are the size of x-ray beam and source, the motion artifacts, and the quantum noise. These factors influence the resolution and quality of all x-ray imaging technologies regardless of the specific technology used for detection and image processing.

The x-ray focus is the momentarily active section of the rotating anode that is emitting x-ray radiation. In the mathematical analysis (in particular, in CT), the x-ray focus should be a point source, providing a single source–image relationship. In other words, almost all mathematical formulations of x-ray imaging assume that the source creates infinitely narrow x-ray beams. In reality, the x-ray source, having finite dimensions, produces a cylindrical beam that irradiates all points from one edge of the irradiated object to the opposite edge in a single illumination, thus smearing the shadow image out over a finite width or breadth. This smearing effect of wide x-ray sources is illustrated in Figure 14.9 that describes a more realistic diagram of x-ray image formation using practical nonpoint x-ray sources. As can be seen in Figure 14.9, geometric distortions and shadowing artifacts are primarily caused by the fact that the source is not a point source.

The finite width source can be considered as an array of an infinite number of point sources strung together. The beam overlap between these point sources can be minimized by reducing the distance from source to object as much as possible without significant loss in intensity. In addition, placing the detector as close to the object as possible reduces diffraction and divergence. An additional measure is to place the source at an angle to the line connecting the source to the object, thus reducing the source dimensions by multiplication with the sine of the angle of the normal of the source surface with the connecting line. By rotating the anode disk, the exposure of the target area of the anode can be reduced without risk of overheating.

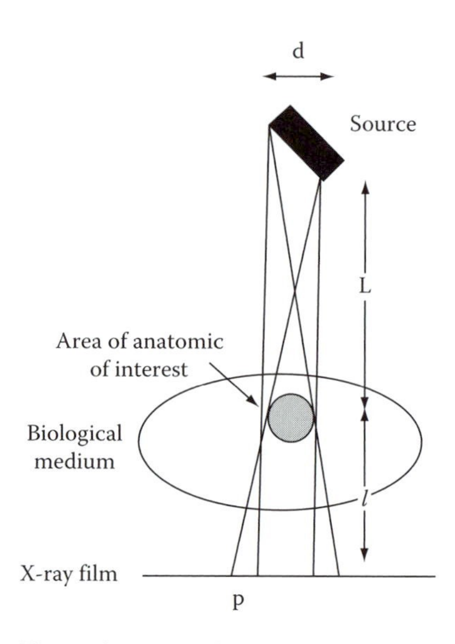

FIGURE 14.9 Diagram illustrating one of the artifacts that affect the sharpness of the image recorded on the photographic plate in conventional x-ray radiography. (Courtesy of Dr. Bob Jones, Lancaster University, Lancaster, United Kingdom. http://www.lancs.ac.uk/depts/physics/physics.htm)

Motion artifacts, caused by the motion of the object during the x-ray exposure time, are other sources of noise in images that are often unavoidable. Two main sources of motion artifact are the heart motion and breathing. The heartbeat is too fast to be eliminated during the imaging process. In addition, the patients cannot be told to stop their heart motion for the sake of imaging! On the other hand, the breathing motion can, in most cases, be avoided by requesting the test subject to refrain from breathing for a few seconds. Other sources of motion artifacts may be introduced by the intestinal motions that are again involuntary. A direct approaching for minimizing motion artifacts is shortening the exposure time; however, this will require an increased dosage, which is obviously not advisable.

Quantum noise is a typical problem for x-ray images (especially in image intensifiers). Quantum noise is a characteristic that is inherited from the quantum nature of the x-ray photon generation principle. Quantum noise is proportional to the square root of the signal amplitude. One way of improving signal-to-noise ratio is by increasing the signal strength; however, this increases the risks to the patient due to radiation damage of the DNA. A second means of increasing signal-to-noise ratio is in the detection side, simply by improving the detection efficiency.

14.6 COMPUTED TOMOGRAPHY

CT, also referred to as CAT, uses scintillation counter arrays or CCD-fluorescent plate array to collect the data to reproduce 3-D representations of the biological medium. CAT has significantly better resolution in imaging and discrimination of soft tissues. In addition, unlike the conventional x-ray imaging that produces the shadow of the objects, CT constructs images showing the slices of the irradiated tissues or objects in the imaging plane.

In addition, unlike the conventional x-ray where in order to form an image, only a single x-ray scan from only a single angle is conducted, in CT, several scans from many angles are taken to form a single image. This process was described in Chapter 13.

CT scanning exposes the patient to moderate to high levels of radiation, mostly due to the extended exposure time. In CT, a repetitive procedure is followed that scans the biological tissues from many directions by revolving both the source and the scintillation counter detectors around the body in a circular motion.

Figure 14.10 describes a very simplified diagram of CT imaging. As can be seen in Figure 14.10, in CT, a scanner takes a series of x-ray scans at various angles positioned in cylindrical symmetry with the body. Information on the attenuation of x-rays is recorded for the projection of a plane of interest in the patient along a line, and this is repeated for a series of small rotations. Then, a computer algorithm processes all these scans together to form a 2-D image using the principles of CT. The attenuation values at the points of interest reveal the local density distribution of the cross-sectional plane in two dimensions. The computer algorithm also stacks the slice images on top of each other to reconstruct 3-D images of the body.

The mathematical description of the image formation protocol applied in CT imaging was presented in Chapter 13. The tomographic methods are used to estimate the integrand of a series of line integrals that are calculated in several directions. More specifically, the objective of x-ray attenuation tomography is to the attenuation coefficients $\alpha(x, y)$ from the ray integral of the following format:

$$\int_{l_i, \theta_i} \alpha(x, y)\, dl_i = p_{l_i, \theta_i} \tag{14.10}$$

where projections are created for all rays l_i and all angles θ_i. As discussed in Chapter 13, the scans for different rays are achieved by translation of the transmitters and detectors. Similarly, the scans at different angles are obtained by rotation of the transmitters and detectors.

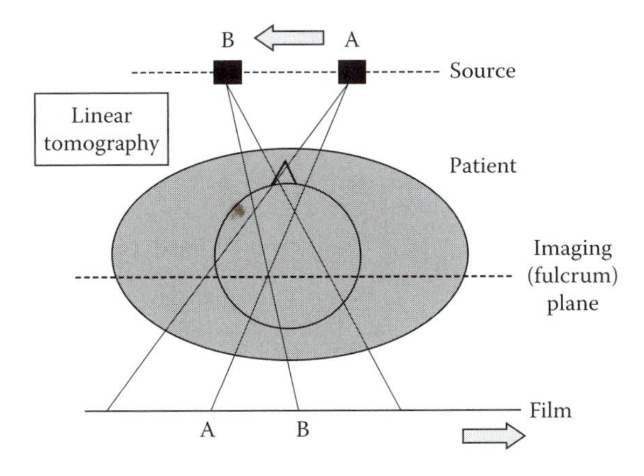

FIGURE 14.10 X-ray scanning to form a cross-sectional slice. (Courtesy of Dr. Bob Jones, Lancaster University, Lancaster, United Kingdom. http://www.lancs.ac.uk/depts/physics/physics.htm)

The computational techniques in x-ray attenuation tomography, such as the ones based on Fourier slice theorem, estimate $\alpha(x, y)$ and then use the discriminative power of the attenuation coefficient to create an image of the body.

Next, we review some specific CT technologies used in biomedical imaging and diagnostics.

14.7 BIOMEDICAL CT SCANNERS

Two general types of medical CT scanner technologies can be distinguished: fan-beam and parallel scanning. These commercial technologies are often a combination of the parallel and fan-beam scanning technologies described in Chapter 13.

The first type of fan-beam technology exploits the naturally occurring divergence of the x-ray sources for delivery and detection. First, the beam divergence is collected by an array of detectors. Then, the detector undergoes a linear translation in the radial direction. After completion of the entire width of the medium, the entire transmitter/detector system is slightly rotated and the scans are repeated. An illustration of the scanning principle is shown in Figure 14.11. A typical array of detectors contains 30 detectors.

Another fan-beam scanning system makes the divergence of the source beam fan out across the width of the patient, covering a large number of detectors simultaneously. This way, the overlap that is unavoidable in the first type of scanning system can be eliminated. Total exposure is also concurrently reduced. The entire set of source and detectors still require rotation to complete the data acquisition for a substantial image reconstruction algorithm. Figure 14.12 provides an illustration of the functional schematics of this type of scanners.

In the more current generation of scanners, a very large number of stationary detectors are arranged in a ring surrounding the patient. The total number of detectors now surpasses 1000. Only the source with diverging beams rotates in this configuration.

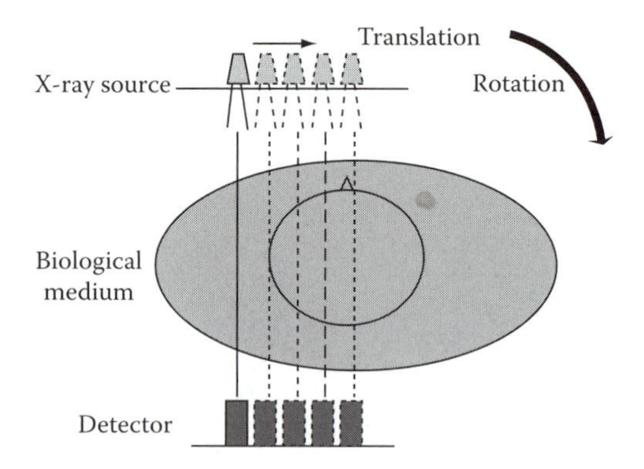

FIGURE 14.11 Diagram of first-generation of tomography scanners; linear motion of both source and detector scan a slice of the body, followed by rotation over several degrees. (Courtesy of Dr. Bob Jones, Lancaster University, Lancaster, United Kingdom. http://www.lancs.ac.uk/depts/physics/physics.htm)

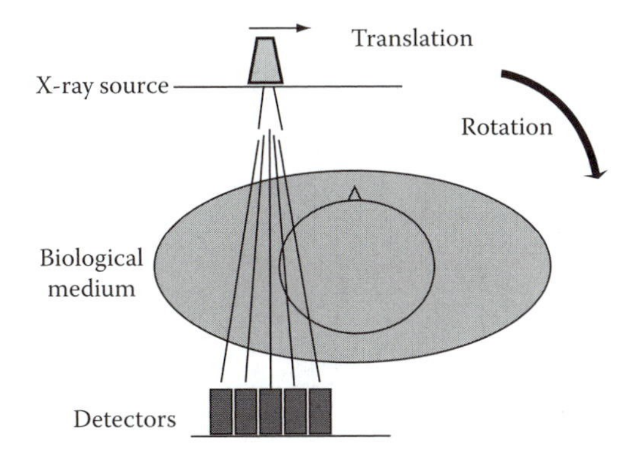

FIGURE 14.12 Diagram of second-generation tomography scanner utilizing the fan-beam scanning principle, initially repeating the same linear scanning motion followed by rotation as the first-generation tomograph. The fan beam however allows for a smaller dose due to the collection of all transmitted radiation. (Courtesy of Dr. Bob Jones, Lancaster University, Lancaster, United Kingdom. http://www.lancs.ac.uk/depts/physics/physics.htm)

A single slice of patient now takes <1 s. The method of operation is illustrated in Figure 14.13. This typical operation in the medical literature is often illustrated in more concise diagram as in shown in Figure 14.14. A modern spiral CT machine rotates the x-ray source along a spiral path, thus enabling the imaging of several cross sections in a much shorter period of time.

Points from adjacent layers and adjacent points within a single layer can be correlated to each other by interpolation to increase the display accuracy artificially by pattern recognition. Combining many adjacent layer 2-D scans allows the computer to calculate a high-resolution 3-D density distribution volumetric display of the internal organization of tissues.

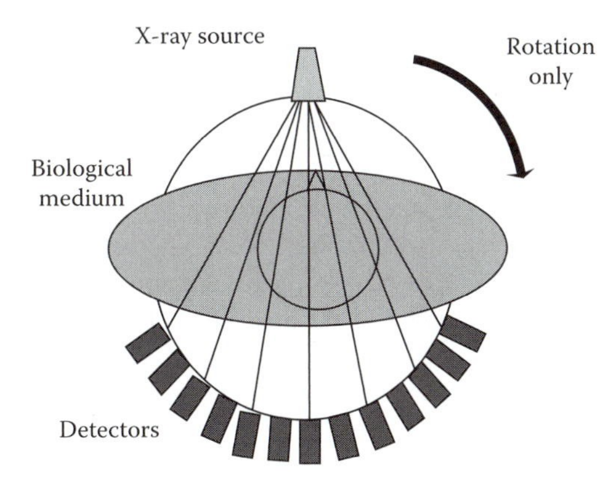

FIGURE 14.13 Diagram of ray deployment in third generation of tomographic scanners. Wide fan beam and elimination of the linear scan reduce the exposure even further and yield more detail. Both the source and an array of multiple detectors move jointly over a small angle each scan. (Courtesy of Dr. Bob Jones, Lancaster University, Lancaster, United Kingdom. http://www.lancs.ac.uk/depts/physics/physics.htm)

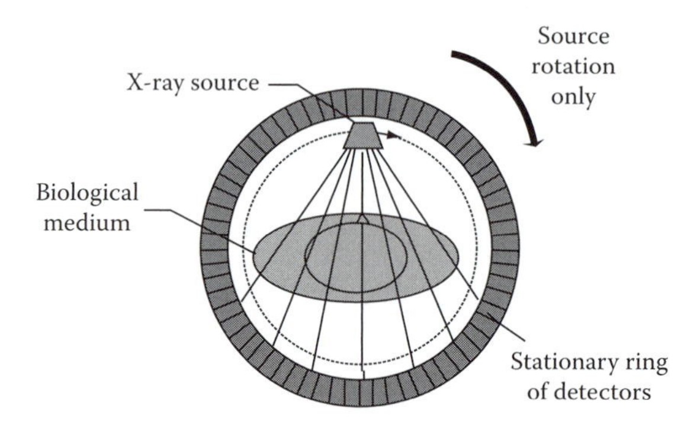

FIGURE 14.14 Diagram of fourth-generation tomography scanners, representing the present-day most commonly used outline. A large array of detectors form a closed circle around the patient, only the source moves in a circular motion. (Courtesy of Dr. Bob Jones, Lancaster University, Lancaster, United Kingdom. http://www.lancs.ac.uk/depts/physics/physics.htm)

14.8 DIAGNOSTIC APPLICATIONS OF X-RAY IMAGING

X-ray imaging is used for various diagnostic applications. For instance, a high-density tumor in an air-filled lung will look like a gray mass on black background. Low-density cyst in radiopaque bone will look like a gray mass on white background on film. Currently, undetectable by x-ray imaging are most soft tissues: liver metastasis, colon cancer, and infections.

Some of the main applications of x-ray imaging in coronary obstruction visualization and the classic x-ray image of the broken bone are briefly described in the following.

A typical usage of the x-ray imaging is the detection of coronary obstruction. During or as a precursor to a heart attack, coronary blood vessels will become occluded. Only with the aid of contrast fluid injected in the coronary arteries can these arteries be visualized under fluoroscopy while a catheter is positioned in a feeder artery to the suspected area of the heart. Blood flow can be seen to either completely avoid a certain perfusion area of the heart, or it will expose a narrowing of a vessel by contrast.

When a bone is broken, it produces a distinctive look under x-ray imaging. Conventional x-ray imaging of the extremity or whole body will reveal discontinuities in the standard anatomic geometry of bone structures at places where the bone is broken or even dislocated. Based on the known geometry of the bone structure, discontinuities will show up irrespective of prior anatomical knowledge. Anatomical knowledge will however confirm any other bone structures that may be in a different plane of the body, and thus may appear as discontinuity in a compressed 3-D display and only show a 2-D outline of all information in between the camera or photographic plate and the x-ray source.

A major application of CT is detection of brain and other types of tumors. Due to high resolution of the CT, these images are significantly more informative than the conventional x-ray and provide the physicians with accurate geometric information such as the volumetric measurements of the tumor. During the last couple of decades, MRI technology has replaced CT for such applications, primarily due to its higher resolution as well as the fact that MRI is not harmful to biological tissues.

One of the most exciting applications of x-ray is in whole-body CT. This system creates a complete 3-D visualization of the human body in a very high resolution. The 3-D image can be easily rendered and investigated for tumors or any kind of abnormalities such as enlargement of otherwise healthy tissues. The capabilities of the whole-body 3-D x-ray tomography had made it a candidate for a major checkup system. The main drawback of such systems is the x-ray dosage of a relatively long exposure to x-ray that can cause damage in biological tissues.

14.9 CT IMAGES FOR STEREOTACTIC SURGERIES

The stereotactic surgeries eliminate the need for major neurosurgical procedures. The typical procedures such as biopsy can be performed through a hole in the skull of only 5 mm diameter. This calls for accurate positioning of the probe and other smaller surgical tools. The combination of a reference system and CT provides an invaluable image registration system that allows stereotactic neurosurgery.

The stereotactic devices provide a reference system (typically a frame) that is fixed to the skull. Figure 14.15 shows the Cosman–Roberts–Wells System (CRW-System) made by Radionics. The stereotactic localization device is mounted on the head of a patient by means of a base ring on which various surgical tools and reference markers can be positioned. The patient can be imaged with the device in place to provide a frame of reference.

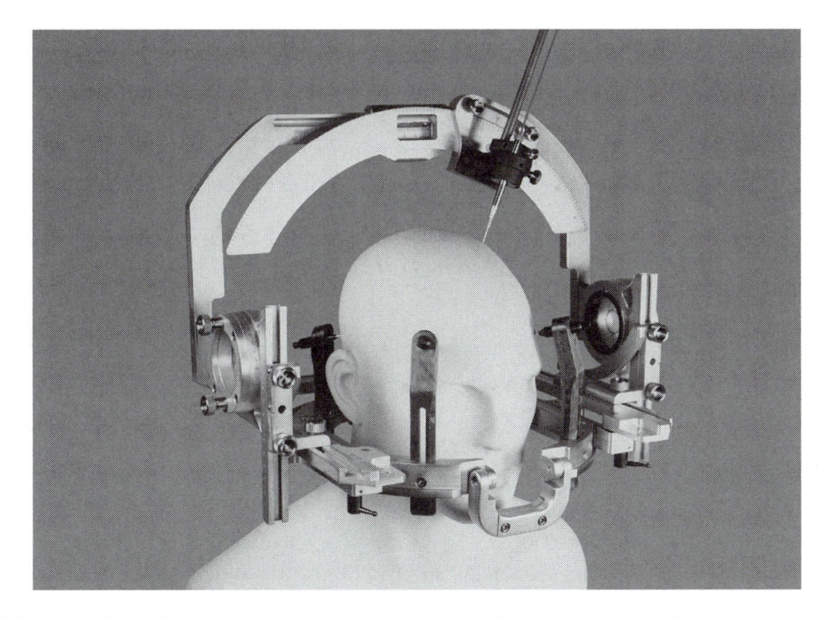

FIGURE 14.15 CRW stereotactic device by Radionics, as used in registration and image-guided surgery. (CRW™ is a trademark of Radionics. Copyright © Radionics. All rights reserved. Reprinted with the permission of Radionics, a division of Tyco Healthcare Group LP.)

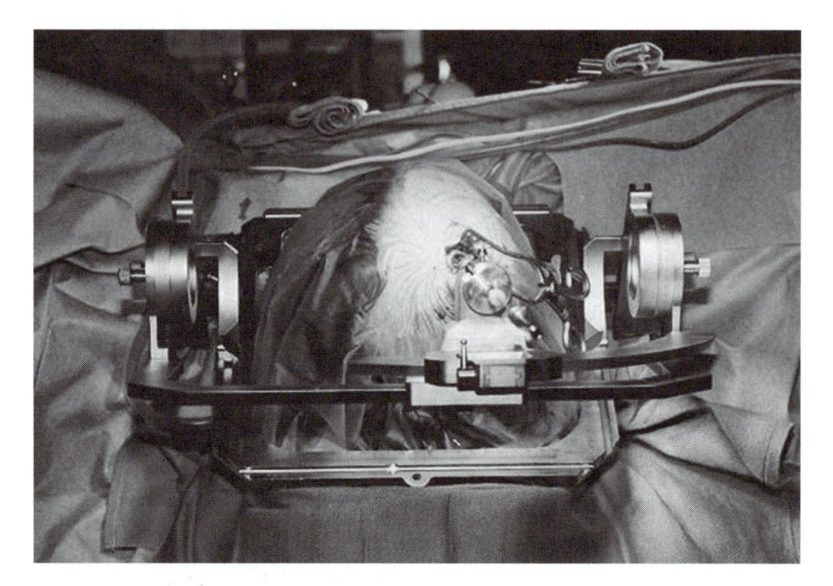

FIGURE 14.16 CRW stereotactic device by Radionics mounted on a patient's head during image-guided surgery. (CRW™ is a trademark of Radionics. Copyright © Radionics. All rights reserved. Reprinted with the permission of Radionics, a division of Tyco Healthcare Group LP.)

The stereotactic device, as shown in Figure 14.16, illustrates the surgical accessories in place while the patient is undergoing a procedure. The device is used under imaging to provide registration of a brain tumor or other pathological conditions against the reference frame of the CRW system prior to the start of a minimally invasive surgical procedure. Surgical interventions can then be guided accurately and unequivocally for various delicate neurosurgical procedures or biopsies.

14.10 CT REGISTRATION FOR OTHER IMAGE-GUIDED INTERVENTIONS

While stereotactic surgeries are among the most commonly used applications of CT-based registration and image-guided interventions, there are a number of other procedures exploiting CT images.

As in stereotactic surgeries, in other image-guided interventions, correspondence is established between image and the physical space of the patient during the intervention. Establishing this correspondence allows the image to guide, direct, and monitor therapy, akin to providing a 3-D map for navigation. The main objective is to make the intervention more accurate and hopefully safer while becoming less invasive for the patient. In the last few years, image registration techniques have been introduced routinely in clinical procedures for image-guided neurosurgery systems and in computer-assisted orthopedic surgery. In CT registration, it is important what the topic is for the registration exercise. When monitoring changes, the changes can be either in intensity or in volume. Changes in intensity can be minimized by normalization. Volume changes will rely on the location of boundary outlines as described in Chapter 4 and to some degree in Chapter 3.

Most registration applications rely on correspondence for comparison, such as the position, shape, and size of the eye, nose, and particular bones. When analyzing correspondence in image changes over time, such as tumor growth over a period of several months, the algorithm may require scaling based on anatomical and geometric landmarks.

An entirely different class of registration is recognition of correspondence between different individuals. On a coarse scale, the images may correspond after appropriate nonrigid transformations have been made to the images. However, under higher-resolution observation, they may not give the conclusive evidence needed for pathological evaluation.

14.11 COMPLICATIONS OF X-RAY IMAGING

Some of the biological effects of x-rays resulting from the high energy interaction with molecules and atoms in the biological medium, respectively, may cause ejection of one or more orbital electrons by a photon that creates an ion pair; ions are unstable and give rise to free radicals. These free radicals are chemically aggressive and may have undesirable consequences since they are mutagenic (cause changes in the DNA structure), teratogenic (x-ray radiation may be life shortening), and even lethal. The most prominent complication is the fact that x-ray radiation has carcinogenic consequences.

14.12 SUMMARY

The advantage of radiography is the fact that it is relatively cheap, in addition to the fact that it reveals ample contrast between bone, soft tissue, and lung. Some of the disadvantages are poor soft tissue contrast in addition to the fact that it has not much use for distinguishing adjacent healthy and diseased soft tissues. One major disadvantage is the radiation hazards and epidemiological effects of x-ray radiation.

PROBLEMS

14.1 Read image file "p_14_1.jpg." This is an x-ray film image of the left and right breast combined.* The right breast shows asymmetric changes. Compare the left breast (LMLO) with the right breast (RMLO) and locate the region of change. Pick a convenient location in the region of asymmetric change and use seed growing to find the outline of the suspected area.

14.2 Read image file "p_14_2.jpg." This image shows a fracture of the fibula and medial malleolus.*

* Courtesy of MedPix. http://rad.usuhs.mil/medpix/

TABLE 14.1
T-Score Criteria for Osteoporosis in Women

Normal	BMD > −1.0 below the young adult reference range
Low bone mass (osteopenia)	−1.0 > BMD > −2.5 standard deviations (SD) below the young adult reference range
Osteoporosis	BMD < −2.5 SD below the young adult reference range
Severe osteoporosis	BMD < −2.5 SD below the young adult reference range, often associated with one or more fractures

Source: Courtesy of David Holdsworth, Robarts Research Institute, London, Ontario, Canada.

a. Use edge detection methods (in particular, region growing technique) and display the discontinuity of the broken bone.
b. Choose some seed values in the middle of each region to start the region growing process.
c. Find the maximum length of the gap.

14.3 Osteoporosis is often indicated by loss of bone density. Several methods are available to measure bone density, but, currently, the most widely used technique is DEXA (dual energy x-ray absorptiometry). The bone mass density (BMD) is often the accepted indication of osteoporosis (Table 14.1). Read image file "p_14_3.jpg." Image "p_14_3.jpg" is an image of the lumbar spine of a patient with severe osteoporosis with multiple fractures.* The BMD is approximately 10 mg/cm^3, with a T-score of −6.
a. The file contains two images attached to each other. Use MATLAB® to separate the two images and display the images separately.
b. Design a thresholding method to determine the most obvious locations of osteoporosis outlined by the red ellipse. Osteoporosis is determined based on the increased x-ray transmission and the scale of apparent bone thickness illustrated in the insert (darker image tone due to increased oxidation of the photographic plate). *Hint:* You can start with creating the histogram and identifying the range of gray levels corresponding to oxidation.
c. The angle between vertebrae is an important indicator for spine problems. Use edge detection to find the outline of the vertebrae. Determine the angle between the three lower vertebrae of the lumbar spine in the image.
d. Fractures in the bone resulting from osteoporosis are also visible. Use thresholding techniques to locate the fracture sites.

14.4 Read image file "p_14_4.jpg" and display the image. Image "p_14_4.jpg" shows the axial, sagittal, and coronal views of the lumbar spine region (L1 and L2) of a patient with relatively normal bone mass density.* However, the trabecular bone is inhomogeneous and there is significant mineralization between L1 and L2 (indicated by the blue arrows). Other abnormalities in the bone structure are the

* Courtesy of Mindways Software, Inc., San Francisco, CA; Courtesy of Keenan Brown.

somewhat irregular bone density distribution and, more prominently, the worn edges of the vertebrae.

a. Using MATLAB, split the image into three separate images, each showing the vertebrae from one specific angle.
b. Design a thresholding method to determine the most obvious locations of osteoporosis outlined by the red ellipse. Osteoporosis is determined based on the increased x-ray transmission and the scale of apparent bone thickness illustrated in the insert (darker image tone due to increased oxidation of the photographic plate).
c. In each image, find the major and minor axis of each vertebra. The length of these axes identifies a potential deformation of the vertebrae. Find eccentricity of each vertebra.
d. The angle between vertebrae is an important indicator for spine problems. Use edge detection to find the outline of the vertebrae. Determine the angle between the three lower vertebrae of the lumbar spine in the image.

14.5 Read image file "p_14_5.jpg." Image "p_14_5.jpg" shows the axial and sagittal views of the lumbar spine region (L1 and L2) of a patient with relatively normal bone mass density.* This region of the spine is predominantly of interest in the determination of bone QCT of DXA in the assessment of bone mass measurement. DXA measures total bone (cortical and trabecular) as well as extraosseous mineral, which is visible in the image. This patient exhibits aortic calcifications that would also be misclassified as bone in DXA; however, the locations would indicate the lack of structural benefit in spinal bone formation and can be excluded.

a. The file contains four images. Use MATLAB to separate the four images and display the images separately.
b. In each image, find the major and minor axis of each vertebra. The length of these axes identifies a potential deformation of the vertebrae. Find eccentricity of each vertebra.
c. The angle between vertebrae is an important indicator for spine problems. Use edge detection to find the outline of the vertebrae. Determine the angle between the vertebrae.
d. Design a thresholding method to determine the most obvious locations of osteoporosis outlined by the red ellipse. Osteoporosis is determined based on the increased x-ray transmission and the scale of apparent bone thickness illustrated in the insert (darker image tone due to increased oxidation of the photographic plate).

14.6 Read image files "p_14_6_a.jpg" and "p_14_6_b.jpg." Image "p_14_6_a.jpg" is an x-ray film image of a 62 year old male pelvic bone, and "p_14_6_b.jpg" is the x-ray film image of a 21 year old female pelvic bone.† Use edge detection methods to outline the pelvic bone structure, scaling, and nonlinear deformation to register the male pelvis with the female pelvis.

---

* Courtesy of Mindways Software, Inc., San Francisco, CA; Courtesy of Keenan Brown.

† Courtesy of MedPix. http://rad.usuhs.mil/medpix/

14.7 Can the relative body-fat-to-muscle ratio of an arm of a grown man be determined from x-ray imaging and under what conditions?

14.8 Read image file “p_14_8.jpg” and display the image. Image “p_14_8.jpg” is an x-ray fluoroscopy image of a heart with a catheter in the coronary vessel indicated by the blue arrow. The apex (bottom tip) of the heart is indicated by the red arrow, and one of the ribs is marked with a yellow arrow.

a. Use thresholding and edge detection techniques to find the outlines of the heart.
b. Choose some seed values in the middle of the heart to start the region growing process to outline the heart.
c. Apply Canny edge detection technique to find the outlines of the catheter.
d. Apply Canny edge detection techniques to find the outlines of the ribs.

15 Magnetic Resonance Imaging

15.1 INTRODUCTION AND OVERVIEW

Magnetic resonance imaging (MRI) is an imaging technique that makes use of the phenomenon of nuclear spin resonance. The principle idea of MRI is based on the fact that when a magnet is exposed to an external magnetic field, it tries to orient itself to align with the external magnetic field. This idea explains that the spin axis of the protons in the atoms of the biological tissues exposed to the MRI's large magnetic field will orient itself in a direction parallel to the magnetic field lines. In the majority of cases, the magnetic resonance is tuned to imaging of the magnetic spin of the hydrogen nuclei in water molecules. Measuring the spin information for a group of molecules provides the means of creating an MR image of the biological tissue under study.

The possibility of using the nuclear magnetic resonance (NMR) was discovered in the 1940s when the discovery was made that certain substances absorb and emit radiofrequency electromagnetic radiation when placed in an alternating magnetic field. The initial applications were in the molecular analysis of the chemical and physical properties of single-element liquids or solids. In the early 1970s, the biological applications of NMR imaging were first proposed by Raymond V. Damadian. He recognized a difference in nuclear magnetic relaxation times of healthy and cancerous tissues. This was the first indication that MRI could be applied to collect information about the tissue physiology.

Further improvements were incorporated by the chemist Paul Lauterbur. His technique was still able to generate only two-dimensional (2-D) images. Later on, Peter Mansfield extended MRI capabilities by introducing the techniques to produce a full three-dimensional (3-D) rendering of biological tissues. The latest major discovery in MRI was functional magnetic resonance imaging (*f*MRI). Unlike MRI that focuses on the anatomical details of the tissue, *f*MRI is designed to create images showing the functional activities of the tissue. For instance, *f*MRI techniques measure the blood oxygenation levels in the brain to monitor the brain functions.

Since the discovery of MRI, this technology has been used for very many medical applications. Due to the resolution of MRI and the fact that as far as we know this technology is essentially harmless, MRI has emerged as the most accurate and desirable imaging technology. It is anticipated that as the price of MRI technology reduces, many currently used technologies such as x-ray CT scans will be replaced

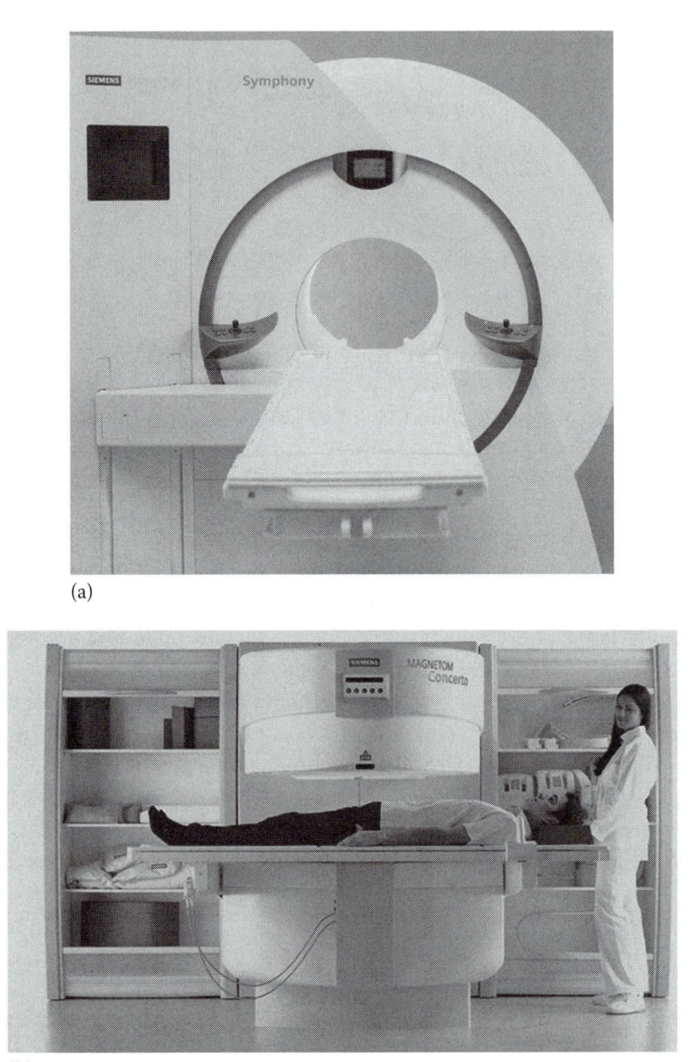

FIGURE 15.1 Pictures of two different types of Siemens MRI machines. (a) Conventional MRI from the Symphony series, MAGNETOM Symphony 1.5 T and (b) open MRI MAGNETOM Concerto 0.2 T. (Courtesy of Siemens AG, Medical Solutions, Magnetic resonance; brochure: Magnets, flows and artifacts and Siemens CD.)

by MRI. A picture of a representative configuration of a conventional MRI machine and an open MRI machine are shown in Figure 15.1.

This chapter first focuses on the principle physics of MRI and then discusses the MRI technology. We also discuss the principle ideas as well as the applications of *f*MRI. The use of MRI for medical diagnostics will also be given in this chapter.

15.2 PHYSICAL AND PHYSIOLOGICAL PRINCIPLES OF MRI

While for the purpose of imaging, only the net result of a group of protons will be sensed for NMR imaging, the principal mechanism of NMR imaging is based on the spinning of a single neutron in the presence of an external magnetic field. The protons in the nucleus of atoms have an intrinsic rotation around a central axis. This rotation resembles the spinning of an off-balance spinning top as illustrated in Figure 15.2. The angle and the annular velocity of the rotation, ω, are both intrinsic properties of each particle. The magnetic field **m** is also specific to each particle or element. This means that a moving charge, such a proton, produces its own magnetic field, which is a function of the charge and speed of the motion.

The interaction between the magnetic fields of the moving charges inside a tissue and an external magnetic field provides the means of NMR imaging. Next, we focus more closely on the magnetic field generated by the macroscopic objects and the interactions between the magnetic field of the particles and the external magnetic field. A nucleus that has these qualities can be seen as a rotating, electrically charged object causing a magnetic moment and, as a result, a magnetic dipole. These atoms are nanoscale magnets that behave just like large magnets. At the macroscopic level, magnetic dipoles generated by atoms can group together to form an ensemble. These types of ensembles are composed of atoms that have an odd atomic number or an odd atomic weight that can produce a nuclear spin.

The sum of the magnetic moments of these dipole groups, i.e., the sum of all individual **m**'s, is called the nuclear magnetization **M**. The nuclear magnetization is typically zero, provided that there is no exterior magnetic field. In human tissues, there are a large number of such dipoles that essentially cancel the magnetic effects

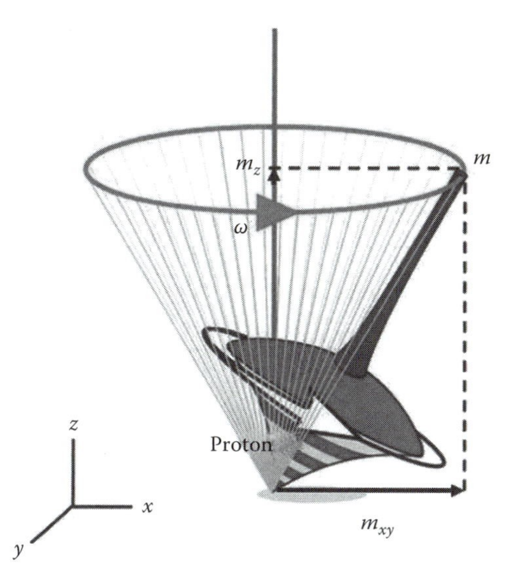

FIGURE 15.2 Proton spin. (Courtesy of Siemens AG, Medical Solutions, Magnetic resonance; brochure: Magnets, flows and artifacts.)

of each other. However, if the human body is exposed to an external magnetic field, these ensembles start showing measurable magnetic effects.

In NMR imaging, all nuclei with an odd number of protons are immersed in a static magnetic field, H_0, in the z-direction. In MRI technology, a very strong constant magnetic field with a typical magnitude between 0.2 and about 3 T is used as H_0. Knowing that the earth's magnetic field is approximately 5×10^{-5} T, it can be seen that the applied magnetic field is very strong. The presence of this strong external magnetic field creates a net magnetic field in the microscopic elements. The resultant nuclear magnetization, **M**, is the total magnetic moment of all the microscopic units, e.g., elements with an odd number of charged particles in the nuclei. The alignment of the individual magnetic dipoles in the external magnetic field is illustrated in Figure 15.3. This nuclear magnetization is oriented in the direction of the external field, either parallel to the external field or in the exact opposite direction (antiparallel).

Due to energy considerations, the microscopic spins cannot orient themselves instantaneously from their random direction to align with the external field lines. Rather, these small magnetic spinning tops need to spiral down to the energy content of the forced direction. The process of spiraling down from one direction to another direction is called precession. The precession process plays an important role in magnetic imaging. The proton spin in the process of precession is illustrated in Figure 15.4. This precession motion is analog to the motion and orientation of a gyrocompass adjusting to the earth's magnetic field, which also takes some time to happen. The alignment of proton magnetization vector due to an external magnetic pulse is illustrated in Figure 15.5. As can be seen in the figure, a radio frequency (RF) pulse causes a series of fluctuations on the magnitude of the proton's magnetization vector.

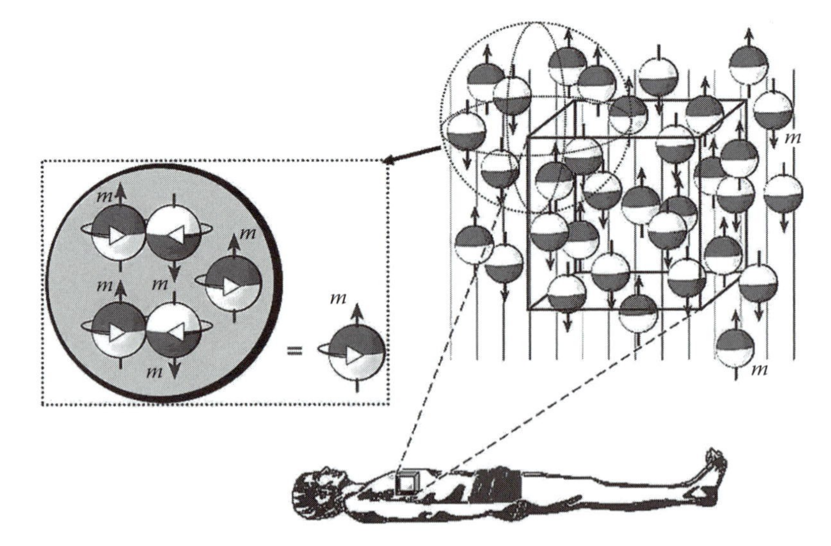

FIGURE 15.3 Schematic representation of the distribution of the spin magnetization orientation in a whole-body scan with respect to external magnetic field. (Courtesy of Siemens AG, Medical Solutions, Magnetic resonance; brochure: Magnets, flows and artifacts.)

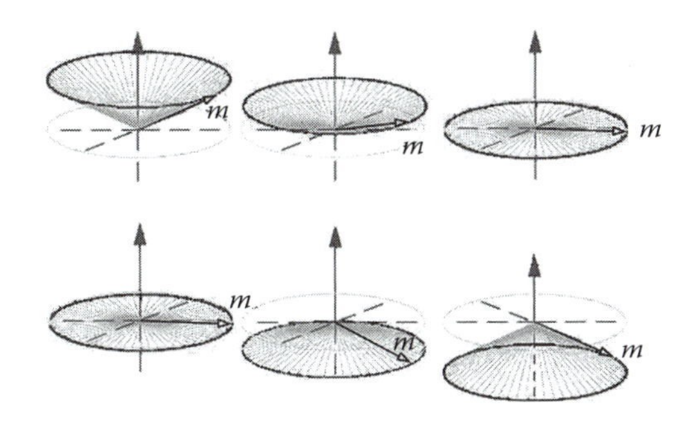

FIGURE 15.4 Precession of proton in attempt to align with external magnetic field. (Courtesy of Siemens AG, Medical Solutions, Magnetic resonance; brochure: Magnets, flows and artifacts.)

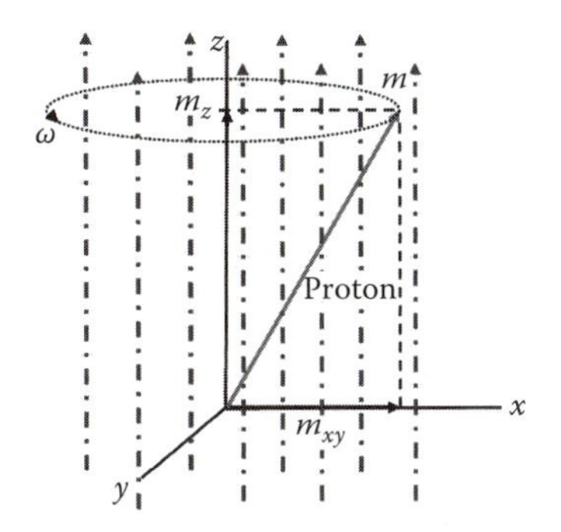

FIGURE 15.5 Principle of field application and alignment. (Courtesy of Siemens AG, Medical Solutions, Magnetic resonance; brochure: Magnets, flows and artifacts.)

The resulting magnetization vector of the proton **M** will swirl around the external magnetic field vector **H** in a spiraling motion moving closer to the direction of the external field vector with every rotation until it is aligned. This precession takes place with a particular frequency called the Larmor frequency, f_{Larmor}. The Larmor frequency is directly correlated to the magnitude of the external magnetic field expressed in units Tesla. For instance, the Lamar frequency of the aligning of hydrogen nucleus can be approximated as follows:

$$f_{Larmor} = 42.85|\mathbf{H}| \tag{15.1}$$

The Larmor frequency is specific to each element. Since hydrogen is abundant in tissue, water, and other biological molecules, hydrogen is the main element studied in NMR imaging, and the Larmor frequency of hydrogen plays a central role in NMR imaging.

During the decaying swirl, the energy difference between the natural spin orientation and the forced orientation is emitted as energy in the form of electromagnetic waves with the Larmor frequency. This electromagnetic radiation is a critically damped oscillation, as shown in Figure 15.5, giving an exponentially decaying sinusoidal wave train. The electromagnetic radiation pulse results in a magnetization alignment that emits a RF pulse of its own, which is referred to as the free induction decay (FID). This pulse can be used to identify the magnetic characteristics of the tissue under investigation.

Before discussing the image formation in MRI, we briefly describe the chemical elements that can be used as the basis for MRI. Every element with an odd number of protons produces a small magnetic field around itself. The MRI technology uses the nuclear spin of atoms with hydrogen (^1H) as the most common element. Other odd number elements that can be used in NMR imaging are sodium (^{23}Na), fluorine (^{19}F), carbon (^{13}C), phosphorus (^{31}P), potassium (K), and lithium (Li). Each atom has a nuclear spin, which is proportional to the mass and therefore the angular momentum of the nucleus. Even though the charges in larger atoms still respond to the external magnetic field, their relatively large mass can restrict their agility needed for the imaging applications. The proportionality between the charge and mass is often measured by a quantity called the gyromagnetic ratio, γ. The gyromagnetic ratio is defined as follows:

$$\gamma = \frac{q}{2m} \tag{15.2}$$

where q and m stand for the charge and the mass of the particle, respectively. Equation 15.2 is used to describe the gyromagnetic properties for hydrogen in which m is replaced by the mass of a single proton. The γ in hydrogen is relatively large, which is another reason supporting the use of hydrogen for MRI.

Due to the small magnitude and short duration of the FID signals generated by the static source, the previously described process cannot produce a practically useful image of the biological tissues. In order to create a meaningful image, another source of magnetic field that exploits the resonance phenomenon is deployed. This secondary magnetic field, which is an alternating field, creates a resonance state that allows a tomographic imaging of the body based on the physical principles of resonance, as discussed next.

15.2.1 Resonance

The static magnetic field discussed in the previous section is typically used as a "bias" field to activate the molecular units and prepare them to be stimulated by an alternating external field. When an external alternating electromagnetic field that alternates with the Larmor frequency is applied, the precession motion of the proton spin will come into resonance, and the microscopic magnetization vector will lose the equilibrium that it would have reached if the units were exposed only to the static external magnetic field.

When the alternating external electromagnetic field is lifted, the protons will realign themselves again, as the static external magnetic field is still active. The subsequent realignment will result in emission of a powerful FID signal that can be easily recorded. The amplitude of the FID signal burst is an indication of the quantity of the protons that are present in every point inside the tissue.

Since each element has its own Larmar frequency, the element that responds to the alternating field is the one whose Larmar frequency corresponds to the frequency of the field. This means that the resulting magnetic resonance happens only in the element with the Larmar frequency corresponding to the frequency of the alternative field. In many MRI systems, the frequency of the alternating field is tuned to detect the Larmar frequency of hydrogen. By scanning a range of frequencies and examining (detecting) the frequency spectrum of the emitted NMR signal or FID, one theoretically can perform a comprehensive chemical identification of the tissue. Spectral imaging will be discussed in detail later in this chapter.

To summarize the resonance process described earlier, the imaging process can be described as the following steps:

Step 1: The tissue is exposed to a homogeneous static magnetic field.
Step 2: After all protons are aligned, the imaging system exposed the sample to a train of RF pulses at the respective Larmor frequency through the tissue. This causes the molecules having protons excited by the RF pulses generate and emit FID signals.
Step 3: The emitted FID signals are collected by the magnetic detectors.

The FID signal collected in Step 3 is used to determine the total number of free protons. While the exact number of free protons in a biological medium is not very informative by itself, the relative volumetric distribution of free protons in the tissue identified by the previously described process is a very informative characteristic. Specifically, since the presence and density of protons in hydrogen and other elements can identify the distribution of molecules in the tissue. This relative volumetric distribution is therefore used to form an image of the tissue. The detection of proton density is performed using the measurement of some time intervals that are described next.

As shown in Figure 15.6, due to the external RF signal, the magnetization **M** changes the alignment and will no longer be parallel to the external field. As can be seen in Figure 15.6, the magnetization vector, instead of aligning with the static magnetic field (in blue), rotate around the z-axis with a frequency corresponding to the frequency of the external alternating field. The magnetization is split into a

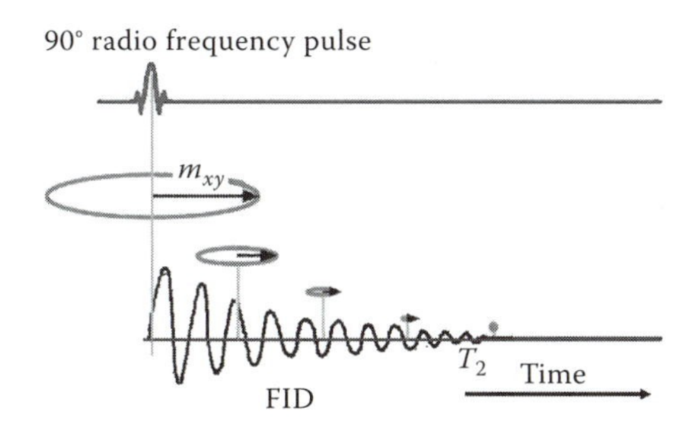

FIGURE 15.6 Disorienting RF pulse that strikes all protons out of alignment from the external magnetic field and the resulting FID RF pulse. (Courtesy of Siemens AG, Medical Solutions, Magnetic resonance; brochure: Magnets, flows and artifacts.)

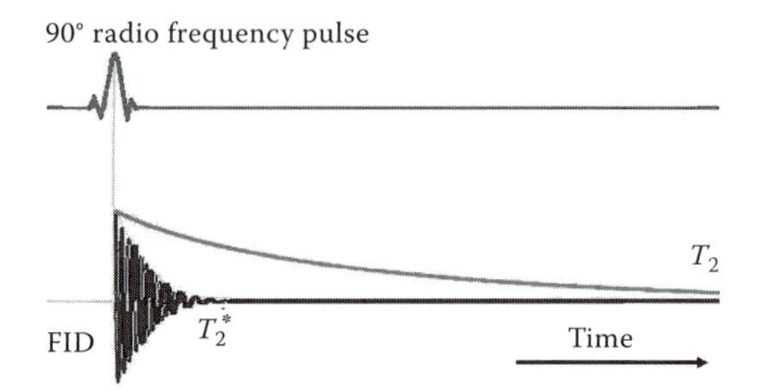

FIGURE 15.7 FID pulse with time constant T_2^* and the decay of the transverse magnetization with time constant T_2. (Courtesy of Siemens AG, Medical Solutions, Magnetic resonance; brochure: Magnets, flows and artifacts.)

transverse component, $\mathbf{M}_{xy}$, and a longitudinal component, $\mathbf{M}_z$, for signal analysis. The resulting angle between the magnetization vector and the z-axis is called the RF flip angle, or the flip angle for short.

As the RF pulse excitation is applied, the transverse component $\mathbf{M}_{xy}$ starts rotating around z-axis at a flip angle and an angular frequency corresponding to the Larmor frequency. As the excitation pulse dies, the deviation angle of the traverse component from the z-axis decreases exponentially with in time. The relaxation time of $\mathbf{M}_{xy}$ vector, i.e., the time it takes for this component to die away, is defined as the transverse relaxation time T_2, or spin–spin relaxation time. This relaxation time is shown in Figure 15.7. The decaying of the traverse magnetic vector induces an oscillating but decaying voltage that is detected by a receiver coil located around the tissue. By registering this voltage, the relaxation time T_2 is registered (Table 15.1).

The longitudinal component $\mathbf{M}_z$ also changes as the RF pulse reaches to the zero state. This component, as illustrated in Figure 15.8, becomes larger and larger until it reaches its maximum when the complete realignment with the static field is achieved. The realignment rate of the longitudinal component $\mathbf{M}_z$ is described by a longitudinal relaxation time T_1, which is called the spin-lattice relaxation time. The voltages detected by the detector coils can also identify the relaxation time T_1.

TABLE 15.1
Longitudinal and Transverse Spin Relaxation Times for Various Tissues

Tissue	T_1 (s)	T_2 (s)
Brain	0.5–1	0.06–0.1
Fat	0.2–0.7	0.05–0.09
Muscle	1–1.8	0.02–0.07

Note: T_1 and T_2 values for tissues at 1.5T Magnetic Field Strength.

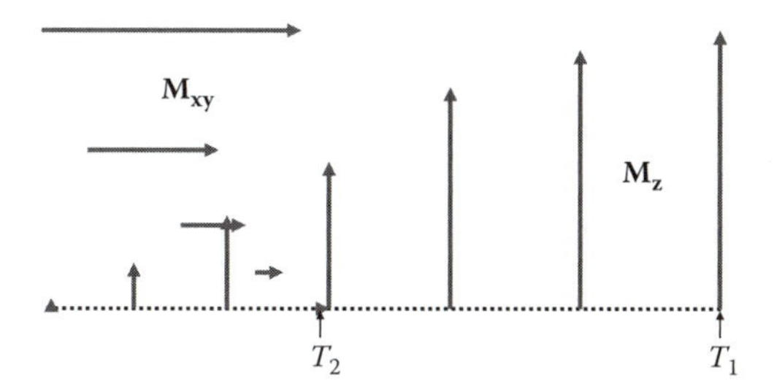

FIGURE 15.8 Schematic representation of the decaying transverse magnetization and increasing axial magnetization.

All time constants and frequencies, as described before, are nucleus specific. Note that there is no direct correlation between the decreasing transverse and the increasing longitudinal magnetization; however, $T_2 \leq T_1$ always holds true.

In many clinical MRI procedures, additional information is retrieved by introducing deliberate inhomogeneities to the tissue to be imaged. It is also customary, especially in research studies, to collect more information about the tissue simply by devising specialized electromagnetic radiation protocols and therefore creating custom-designed external magnetic fields.

15.3 MR IMAGING

In order to create a useful MR image of the tissue, one needs to identify the type of the elements at each location of the tissue by discovering the Larmor frequency of the material at each location. In practical systems, this is achieved by exposing the tissue to an inhomogeneous magnetic field. Since the magnetic field strength in different locations within the tissue volume will be different, the detected characteristic Larmor frequency at each location will identify the type of the tissue at that point. The magnetic field inhomogeneity will need to be identifiable to correlate the particular field strength with a location in the tissue volume. The traceability is accomplished by giving the magnetic field a uniform gradient across one orientation of the radius of the magnetic coil that surrounds the patient.

Assuming the gradient of the magnetic field to be in the radial direction, the magnetic field lines are pointing in the long axis of the cylindrical symmetry or the length of the patient's body. The gradient magnetic field for a typical MR imaging of the human body is illustrated in Figure 15.9. The magnetic field points in the z-direction, and the magnetic field intensity vector is described in magnitude by

$$|H| = H_0 + G_x \tag{15.3}$$

where

$$G_x = k_1 \cdot x \tag{15.4}$$

In the preceding equations, G_x is the magnetic field gradient in the x-direction, k_1 is a constant, and H_0 is the homogeneous external magnetic field. The term $k_1 \cdot x$ describes the gradient in the magnetic field superimposed on the constant field H_0 in the x-direction.

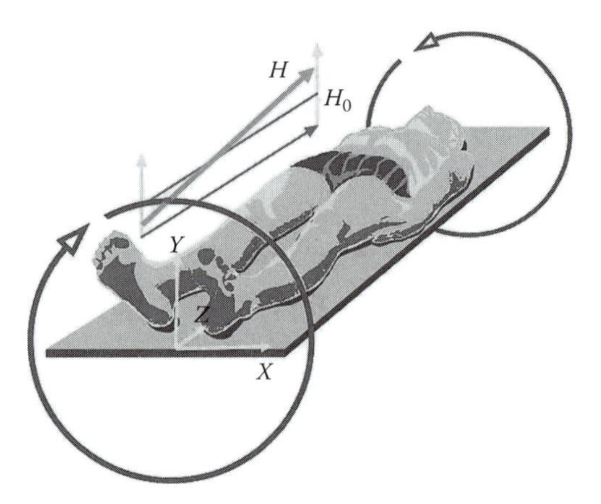

FIGURE 15.9 Magnetic field gradient diagram. (Courtesy of Siemens AG, Medical Solutions, Magnetic resonance; brochure: Magnets, flows and artifacts.)

The Larmor frequency will now be a function of position as expressed by combining Equations 15.5 and 15.6:

$$f_{Larmor} = f_0 + k_2 \cdot x \tag{15.5}$$

where k_2 is a constant.

When an RF pulse with frequency f_R is sent through the patient, only the protons in the locations that obey the following restriction will come into resonance at any given time:

$$x = \frac{f_R - f_0}{k_2} = \frac{f}{k_2} \tag{15.6}$$

where $f = f_R - f_0$.

It has to be emphasized that only the hydrogen nuclei that obey the condition stated in Equation 15.9 will emit the FID signal after the external RF pulse is removed. This will select a slice of the patient's body for imaging based on the frequency f_R, as illustrated in Figure 15.10.

Immediately after the FID signal has been collected, the gradient of the magnetic field is rotated over a 90° angle. A common way of applying the magnetic field is by rotation of the field gradient over 90° and, after a delay time T_D, rotating the field gradient back to the original direction and acquiring the FID signal. This process produces an external magnetic field with the gradient in the direction of the y-axis formulated by Equation 15.11:

$$|H| = H_0 + G_y \tag{15.7}$$

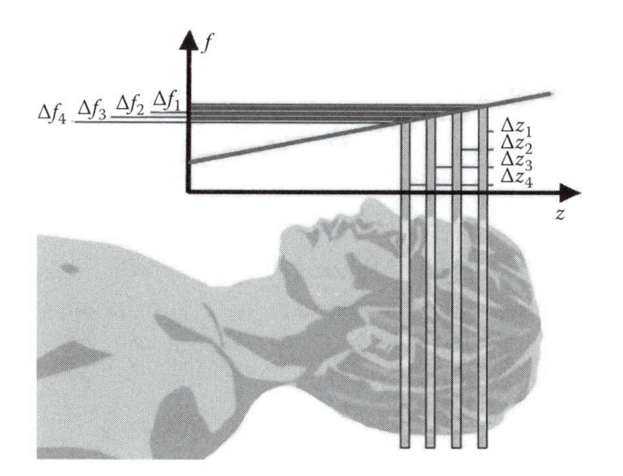

FIGURE 15.10 Slice selection algorithm. (Courtesy of Siemens AG, Medical Solutions, Magnetic resonance; brochure: Magnets, flows and artifacts.)

where the magnetic field gradient in the y-direction is given as

$$G_y = k_3 \cdot y \tag{15.8}$$

This y-direction gradient is also detected using the shift in the Larmor frequency as described for the x-direction gradient. The same procedure is also repeated for a gradient field in z-direction and the FID signal is measured. This procedure is shown in Figure 15.11. Note that the constant homogenous magnetic field, H_0, does not change direction during this procedure, and only the field strength gradient is allowed to change.

In order to utilize the small differences between T_1 and T_2 time intervals to form images with emphasized characteristics, parameters such as repetition time and flip

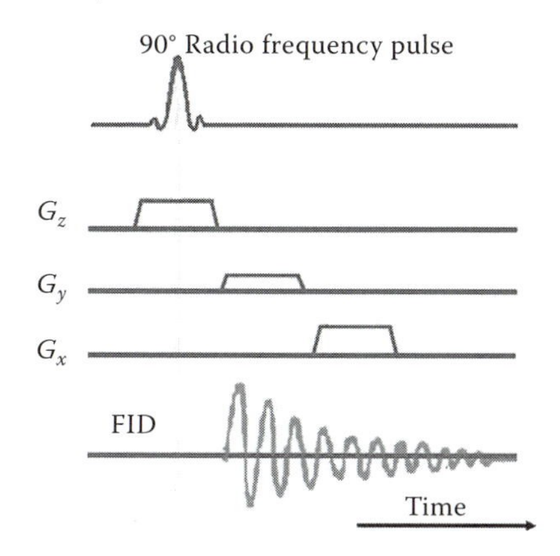

FIGURE 15.11 Phase coding of various magnetic field gradients to produce a FID signal that can be traced to a particular location. (Courtesy of Siemens AG, Medical Solutions, Magnetic resonance; brochure: Magnets, flows and artifacts.)

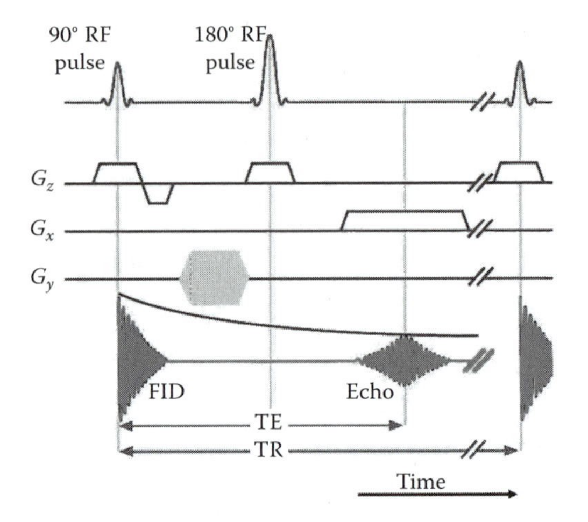

FIGURE 15.12 Pulse resonance imaging algorithm. (Courtesy of Siemens AG, Medical Solutions, Magnetic resonance; brochure: Magnets, flows and artifacts.)

angle (α) can be applied to create images referred to as T_1-weighted imaging and T_2-weighted imaging. T_1-weighted imaging can be used to obtain images of a relatively high anatomical definition, while T_2-weighted imaging is a sensitive method for pathology and disease detection based on the metabolic feedback through the decay of the perpendicular magnetic component. Many disease states are characterized by a representative change of the tissue's transverse relaxation time value.

By repeating the same procedure after rotating the magnetic field gradient over a few degrees each time, the details at the intersections of the various gradient vectors can be retrieved. A schematic representation of this principle is outlined in Figure 15.12. The acquired RF FID signal will need to undergo spectral analysis to correlate all the different frequencies emitted from the different locations to the coordinates within a slice of the body. The image derived from the spectral signal distribution represents the localized proton distribution in a 2-D cross section. In the resulting image, the hydrogen proton distribution will outline the water concentration dissemination within the biological organism. Bone will generally not show up in NMR imaging.

The magnetic gradient, e.g., the gradient in the y-direction, is always applied in pulsed format. The pulse is amplitude or duration modulated in 256 discreet stages to acquire a representative FID. The discretization of the magnetic gradient in fact labels the spins by phase information. Due to this labeling, the position information can be extracted in a unique fashion. As the nuclear spins revert to the same frequency along the y-direction after the short gradient pulse, the phase difference at each discrete point is recorded and compared. As a result, there will be 256 FIDs each with 256 sampling points, which provide 256^2 pixels. Subsequently, this process is repeated a specific number of times to filter out physiological artifacts and noise.

If the RF field is applied for a finite time (pulse) the magnetization vector can be tipped through any desired angle. The angle the magnetization vector **M** makes with the magnetic field vector H depends on the product of the magnetic field intensity and the time frame of interaction (the pulse duration). Most commonly, the angles are perpendicular or antagonistic: $\alpha = 90°$ or $\alpha = 180°$, which are appropriately referred to as 90° pulse and 180° pulse, respectively. Note that the radiofrequency coils in the NMR devices are designed to produce magnetization only in the *x–y* plane and only detect magnetization in the *x–y* plane as well. The key to MR imaging is the design of pulse sequences, which are applied in order to obtain images with desired contrast.

If a 90° pulse followed by an 180° pulse produces an entirely different spectral profile. The detected spectrum will be observed at a characteristic echo time delay, *TE*, which is twice the time interval between the two respective pulses. The sequence of RF pulse delivery and FID acquisition is illustrated in Figure 15.12.

While MRI is often used to create images identifying the anatomical features of the biological tissues, it has the potential to image metabolic activities. Such a specialized MR imaging is called functional MRI (*f*MRI). *f*MRI is typically used to generate maps of brain function and localize regions with increase metabolic activity such as tumors. We will discuss *f*MRI and its applications after reviewing the reconstruction methods used to form MR images.

15.4 FORMULATION OF MRI RECONSTRUCTION

An MR image is generally reconstructed using the Fourier slice theorem described in the previous chapters. During the tomography process, the signals produced by the inhomogeneity of the tissues are processed using signal processing methods. This process creates an image of the tissue as function of space. As described in the previous chapters, the computational processes involved in the Fourier slice theorem are primary performed using the discrete Fourier transform or DFT.

Following the 90° shift in magnetic field gradient, the characteristic FID pulse can be acquired. At time $t = 0$, the nuclear spins will be aligned with the magnetization M along the *z*-direction. This condition is referred to as thermal equilibrium. During the pulse, the magnetization vector will be tipped into the *x–y* plane by an oscillating field: $H = H_0 \cos(\omega t)$. When the RF pulse is switched off, the magnetization will precess and the measured value in the *x–y* plane will exhibit a damped oscillation type signal. The *x–y* projection of the magnetization as a function of time is the FID signal. The FID signal is the result of many nuclear spins decaying simultaneously while observing their projection in the *x–y* plane, which converges to zero. This net *x–y* projection is inherent to the fact that all nuclei will experience a slightly different magnetic field and will thus experience a different precession frequency. Additionally, the magnetization will attempt to return to its prior equilibrium that was at zero net magnetization. Using the rotating frame of reference, where the reference frame rotates with the RF frequency, the magnetization spins will have a frequency that is slightly off from this RF frequency. By measuring the difference in frequency, the detection process is simplified dramatically. The magnetization can now be written for both the *x–y* and *z*-projections using the time constant of the transverse component of the magnetic field, T_2^*. In the x–y plane, the magnetization is expressed in Equation 15.9:

$$\mathbf{M_{xy}} = \mathbf{M_0} e^{-t/T_2^*} \tag{15.9}$$

The declining axial magnetic moment is expressed similarly, except with the time constant of the relaxation of the longitudinal field, T_1. The difference between the steady-state magnetic field and the changing axial component is provided in Equation 15.10:

$$\mathbf{M_0} - \mathbf{M_z} = \mathbf{M_0} e^{-t/T_1} \tag{15.10}$$

In general, the following holds true: $T_1 > T_2^*$. This means that the x–y projection of the magnetization decays faster than the difference.

Based on this information, it is clear that the FID contains all the information of the NMR signal.

The RF pulse is repeated many times, which provides a platform for averaging. The averaging process will increase the signal-to-noise ratio and will give a representation that is relatively true to the process of what the signal should look like, since physiological effects are canceled out this way as well. The frequency spectrum of the MRI signal will have two characteristics of importance: line width and chemical shift.

One particularly interesting spectrum arises from water molecules in the neighborhood of proteins or other large molecules, commonly found in biological media. The water with large molecules gives a very broad frequency spectrum. In addition, the precession of the magnetization vector in the y-direction can be written as the result of two influences acting on it:

$$\mathbf{M_y} = \mathbf{M_0} e^{-t/T_2^*} \tag{15.11}$$

and

$$\frac{1}{T_2^*} = \frac{1}{T_2} + \frac{\gamma \Delta H_0}{2} \tag{15.12}$$

The term $1/T_2$ represents the dephasing of spins as a result of the local magnetic fields produced by neighboring spin systems, and the term $\gamma \Delta H_0/2$ represents the dephasing due to the localized inhomogeneous magnetic field across the biological sample.

An exponentially decaying magnetization vector in the time domain will display a single broad frequency band in the frequency domain. A damped harmonic oscillation in the time domain will have a spectrum of two broad peaks in the frequency domain. This can be seen from the complex FT:

$$f(t) = \int F(\omega) e^{-i\omega t} d\omega \tag{15.13}$$

Here, we briefly present a simplified version of the reconstruction method, specialized toward the MR images. To have a simpler notation, we restrict ourselves to the one-dimensional (1-D) case where we would like to find the proton density along a line. Note that the time frequency of the precision in the FID signal is directly proportional to the magnetic field strength, where the angular frequency and the standard frequency are linked as described in Equation 15.15:

$$\omega = 2\pi f \tag{15.14}$$

specifically,

$$\omega_x = \gamma x G_x \tag{15.15}$$

Now, if the density of the proton at each point is shown as $\rho(x)$, the measured signal $f(t)$ is related to this intensity according to the following simplified line integral:

$$f(t) = \int_x \rho(x) e^{-i\gamma x G_x t} dx \tag{15.16}$$

This is a typical tomographic equation. In the previous chapter, we described how the Fourier slice theorem can be used to solve such equations. The preceding equation can be interpreted as a Fourier relationship between FID in the time domain $f(t)$ and a spin density profile along the x-direction.

Typical MR images files are often limited to 256 × 256 pixel matrices. In these cases, the pixel size is in the order of 1 mm. The third dimension introduced by the slice thickness can range from 1 to 10 mm. Larger matrix arrays are becoming available in the order of 512 × 512 pixels that provide better resolution. Image resolution is steadily falling below 1 mm. Under MRI, the gray matter appears in the medium range of gray values on T_1-weighted images. Under MRI, the white matter then has higher amplitudes than the gray matter.

Knowing the physical concepts of MRI and the general reconstructions methods applied to form the images, we will next focus on *f*MRI and its applications.

Examples of various imaging techniques and 3-D rendering of the inner ear are illustrated in Figure 15.13.

15.5 FUNCTIONAL MRI

A major field of study in medicine is the study of the function(s) of each part of the brain. The "brain mapping" has been the main ultimate goal of neuroscience as well as cognitive science. While sometimes researcher would like to know the functions of a specific part of the brain, the reverse question has been more intriguing: If we focus on one specific function, such as visual recognition, how can we identify the parts of the brain that are directly involved in the process?

The *f*MRI is in principle the best tool available to perform brain mapping. This technology allows observing the brain while a certain task is performed. The parts

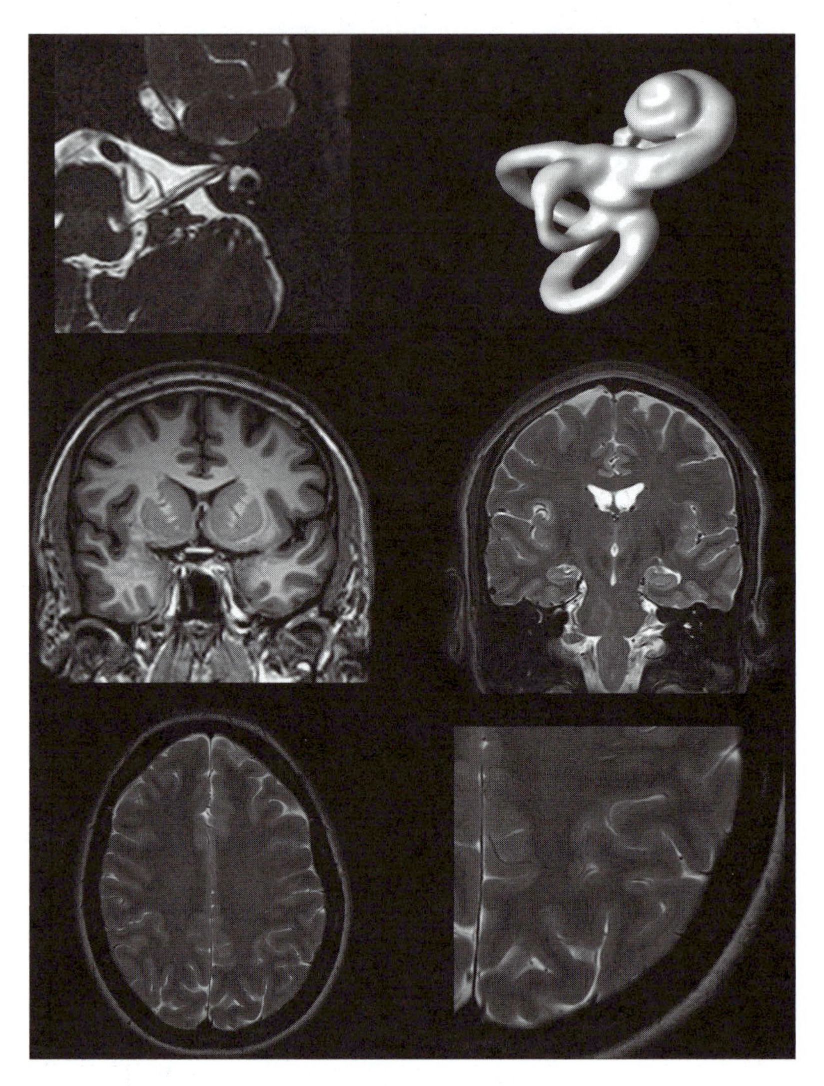

FIGURE 15.13 Examples of sections of brain and head and neck scans including 3-D rendering applied to the inner ear. (Courtesy of Philips Medical Systems.)

of the brain that are activated in the collected MR images are then associated to the performed task. Since any function in all cells including neurons is associated with the consumption of the oxygen contained in blood, the monitoring of the functional activities of the neurons is in principle equivalent to the detection of oxygen consumption. In the early 1990s, it was discovered that the oxygenation level of blood will act as a contrast agent in MRI. This discovery forms the basis of *f*MRI as it is used in present day.

The MRI contrast around blood vessels can be attributed to the state of oxygenation. Specifically, deoxyhemoglobin is more paramagnetic than oxyhemoglobin, which has almost the same magnetic susceptibility as most tissues. This observation led to the use of deoxyhemoglobin as a contrast agent for most *f*MRI methods.

The reason functional imaging can be achieved by detecting the oxygenated blood roots in the physiology of the biological tissues. For instance, neuronal function has a metabolic activity that is directly related to changes of the oxygenation state of the neurons as follows. The oxyhemoglobin carries the oxygen to the neurons, and, during the metabolic activity of the nerve cells, the oxygen uptake by the neurons causes oxyhemoglobin to change into deoxyhemoglobin. In addition, neurons require glycogen, obtained from the red blood cells, for their metabolic processes during electric activity. The glucose uptake can be measured with the chemical fluorodeoxyglucose (FDG) that has an intrinsic magnetic moment and is incorporated in the cellular metabolism as regular glucose. The oxygen and glucose requirement by the neurons during cellular depolarization activity has as a direct consequence an increased blood perfusion in the capillaries surrounding the nerve cells.

The exact *f*MRI procedure is designed based on the functional characteristics to be evaluated to ensure that there is a reasonable correlation between these characteristics and certain traceable metabolic aspects. For instance, if the motor-control activities of the brain need to be evaluated, the patient will be asked to move a toe or a finger while the system collects data.

One issue in the task design is the concern that the sequence of the tasks assigned to the patient must be in a specific order to derive a correlation between the brain activities and a particular cognitive or motor task. An additional requirement is that any inappropriate and unrelated actions must be filtered out by this methodology. Other typical examples of specific tasks involve audio or visual input stimuli to evoke a cognitive response in the brain.

Two commonly used methods apply a fast data acquisition protocol to reduce the errors from lapses in attention or motion artifacts. The first method is called fast low angle shot (FLASH). During FLASH imaging, there is a short interval between the *f*MRI RF pulses. This short interval reduces the flip angle and consequently reduces the realignment rate, T_1. As a result, the acquisition sequence can be accelerated. The second method is echo planar imaging (EPI). EPI applies small amplitude RF pulses combined with a high gradient in the magnetic field. The steep gradient provides better contrast and faster acquisition with typical acquisition times under 100 ms. The low intensity and high gradient have the disadvantage of introducing distortions and a low signal amplitude. In particular, in the brain, the magnetic inhomogeneities start playing a significant role in the image formation. However, due to EPI's speed, it is one of the most commonly used techniques in *f*MRI.

15.5.1 BOLD MRI

The oxygen consumption increases only slightly during the metabolic activity of neurons. This means that in such cellular activities the oxyhemoglobin-to-deoxyhemoglobin ratio changes only marginally. This has led to more specialized versions of *f*MRI procedures for functional brain imaging. This type of imaging falls in a class of its own that is named after the principles of the technique. Blood oxygenation level dependent (BOLD) contrast imaging uses the disparity in magnetic properties of oxygenated (diamagnetic) and deoxygenated (paramagnetic) blood.

The BOLD technique relies on the fact that a localized change in blood flow is observed when the brain neurons are activated and, consequently, the local oxygenation levels change. This increase in oxygenation and hence a decrease of deoxyhemoglobin level results in a change in the MR decay parameter, T_2^*, that can be measured. These blood flow and oxygenation changes on both vascular and intracellular level have a temporary delay with respect to the neural depolarization sequence of the cell. This time lag between the physical change in oxygenation level and actual neural activity is identified as hemodynamic lag.

A BOLD MRI representation of vascular imaging is shown in Figure 15.14.

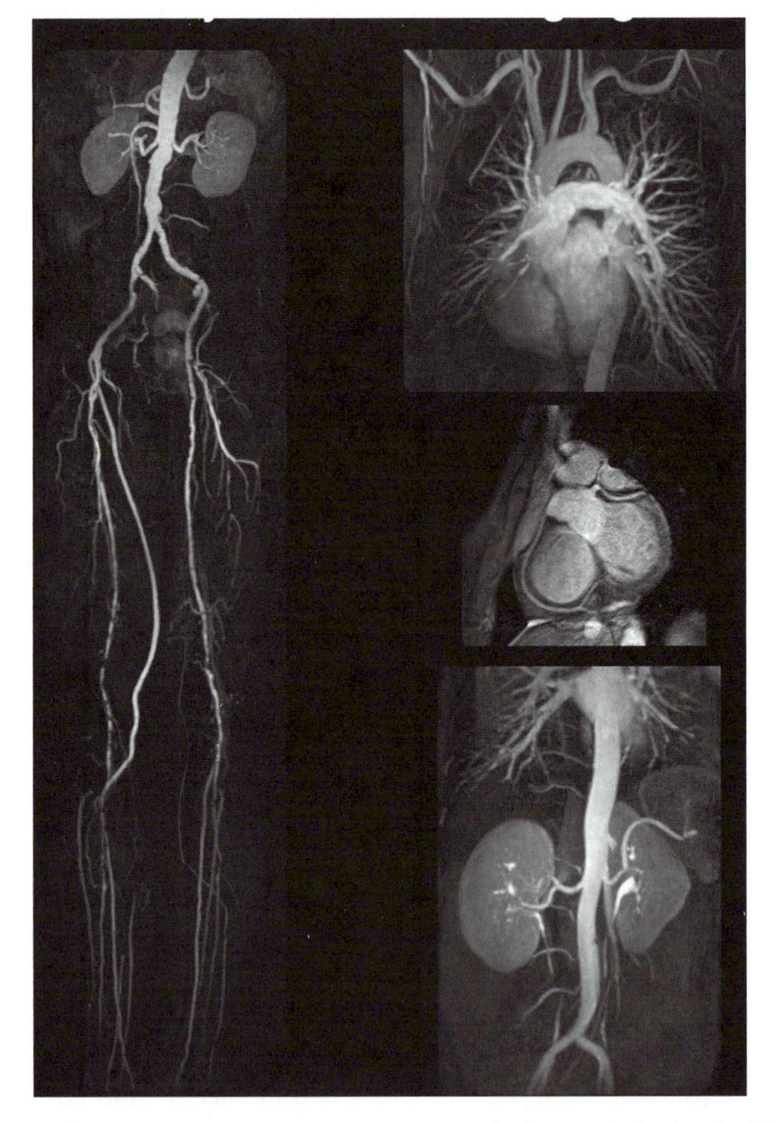

FIGURE 15.14 Spectroscopic MRI whole-body vascular image obtained under 3 T magnetic field strength imaging conditions. (Courtesy of Philips Medical Systems.)

15.6 APPLICATIONS OF MRI AND *f*MRI

Pathological conditions and injuries can be revealed with great detail based on T_1 and T_2 weighing. Some examples of the diagnostic use are the localization of tumors and identification of internal hemorrhaging. Knowing that MRI is rather harmless, this technology can be used for practically all applications described for x-ray CT and many applications in which ultrasound imaging is used for. However, the cost of performing MRI and the fact that during the acquisition of MRI, the patient is expected to stay still are limiting the actual usage of this technology.

Another factor that limits the use of MRI for certain applications such as intraoperational imaging is the fact that ferromagnetic tools cannot be used in the MRI room. In other words, while it is desirable to conduct MRI while the surgery is performed, the typical tools used in surgery cannot be used in the same room MRI is taken. Surgery tools made of titanium can be used in the MRI room, but due to the high cost of such tools, they are not used in typical surgeries.

Due to the substantial similarities between the applications of x-ray CT and MRI, the specific applications of MRI in acquiring anatomical information are not described in detail, and, rather, we focus on the main applications of *f*MRI.

Typical examples of the clinical applications of *f*MRI predominantly revolve around the detection of focal neuron depolarization in the brain. Specific conditions involved with focal neuronal activity are in visual, auditory, sensory motor, and language activities. For most of these functions, the typical locations of the cortical activity are known. *f*MRI is used to aid the diagnosis of certain diseases such as epilepsy, schizophrenia, Alzheimer's, Parkinson's, intracranial lesions, depression, and hearing impairment. Location and identification of brain tumors is also a clinical issue that can be resolved with *f*MRI. Some of the activities are further described in the following.

A representative NMR image of the neurovascular activity is presented in Figure 15.15.

15.6.1 *f*MRI for Monitoring Audio Activities of Brain

Specific auditory tasks are presented while a subject is inside the MRI machine, and the changes in blood supply to the areas of the brain that apparently are active in data processing will become evident.

Auditory stimuli can be voice or language recognition or purely sound perception. Examples of auditory tasks are the delivery of sound burst with a particular frequency pattern (tonotopic), sound burst with amplitude variations (amplitopic), evoked response type of stimuli using short sentences with or without rhyme, and additional audio–speech combination assignments. Images will need to be obtained in a relatively fast algorithm in the order of five images per second to be able to recognize significant differences in the cortical activity. A period of rest with no input is required between each assignment for calibration purposes, while the data acquisition is maintained at the same rate.

The auditory region of the cortex is predominantly located in the frontal section of the brain and in the temporal section in a lesser degree. The studies of the auditory

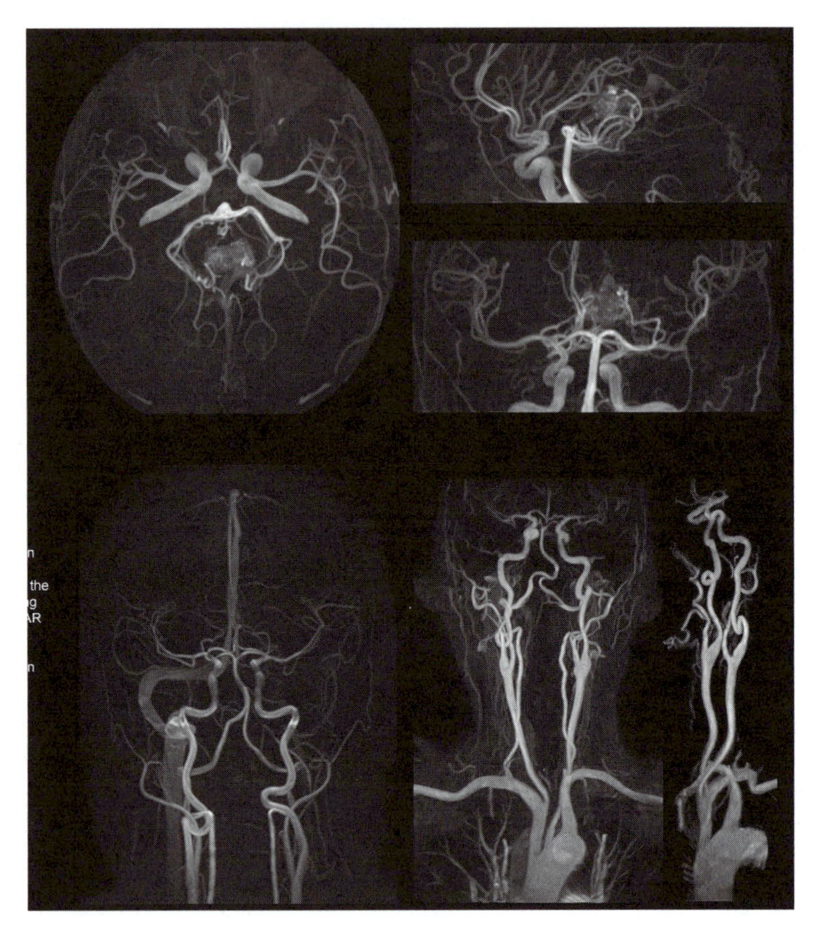

FIGURE 15.15 Spectroscopic neurovascular MRI scan under 3T magnetic field strength imaging conditions. (Courtesy of Philips Medical Systems.)

cortex will not only help identify hearing impaired–related problems but also aid in the diagnosis of certain types of dyslexia.

In dyslexia studies, the regions of the cortex under investigation are focused on the frontal and temporal cortex. The temporal cortex is more involved in the data processing part of the auditory input, and this is where the *f*MRI changes will show significant differences when compared to the *f*MRI scans of control subjects.

15.6.2 *f*MRI for Monitoring Motoneuron Activities of Brain

As in other cortical monitoring, *f*MRI is the most appropriate way to obtain any significant information on the motor cortex activity of the brain.

The motor neuron activity can be determined by means of evoked potential recordings resulting from specific motor tasks. These tasks are designed based on the clinical concerns about the patient. Assignments would involve, for instance, hand, foot, finger, or two motions in a predetermined grid pattern with one or two

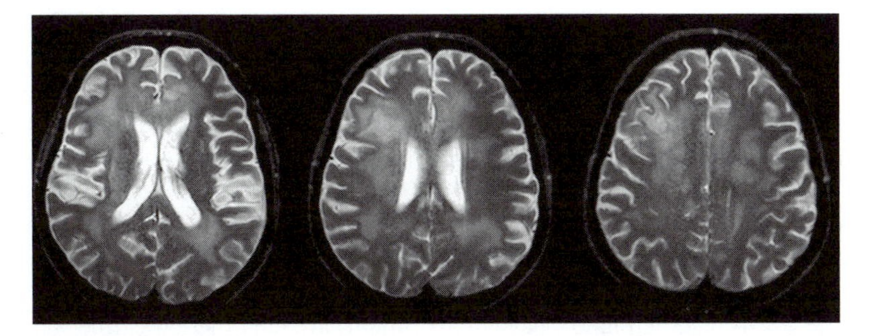

FIGURE 15.16 Nuclear isotope MRI brain slice selection, showing temporal lobe activity related to the jaw, mouth, and throat. (Courtesy of Philips Medical Systems.)

degrees of freedom. The recorded *f*MRI scans will indicate the cortical activation and identify the root of the problem.

Figure 15.16 illustrates the cortical activity following an evoked response resulting from swallowing; no other regions of the brain appear to be active, which excludes speech.

15.6.3 *f*MRI for Monitoring Visual Cortex Activities

In *f*MRI of the visual cortex, it is customary to provide the patient with a checkerboard of black and white squares that can change pattern configuration to examine the changes in the activities of the voxels in the posterior side of the brain. The cortical region on the occipital lobe of the brain that is involved in visual perception is often referred to as the visual cortex.

Depending on the clinical status of the patient, other types of stimuli are used to evaluate the response of the visual cortex. Different levels of visual impairments and their neuronal roots are identified using such test. The *f*MRI of the visual cortex is the typical next clinical diagnostic stage after applying the evoked potential EEG studies described in Chapter 10.

15.7 PROCESSING AND FEATURE EXTRACTION OF MRI

All image processing features described in Part I of the book are applied for analysis of the regions identified in typical MR images. The majority of these methods are the same methods used in the analysis of x-ray CT images. The only difference is that MR images have much higher resolution and are much less noisy compared to typical x-ray CT images.

As mentioned earlier, the resolution of MR images in the z-direction is much less than the planar resolution. This is due to the fact that after taking each slice image, the patient bed is moved slightly and a new slice image is captured. Due to physical size of the sensors as well as the dimensions of the bed, the fineness of the bed movement is limited. This in turn limits the z-direction resolution. In MR image processing, it is common practice to use interpolation methods to use the information contained in two neighboring slice to estimate a slice between the two slices.

Even though the estimated slice is not truly measured during the data acquisition process, if the estimation is a reliable one, this process doubles the resolution in the *z*-direction. A common estimation method use for MR image interpolation is the simple averaging of the pixels in the two slices around the estimated slice.

Another commonly used group of MR image processing methods are the algorithms used to register MR images with the images captured by other modalities such as positron emission tomography (PET). The registration process between MRI and other image modalities is described in more detail later in this chapter.

Processing of *f*MR images are often not based on the image regions. Rather, when the voxels responding to a particular stimulus are identified, the time signals of these voxels collected throughout the experiment are treated as 1-D signals and are analyzed using methods such as DFT and discrete wavelet transform (DWT). The feature extraction methods applied for the analysis of these time signals are exactly the same as those applied for processing of the evoked potential EEG recordings.

15.7.1 Sources of Noise and Filtering Methods in MRI

Even though the overall resolution and signal-to-noise ratio of the MR images are very high, there are several distinct sources of noise that can be identified in MRI technology. These sources are thermal noise, subject motion, physiological activity, low frequency drift, spontaneous neural and vascular fluctuations, shear and strain noise, and artifacts arising from rapid imaging methods.

Thermal noise results from the fact that temperature is a form of kinetic energy of atoms and molecules. The nuclear spin orientation of certain individual molecules and atoms may, as a result, be affected by the heat produced by the MRI machine and the fact that the patient is enveloped by the MRI machine, retaining some heat produced by the patient's body.

The scanning process relies on the assumption that detected spins stem from one particular location that does not change in time. Any motion by the patient will disturb the location registration algorithm and will produce a motion artifact. The main noise and artifacts that need compensation are often motion artifacts. When MRI is taken, patients are supposed to stay still, but, in reality, it is often the case that during the long duration of the data acquisition process, patients do move. This is more significant in children or claustrophobic patients who are not comfortable inside the MRI machine. This makes motion artifacts the main sources of noise in MRI. Motion artifact is often removed using deblurring filters described in Part I of the book as well as more specialized filters designed for this purpose.

The main share of the physiological noise originates from breathing, additionally heartbeat, and peristaltic motions. A rather more fundamental source of noise deals with the way the actual readings are collected. As a general rule, when scanning thinner slices of the tissue, higher levels of noise are registered by the detectors. As a result, if thin slices of images are needed, often the dose of the enhancer agents needs to be adjusted. In many applications, image improvements must be obtained by using an experimentally optimized dose that balances contrast and saturation.

Nerve tone changes and nervous twitches can result from adaptation and irritation and may not be avoided. This type of noise will need to be recognized as spontaneous neural fluctuations during diagnostic measurements. Fat tissue can be a source of shear and stress, which momentarily result in a change in magnetic spin orientation. This phenomenon is referred to as shear and strain noise. Rapid imaging will put a strain on the Nyquist theorem resulting in image distortions resulting from slow magnetic orientation response and slow sampling rate.

The main methods used for denoising of the MR images are soft and hard thresholding of the wavelet coefficients as introduced in Part I of the book. Another popular filtering method of the wavelet coefficients applies statistical methods. Filtering of the wavelet coefficients using statistical analysis is frequently performed in two stages. The first stage detects the presence of the signal by applying a χ^2-test. The second stage entails thresholding of the individual coefficients of the remaining subbands by applying a two-tailed Z-test. Wavelet transform (WT) of *f*MRI signals in the time domain can selectively remove unwanted introduction of temporal autocorrelations.

15.7.2 Feature Extraction

Geometrical features of an object in MR images can be easily captured using measures such as area, eccentricity, compactness, and so on. Since MR images have texture details of objects such as tumors, several texture measures as the variance of the gray levels of the pixels within the object can be used to represent texture. Geometrical features together with texture measures are often sufficient to identify the majority of malignant and benign tumors from MR images.

All DFT, DCT, and DWT decomposition methods discussed in the previous chapters are used for feature extraction from MR images. DFT coefficients in high frequencies are used to capture the texture of the objects under study. Wavelet methods are heavily used for both MRI filtering and feature extraction. The wavelet features are often the wavelet coefficients (or the second power of the coefficients) at different scales. These coefficients, however, need to be selected to represent the true information in the image and not the additive noise.

15.8 COMPARISON OF MRI WITH OTHER IMAGING MODALITIES

As mentioned earlier, the resolution of MRI is relatively higher than other image modalities. In addition, MR technology allows both anatomical imaging (regular MRI) and functional imaging (*f*MRI) of the biological tissues. Other technologies often are used either for anatomical imaging or for functional imaging. Moreover, unlike some other technologies, including x-ray CT, MRI is known to pose to harm on the biological tissues.

Another difference between MRI and CT imaging is the fact that MRI can be performed in any arbitrary slice orientations, while CT imaging is performed in axial direction only. This difference has an impact on image registration. For registration purposes, the CT and MRI scan will need to be in the same field of view to assure the best possible matches. Frequently, this can only be accomplished if the decision to perform both CT and MRI is made in advance. MRI does not image bone, while x-ray CT will image predominantly bone tissues.

15.9 REGISTRATION WITH MR IMAGES

The registration with MR images can be done for two purposes. Frequently, patients are imaged with various image modalities for one single diagnostic application. The first reason for registration roots in the fact while MRI provides some functional information, there are as significant amount of functional information captured by other modalities such as PET that need to be superimposed on the anatomical images. As a typical example, it is known that the anatomical details as well as the resolution of PET images are very limited, and, often, it is necessary to superimpose the functional information of PET on MRI or CT.

The second reason to perform registration is the need to register different MR images captured with different MR machines or even with the same machine at different times. More specifically, sometimes multiple imaging sessions on the same or different MRI machines are scheduled to track progress and document changes following a treatment. In *f*MRI, it is also customary to acquire a series of images in one session under different conditions (e.g., investigating evoked responses or metabolic parameters). Knowing that each time the exact position of the patient as well as the exact calibration of the machine might be different, one needs to register these multiple images with each other. In order to do so, often the polynomial registration methods, as explained in Part I of the book, are used. These methods often require tie points to calculate the mapping between the two images.

One popular method in providing the tie points is through the use of external markers. However, external markers may sometimes interfere with the coils in the MRI device. An additional factor of concern is the external markers' position with respect to the biological medium that is being imaged. Specifically, the MRI machine has a limited field of view, and the markers may fall outside this view. Other issues are distortion of the markers due to the location with respect to the sensors and shadow imaging of the markers, which may hide biological points of reference.

In the cases where the use of external markers may not be a feasible option, computational registration methods are applied that apply the counter of solid objects such as the skull for registration. In such a procedure, the corresponding locations on the skull bone in both imaging modalities are identified and registered. Then, the rest of the pixels in the two images are registered using the same mapping that maps the contour of the skull in the two images.

When registering MRI with PET, the image sizes play an important role. The typical MRI machines usually generate 256 × 256 image matrices, and the more advanced MRI systems even produce 512 × 512 matrices. PET, on the other hand, typically has image of 128 × 128 pixels. Each pixel in PET slices often represents a region with the areas of 2–8 mm^2. The PET slice thickness depends mostly on the hardware used. The gray-level range of PET is also significantly less than that of MRI. These differences call for registration methods to superimpose PET on MRI that address the differences of the two technologies both in the special and gray-level resolutions. Such registration methods are often specialized to accurately map certain objects in the brain in the two modalities. One biological object of interest in registration is the gray matter of the brain.

Another image registration technique used for comparing PET and MRI relies on physiological matches, since both MRI and PET have the capability to extract certain physiological data. Especially in tumor location, the MRI and PET can identify malignant tumors from healthy tissue, although PET is known to have a slightly better confidence rating in malignancy determination.

15.10 SUMMARY

MRI relies on the free movement of odd protons in a nucleus. MRI provides the highest resolution among all imaging modalities used for biomedical applications. The use of deoxyhemoglobin as a marker is used in an imaging technique called BOLD contrast imaging. This method is very useful in mapping brain activity and constitutes the fundamental idea of *f*MRI. MR images are often registered with images captured with other modalities such as PET to provide the anatomical resolution to the functional information of other modalities.

PROBLEMS

15.1 Read the image in file "p_15_1.jpg" and display the image. This is a dorsal look of a frontal plane view of a chest MRI showing a section of the heart. The heart is indicated by an arrow.

   a. Improve the quality of the image using a high-boost filter.
   b. Choose a convenient location in the region the heart and use seed growing to find the outline of the heart.* Start with a seed in the center of the supposed structure of the heart.

15.2 Read the image in file "p_15_2.jpg" and show the image. This is a dorsal look of a frontal plane view of the heart.* This image is taken from the same patient during the same imaging session as "p_15_1.jpg," approximately 7 mm posterior.

   a. Use seed growing to outline the bone structures in both images. Start with a seed in the center of the supposed bone structure.
   b. Select some tie points in the two images and register image "p_15_2.jpg" with respect to image "p_15_1.jpg."

15.3 Read the image in file "p_15_3.gif" and display it. The file contains MR images of the spine from various angles and cross sections.†

   a. Split the six images.
   b. Use a high-boot filter to improve the quality of the images.
   c. In the two images where the spine and the vertebrae are most visible, choose a seed point in the middle of the vertebrae for each disk to start the region growing process.
   d. Calculate the size of the gaps between the vertebrae in the same manner.
   e. Find the angle between the disks in the lower section of the image. The vertebrae interdisk angle has important clinical applications for diagnosing certain back problems and herniated disks.

---

* Courtesy of Dr. Godtfred Holmvang, posted on PhysioBank. http://www.physionet.org/physiobank/
† Courtesy of Philips Medical Systems.

15.4 Read the image in file "p_15_4.jpg" and display it. The file on the left contains MR images of the feet, and the right side shows the ankle.*

a. Split the two images.
b. Use both Canny and the Laplacian of Gaussian edge detection method to find the boundaries of the femur. Compare the edge detection results.
c. Choose a seed point in the middle of the bones in the foot each region to start the region growing process.
d. Find the spaces between the bones in the same manner.

15.5 Read images "p_15_5.jpg" and display it. Image "p_15_5.jpg" is an MR image of the brain with activity in the visual cortex of the brain.* The left side is a posterior view, and the image on the right is an axial view in the caudal direction with the eyes on top.

a. Split the two images.
b. Use the Laplacian of Gaussian edge detection method to find the boundaries of the active region indicated by the blue arrows (the BOLD section).
c. Choose a seed point in the middle of the visual activity section to start the region growing process.

15.6 Read the image in file "p_15_6.jpg" and display it. The file contains MR images of the knee, with a detail of the meniscus on the left.* Both images are axial views.

a. Split the two images.
b. Use the Laplacian of Gaussian edge detection method to find the boundaries of the meniscus.
c. Choose a seed point in the middle of the bones in the knee each region to start the region growing process.
d. Find the spaces between the bones in the same manner.

---

* Courtesy of Philips Medical Systems.

16 Ultrasound Imaging

16.1 INTRODUCTION AND OVERVIEW

Ultrasound is a method that uses sound waves to interact with tissues and act as the energy source for image formation. The ultrasound interaction in this manner determines specific characteristics of the tissue response to sound waves. Sound waves are mechanical, longitudinal waves that travel through matter. In longitudinal waves, the motion of the mechanism that forms the wave (e.g., particles and molecules) is parallel to the direction of wave propagation.

The motion of sound waves is in sharp contrast to electromagnetic waves (e.g., light, x-ray, and radio waves). In electromagnetic waves, the electric field and the magnetic field that provide the wave mechanism are perpendicular to each other and perpendicular to the direction of propagation. These kinds of waves are called transverse waves. Unlike electromagnetic waves, sound cannot travel in a vacuum; its energy is propagated by the motion of the particles in the medium that it is traveling through. Ultrasound waves are represented by pressure waves; compression and expansion form the crests and valleys, respectively, in the wave description.

One way to classify sound waves is based on the frequency of the waves. Because sound waves less than 20 Hz cannot be heard by humans, they are referred to as infrasound waves. Audible sound waves are between 20 and 20,000 Hz, whereas any sound waves above the limit of human hearing are called ultrasound. For diagnostic ultrasound, frequencies ranging from 1 up to 100 MHz are routinely used.

In this chapter, we first describe the physics of ultrasound and the interaction of ultrasonic waves with biological tissues and then introduce some of the main medical ultrasound technologies. We also discuss in detail the signal processing methodologies used to create and analyze medical ultrasound imaging technologies.

16.2 WHY ULTRASOUND IMAGING?

We can ask ourselves why ultrasound is such a popular and invaluable diagnostic tool in medical disciplines such as cardiology, obstetrics, gynecology, surgery, pediatrics, radiology, and neurology. One of the main advantages of ultrasound is that this technology is relatively inexpensive, mainly due to the relatively "low-tech" equipment needed in this modality. Ultrasound imaging produces relatively high-resolution images that rival other relatively common imaging modalities such as x-ray imaging, plus it provides soft tissue information. The axial resolution is in the order of millimeters, while the radial resolution depends on the beam diameter.

Moreover, unlike technologies such as x-ray where the applied energy is ionizing and therefore harmful to biological tissues, the sound waves used in ultrasound are harmless. Almost all ultrasound systems can produce images in real time, which is a major advantage for medical imaging. Furthermore, due to the portability of most of ultrasound units, they can easily be used for various purposes in different locations.

Additionally, ultrasound imaging can provide important physiological data such as flow magnitude and direction by applying the Doppler principle, as discussed later in this chapter. A quantitative description of blood flow derived from ultrasound measurements provides vital information to physicians about the local flow characteristics. The flow characteristics will provide indirect information on the tissue metabolism and functionality. This unique capability of ultrasound imaging makes it very suitable for cardiovascular measurements.

Some other unique properties of ultrasound can be better understood when it is compared with x-ray. Ultrasound imaging has reasonable similarities to x-ray imaging as far as the methodology is concerned. Both techniques rely on the assumption of rectilinear propagation for the image formation purposes. Even though ultrasonic waves undergo considerably more diffraction than x-ray, for imaging purposes, the sound waves are often assumed to travel along a straight line in the first-order approximation. On the other hand, ultrasound imaging has considerable differences with x-ray imaging. Ultrasound, as mentioned earlier, has no reported epidemiological side effects on biological tissues under the conditions currently used for imaging. X-ray, on the other hand has been shown to have ionizing effects on biological tissues and can be mutagenic. In many medical diagnostic procedures, such as monitoring of a fetus in the womb, the use of x-ray is strictly prohibited due to the potential mutagenic effects that can permanently alter the genetic makeup of the fetus.

Moreover, while electromagnetic waves only show a relatively negligible different speed of propagation across most biological tissues, the speed of an ultrasound wave is considerably different in different tissues. Informally speaking, wave spends more time passing though one type of tissue than another. These rather small but detectable variations in the speed of sound provide the means to create detailed structural information about the tissue. In addition, the speed of ultrasonic waves in soft tissue is much less than the speed of electromagnetic waves (including x-ray and light), i.e., the typical speed of sound in biological tissues is $V = 1540\,\text{m/s}$, while the speed of electromagnetic waves is $C = 2.9979 \times 10^8\,\text{m/s}$. The fact that the speed of sound is relatively small is heavily used in the determination of the depth of an echo caused by specific tissue inside the body, as explained later in this chapter.

16.3 GENERATION AND DETECTION OF ULTRASOUND WAVES

Ultrasound waves can be produced in two distinctly different modes of operation. One of the mechanisms that can be used for ultrasound generation is magnetorestrictive based. A magnetic material can be made to change its shape under the influence of an external magnetic field. When this magnetic field is a periodically changing field with a constant period, the medium oscillates with the same identical frequency as the driving magnetic field.

The second and most often used mechanism to generate ultrasound is using piezoelectric materials. In piezoelectric ultrasound generation, a class of molecules with an unequal distribution of electric charges can be driven to oscillation by applying an external alternating electric field. As a result, the medium made up of these molecules changes shape in unison at the rhythm of the alternating current through the medium.

Certain commonly used materials for transducers are ceramic, barium titanate, lead-zirconate-titanate, quartz, polyvinylidene difluoride (PVDF). The most commonly used ceramic material is lead-zirconate-titanate. These crystals are sandwiched between two electrodes that are able to apply a voltage across the crystal. The crystals will expand and contract in a sinusoidal fashion under an applied alternating current and will produce sound waves at levels appropriate for diagnostic use with only milliwatts of power. The mechanical wave generation devices are called transducers.

Acoustic waves will partially reflect of interfaces separating two media with different acoustical properties, while the remaining fraction will proceed in the initial direction. Both the reflected and the transmitted signal can be used for imaging purposes. In detecting ultrasound wave, when an acoustic pressure wave reaches a piezoelectric crystal (potentially the same crystal that generated the acoustic wave), the mechanically induced pressure changes the shape of the crystal, which in turn produces a voltage across that crystal. This voltage is detected by the electrodes attached to the crystal. At this point, the pressure signal is converted into a voltage spike whose amplitude is proportional to the mechanical pressure. This analog signal is then converted to a digital signal by an analog to digital converter. The resulting digital signal is then analyzed by the algorithms that extract information such as signal intensity and time interval to form an image of the tissue under study.

In order to better understand both modalities, we need to review some principles of ultrasound physics.

16.4 PHYSICAL AND PHYSIOLOGICAL PRINCIPLES OF ULTRASOUND

In order to better understand the sound wave propagation formation, first, we review some fundamental physics concepts of the ultrasound phenomenon. The concepts reviewed here include the mechanics of sound waves, the frequency of the sound, the frequency content of the emitted and detected ultrasound signal, and the acoustic impedance. We also review the mathematical formulation of acoustic wave propagation and penetration. Knowing these concepts and mathematical formulations of these concepts is essential for understanding and implementation of the tomographic signal and image processing methods.

16.4.1 Fundamental Ultrasound Concepts

In wave theory, the period of a wave, T, describes the time between two consecutive repetitions of an identical pattern in the time domain. The wavelength of the sound wave describes the spatial repetition of pattern sequence. The wavelength λ is coupled to the period of the wave as follows:

$$\lambda = VT \tag{16.1}$$

where V is the local speed of sound. The frequency, f, describes how many times per second a pattern repeats itself. This concept is essentially the reciprocal of the period, i.e.,

$$f = \frac{1}{T} \tag{16.2}$$

The concepts of both wavelength and time periodicity are illustrated in Figure 16.1. Figure 16.1a shows the concept of period in time domain, and Figure 16.1b illustrates the wavelength in the space domain.

Generally, ultrasound is delivered in short bursts to allow discrimination between source and effect and to provide a mechanism to derive additional features from the detected signal. In this method, the piezoelectric crystal will emit an ultrasound beam resulting from an electric impulse from a power source, called a pulser. The pulser will then wait until all of the echoes from that burst of ultrasound are collected before firing another beam. This way, the device has a greater chance of sorting out the chain of echoes while reducing the buildup of echoes on top of each other. An illustration of the pulse train delivery protocol is illustrated in Figure 16.2.

The speed of sound propagation, V, is linked to the elastic modulus of the material, K, and the respective local density of the medium, ρ, i.e.,

$$V = \sqrt{\frac{K}{\rho}} \tag{16.3}$$

The limited speed of sound allows the measurement of the time delay between the transmitter and the receiver of the ultrasound waves, located for instance on two

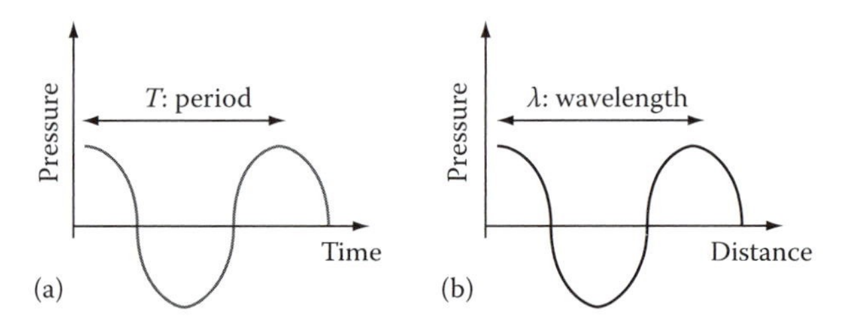

FIGURE 16.1 Concepts of (a) period and (b) wavelength.

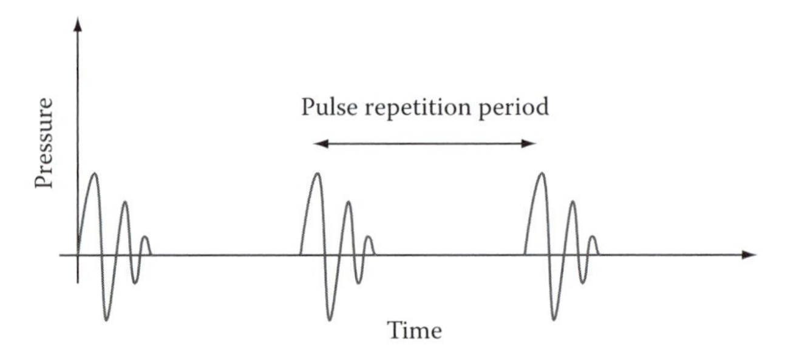

FIGURE 16.2 Ultrasound pulse train delivery protocol.

sides of the tissue. In reflection tomography, the detected signal is collected in the wake of the input pulse and is collected by the same transducer as the one that emitted the ultrasound pulse. The delay between emitted and detected pulsed train is often referred to as "time of flight." As discussed later, one can measure end-to-end delays and use tomographic techniques to calculate the delays in each point of the tissue structure. In other words, once the delay for each tissue is computed, a very informative tomographic imaging technique can be applied, which can reveal invaluable details about the physical properties of the tissues under study.

Another useful concept in ultrasound is the acoustic impedance. In acoustic wave propagation, the factor that limits the speed of the sound is often expressed using a variable called acoustic impedance of a medium, Z_A. The characteristic acoustic impedance depends on the density of the medium and the ease with which motion can be transferred from a point to a neighboring point. This quantity can be related to the speed of the wave as follows:

$$Z_A = \rho V \tag{16.4}$$

The characteristic impedance is often used to describe the mathematical formulation of the wave propagation, as discussed later in this chapter.

16.4.2 Wave Equation

The ultrasound transducer produces a pressure wave that is both a function of location and time, $P(x, y, z, t)$. Acoustic wave propagation in a medium such as a biological tissue is governed by the following wave equation:

$$\nabla^2 P = \frac{\partial^2 P}{\partial x^2} + \frac{\partial^2 P}{\partial y^2} + \frac{\partial^2 P}{\partial z^2} = \frac{1}{v^2}\frac{\partial^2 P}{\partial t^2} \tag{16.5}$$

Often the initial assumption in forming the previous equation is that the wave propagates in the direction of one of the coordinates such as x-direction, while the beam is not confined to one dimension only. The solution to Equation 16.5 can have many different forms, but one typical solution of this equation can be described as follows:

$$P(z,t) = P_0 \sin\left(\frac{2\pi t}{\lambda} - k_x x - k_y y - k_z z\right) = P_0 \sin(\omega t - k_x x - k_y y - k_z z) \tag{16.6}$$

where

$\omega = 2\pi f$ is the angular frequency

$k = \dfrac{\omega}{V}$ is the wave number

Theoretically, the wave number k in the three Cartesian directions can have different values. This is due to the fact that the speed of the sound wave can be different in different directions due to the type of tissues encountered in these directions.

This can potentially cause the wave front to distort during propagation through the tissue; however, the wave number is often assumed to be the same for all directions to simplify the solution.

At this point, it is important to note that even though in the strict theoretical sense, one can attempt to find the wave equation in all points of an inhomogeneous medium such as biological tissue. If such a wave equation was available, one could have used the equation to form very informative images of the biological system under study. However, the trick is in the fact that, in order to generate the wave equation, one needs to know the exact characteristics of all the points in the tissues under study. In reality, if we knew the characteristic information about the structure of the tissue, there was no need for imaging! All tomographic attempts described in this chapter are indeed directed toward finding the acoustic features of the tissue. This means that while knowing the general form of the wave equation might help in understanding the problem, the actual equation is never available, and therefore we need to resort to tomographic methods to analyze the tissue.

Next, the physics of the main ultrasound characteristics that are used for medical imaging applications, i.e., attenuation and reflection, is further described.

16.4.3 Attenuation

Once the sound waves leave the ultrasound probe, they travel through the adjoining tissue in which the waves will be attenuated. Since the ultrasound transducer can only detect sound waves that ultimately reach the crystal, the absorption of sound in the body tissue decreases the intensity of sound waves that can be detected. Hence, the deeper the region of interest is located, the more difficult the detection process becomes. Absorption of sound waves is due to the conversion of the ultrasound energy into motion, which translates into heat energy. This is due to the friction of cells and structures sliding over each other, and the friction of this movement transforms the mechanical energy also into heat energy.

Attenuation in the pressure signal, dP, is directly proportional to the incident pressure, P, the distance over which the absorption takes place, dz, and the tissue-specific attenuation factor, α. In other words,

$$dP = \alpha P dz \tag{16.7}$$

Solving this equation for P in the case of a plane wave, we have

$$P(z) = P_0 \exp[-\alpha z] \tag{16.8}$$

Equation 16.8 is known as the Beer–Lambert–Bouguer law of attenuation. In this equation, the attenuation coefficient α (which is often expressed in neper/m or neper/cm) varies from one tissue to another, and P_0 is the pressure at $z = 0$.

Table 16.1 lists a variety of acoustic properties for some selected tissues. These properties include the speed of propagation, the acoustic impedance, and the attenuation coefficient.

TABLE 16.1
Selected Acoustic Tissue Parameters

Tissue	Speed of Propagation V (m/s)	Acoustic Impedance Z_A (kg/m² × 10⁻⁶)	Attenuation Coefficient α at 1 MHz (dB/cm)	Density ρ (kg/m³)	Propagation Velocity V (m/s)
Water	1540	1.48–1.53	0.002	1000	1480
Blood	1570	1.58–1.61	0.2	1030	1570
Fat	1460	1.37	0.6	900	1450
Muscle	1575	1.68	3.3	1080	1580
Bone	4000	6.0–8.0	12	1850	3500–4300

Acoustic attenuation is notoriously frequency dependent. In fact, the attenuation is almost linearly proportional to the frequency. More specifically, ultrasound attenuation in biological tissues is almost proportional to the wave frequency over the interval of 1–6 MHz, which is the typical range of interest in ultrasound imaging. In other words, the $\frac{\alpha}{f}$ ratio is roughly constant for the typical range of medical ultrasound imaging.

Knowing the frequency-dependent nature of attenuation in ultrasound waves, it can be seen why the higher frequencies resulting from deep reflections will hardly make it back to the piezoelectric sensor/detector. This in effect translates into a low-pass filtering mechanism in acoustic imaging that becomes more visible as the acoustic system needs to penetrate deeper to produce a meaningful image.

Usually one is interested in the ratio of a measured signal, P_1, with respect to the source signal, P_0, and since practical signal ratios often cover a wide range, it is convenient to express ratios in logarithmic form. The intensity ratio of the detected signal, P_1, measured with respect to the input signal, P_0, in logarithmic format yields the decibel expression as formulated in decibels (dB) as follows:

$$\text{dB} = 10\ \log_{10}\left(\frac{P_1}{P_0}\right) \tag{16.9}$$

Note the very high attenuation for bone listed in Table 16.1. This observation shows why one cannot effectively use ultrasound to image the tissues located behind bones. Water, on the other hand, has a very low attenuation coefficient (0.002 dB/cm at 1 MHz), which indicates a relatively low attenuation. Note that air has a high attenuation coefficient (12 dB/cm at 1 MHz). This high attenuation has two practical implications. First, in order to have a meaningful image from biological tissues, one cannot allow any air gap between the transducers and the skin. This is why in ultrasound imaging systems, such sonography, a special gel, which has attenuation levels similar to that of water, is used as the interface of the transducers and the skin to eliminate the possibility of air gaps between the transducer and the human skin. The second observation deals with the inability of ultrasound systems to image the tissues located behind lungs that have air in them. More specifically, almost 99% of the energy incident upon the interface between the lung, which consists of air and soft tissue, is reflected. Practically speaking, in order to create an image of a biological organ using ultrasound, one needs to have a line of sight from the transducer to the tissue without any bones or lungs in the path.

16.4.4 Reflection

The next concept to be discussed is reflection. During propagation, a sound wave often moves through different media. At the interface between two acoustically different media, the path of the sound wave can be significantly affected. Many secondary waves will be generated, one of which is the reflected wave. The angle of reflection is always by definition equal to the angle of incidence (Figure 16.3). The portion of the sound wave that will go through the interface is called the refracted wave, and the part of the wave that gets reflected off the interface is called reflected wave.

In reflection tomography, the creation of echoes in the body by reflection of the ultrasound beam is the basis for all reflected waves. As one can imagine, when the angle of incidence, θ_i, is larger, the deflections from greater depths will have an increasingly higher probability of missing the transducer partially or entirely. In practical applications, the angle of incidence must be kept below 3° ($\theta_i < 3°$) in order for the transducer to receive the information needed to form an image.

Reflection results from a combination of changes in acoustic impedance, usually in the order of the size of the wavelength. Often the reflection on microscopic scale will fall under the principle of scattering in ultrasound imaging. The ratio of reflected to refracted sound waves is dependent on the acoustic properties of both media at either side of the interface. The acoustic impedance of the tissues often characterizes these properties. In order to quantitatively analyze this phenomenon, assume that an incident acoustic wave front hits the interface of the two media with an angle θ_i (with respect to the normal to the interface). In addition, assume the two media to have different acoustic impedances Z_{A1} and Z_{A2}. Further, show the incident pressure as P_i, the reflected pressure as P_r, and the transmitted pressure as P_t. Then, the pressure reflection coefficient, r, and the pressure transmission coefficient, t, are defined as follows:

$$r = \frac{P_r}{P_i} = \frac{Z_{A2}\cos\theta_1 - Z_{A1}\cos\theta_2}{Z_{A2}\cos\theta_1 + Z_{A1}\cos\theta_2} \tag{16.10}$$

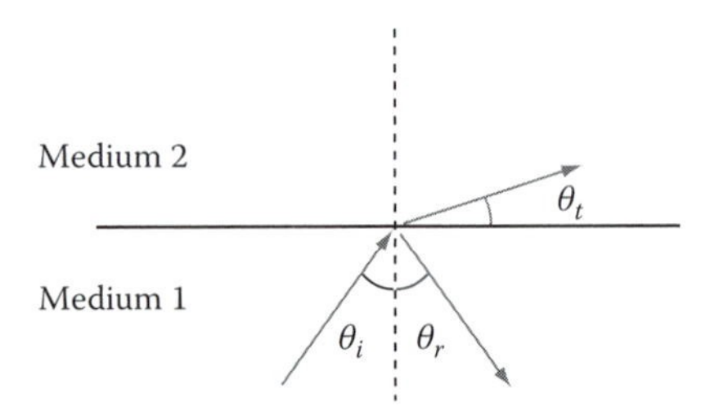

FIGURE 16.3 Definitions at the interface of two media with an incident (i), reflected (r), and transmitted (t) pressure wave front.

and

$$t = \frac{P_t}{P_i} = \frac{2Z_{A2}\cos\theta_1}{Z_{A2}\cos\theta_1 + Z_{A1}\cos\theta_2} \tag{16.11}$$

Equation 16.10 determines how much of the incident pressure wave reflects to the surface, and Equation 16.11 shows the ratio of the transmitted to reflected wave pressures. The previous equations demonstrate that even a fairly small difference in acoustic impedances between both media will still generate enough change in the intensity of the reflected and transmitted signals to be detected during the imaging process.

Since most biological tissues have comparable acoustic impedances, only a small amount of the ultrasound is reflected, and most of the sound is transmitted. Therefore, structures that are relatively deeper can also serve as a reflector and produce echoes. This is why ultrasound can penetrate deep into the body and provide information on interfaces beyond the first reflective surfaces. In fact, ultrasound can "bounce" between interfaces, and the reflections from one surface can reach the transducer multiple times. Obviously, these multiple echoes can complicate the production of an image and act as a source of noise in ultrasound images.

Another source of noise related to reflection phenomenon is caused by the small size of the cells. If the dimensions of reflectors, for example, cells, are smaller than the wavelength of the sound wave, the reflector acts as a scatterer, or as a secondary source. This secondary source is now a point source, radiating spherical waves, in contrast with the incident plane wave front. Specifically, while diffraction is the gradual spreading of a beam of sound, scattering is a form of attenuation in which the sound is sent in all directions. Scattering occurs when the incident sound beam encounters small particles within the tissues. The sound waves interact with these particles, and the waves are reemitted in every possible direction with a certain probability distribution for the scattering angle. The ultrasonic scattering process in biological tissues is very complicated. Tissues have been treated both as dense distributions of discrete scatterers and as continua with variations in density and compressibility. As mentioned earlier, in typical reflection and attenuation tomography using ultrasound waves, scattering acts as a source of noise and causes some complications in the image.

The interface of the transducer and the biological medium (e.g., skin) can also cause interfering reflection. In order to minimize this, as mentioned before, a gel layer with closely matching acoustic impedance is usually placed on the face of the probe between the crystal and the body. This matching layer reduces the difference in acoustic impedance between the probe and the skin. In addition, a copious amount of a coupling agent such as gel or oil must be used on the skin, not only to allow the probe to glide smoothly over the skin, but also to exclude any air (which has significantly higher acoustic impedance) from the probe–skin interface. Several coupling agents are currently available for impedance matching: agar gel, water immersion, and a so-called bladder method, where a water-filled balloon is placed between the ultrasound probe and the surface of the biological medium. This balloon is pliable and conforms to the surface contour.

Next, we study some acoustic properties of biological tissues through an example.

Example 16.1

Note the very large differences between the soft tissues and bone and air. Assuming that the incident wave is perpendicular to the surface of the interface, we use the reflection equation to compare the reflection between two types of soft tissue, i.e., fat and muscle, with the reflection between a soft tissue and a hard tissue, i.e., brain to skull.

The reflection from fat to muscle comes to the following value: $R = \left(\frac{1.7-1.3}{1.7+1.3}\right)^2 = 0.018 \equiv -17.5\,\text{dB}$, or 1.8%, while the reflection from bone to brain gives a much lower attenuation due to the much greater difference in acoustic impedance between bone and brain: $R = \left(\frac{7.8-1.6}{7.8+1.6}\right)^2 = 0.435 \equiv -3.6\,\text{dB}$, or 43.5%. This confirms the fact that the reflection coefficients between soft tissues and bone or air are large. This is in contrast to the signal reflection coefficients at boundaries between soft tissues, which turn out to be relatively small.

Now we are familiar with the main physical properties of ultrasound and before describing the details of the methods used for specific ultrasound tomographic systems, we briefly discuss the practical issues that determine the resolution of such imaging systems.

16.5 RESOLUTION OF ULTRASOUND IMAGING SYSTEMS

Two distinct types of resolution can be distinguished depending on the direction of the scan. The axial resolution is the level of distinction between subsequent layers in the direction of propagation of the sound wave. Lateral resolution is the discrimination between two points resulting from the motion of the transducer signal, perpendicular to the wave propagation.

The axial resolution is a direct function of the wavelength of the sound wave. A wave has a crest and a valley. The crest is maximum pressure (positive peak), and the valley represents minimal pressure (negative peak). Since the measurable reflections are often detectable only when the wave is at the maximal or minimal points, the axial resolution can thus never exceed the distance spanned by half a wavelength. The axial resolution can be maximized by mechanical filtering, thus reducing reverberations from the excitation by the incoming sound wave.

The lateral resolution is often determined by the width of the sound beam traveling through the biological medium. A major factor that influences the beam width and therefore affects the lateral resolution of the system is the physical dimension of the transducer. In general, the transducer sends out a plane wave whose profile is determined by the dimensions of the transducer itself. Since the recorded reflection is also acquired by a transducer with the same cross-sectional area, it is virtually impossible to make any distinction between reflections at the exact locations across the beam profile. In other words, even when the reflections across the beam profile return with different intensities, since the reflections are collected by only a single transducer, the different returned intensities are averaged by the transducer.

One would think that reducing the probe diameter to infinitesimally small dimensions will give the ultimate lateral resolution. However, the smaller transducer dimension will result in a higher divergence of the beam. The divergence of the beam causes greater problems than the initial size of the beam as the returning beam will continue to expand due to diffraction and scattering. Such a broad beam will excite a very large number of transducers upon returning to the ultrasound probe. The lateral resolution will then be lost entirely. In some practical systems, in order to improve the resolution, instead of a single large transducer, an array of medium size transducers is used.

Now we are ready to discuss the main tomographic ultrasound imaging methods used in medical applications.

16.6 ULTRASOUND IMAGING MODALITIES

Three main types of ultrasound imaging can be distinguished: attenuation tomography, reflection tomography, and time-of-flight (TOF) tomography.

One major medical ultrasound imaging system, reflection tomography, relies on the fact that sound waves will be reflected from the border of two different tissues. In reflection tomography, detecting and analyzing the echoes that are reflected or scattered from the different tissues in the biological medium creates an image of the tissue. The intensity of each echo is related to the difference in the acoustic impedances of the respective tissues at that specific interface.

In early ultrasound systems, the transducer would determine whether or not there was an echo, but was not accurate in measuring the intensity of the echoes. These early brightness mode (B-mode) devices could tell that there were interfaces and would display a bright spot on the image that would correspond with that interface. New ultrasound systems can accurately determine the intensity of each echo and therefore determine the characteristics of the interface that has reflected that ultrasound wave. The imaging systems then translate these tissue characteristic specifications into gray scales that can be used in rendering the image. Informally speaking, an intense echo is going to be received by the transducer if there is a large difference in acoustic impedance; therefore, the image for this interface will be brighter than the image of an interface with a lesser difference in acoustic impedance. This technique allows for not only the location of structures but also the characterization of certain material properties of these structures. Since the acoustic impedance is proportional to both the density and the elastic modulus of the medium, these parameters can be derived through inverse solution of the acquired signals.

Attenuation tomography, as another ultrasound imaging modality, uses the fact that the transmitted sound waves will be attenuated to different degrees as they pass through tissues with different properties. This is essentially the same principle used in x-ray attenuation tomography. In attenuation tomography, the attenuation of the sound waves passing through the tissues is utilized to form an image.

The formulation of the TOF tomography is very much similar to those of attenuation and reflection tomography and will be discussed coupled with attenuation tomography. The principle idea of the TOF tomography is based on the observation that the time it takes the sound wave to travel through different tissues varies from one tissue to another.

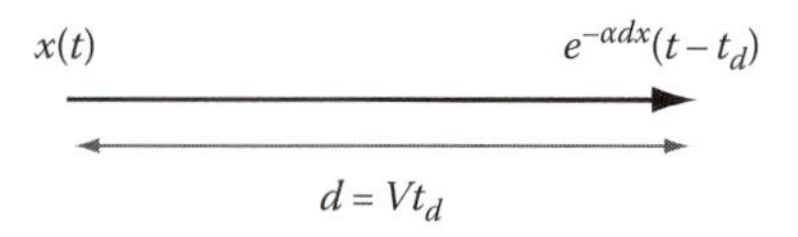

FIGURE 16.4 Modeling of translation distance.

Before formulating these tomographic systems, and in order to see how attenuation and TOF are modeled for ultrasound waves, next we investigate expressing the transmission of an ultrasound pressure pulse $x(t)$ in the Fourier domain. As shown in Figure 16.4, consider a transmitted signal $x(t)$ that is received at a distance d from the point of origination. Based on what was previously mentioned about the physics of ultrasound, the received signal will be $e^{-\alpha dx}(t - t_d)$, which is simply the delayed version of the original signal attenuated by an attenuation factor of α. This means that the measured signal in the Fourier domain will be as follows:

$$\begin{aligned} X_d(f) &= FT\{e^{-\alpha d}x(t-t_d)\} \\ &= e^{-\alpha d}e^{-j2\pi f t_d}X(f) \end{aligned} \tag{16.12}$$

Assuming V as the speed of sound, the distance d can be written as $d = Vt_d$. As a result,

$$\begin{aligned} X_d(f) &= e^{-\alpha d}e^{-j2\pi f\frac{d}{V}}X(f) \\ &= e^{-\alpha d}e^{-j\beta(f)d}X(f) \end{aligned} \tag{16.13}$$

where the time-delay function, $\beta(f)$, is defined as follows:

$$\beta(f) = \frac{2\pi f}{V} \tag{16.14}$$

Propagation time-delay measurement constitutes the fundamental idea of refraction-index tomography and reflection tomography, as discussed later. On the other hand, in inhomogeneous tissues, the attenuation factor changes from one point to another, which makes ideal to form the ultrasonic images using tomographic techniques. In other words, the variations in the attenuation factor provide the basis for attenuation tomography, which is described in the next section.

16.6.1 Attenuation Tomography

A typical setup for ultrasound attenuation tomography is illustrated in Figure 16.5. Before formulating the mathematical equations, we briefly describe the setup and the general function of the elements in the system. As can be seen in Figure 16.5,

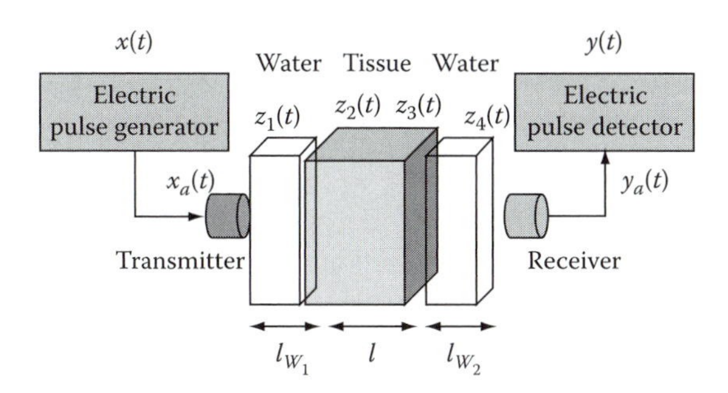

FIGURE 16.5 Diagram of methodology for ultrasound attenuation tomography.

the system is composed of signal generator that produces electric pulses. The electric stimulus signal, $x(t)$, is applied to the transducer that produced the transmitted pressure impulse, $x_a(t)$. The transducer pressure signal then enters the gel or water medium that is used to provide coupling between the transducer and the biological tissue or skin. The acoustic pulse traverses the tissues and at each point within the tissue undergoes attenuation that is proportional to the attenuation characteristics of that point. The attenuated signal then reaches the other side of the tissue and enters the gel on the receiver side. This signal is then converted to an electric signal by the transducer at the receiver side. The comparison of the original electric signal with the electric signal measured on the receiver side quantifies the attenuation characteristics of the tissue.

Knowing the overall function of the system, next we mathematically model the entire process to show how such a system allows tomographic imaging of the tissue. Tracking the signal modifications from the electric generator to electric detector gives the following steps in the image formation that can be identified.

The first step is in the process is the conversion of the original electric signal $x(t)$ to mechanical pressure $x_a(t)$. Modeling this mechanical conversion as a linear process with the impulse response $h_1(t)$, we have

$$x_a(t) = h_1(t) * x(t) \tag{16.15}$$

After applying the Fourier transform on both sides, we can continue our formulation in the frequency domain, i.e.,

$$X_a(f) = H_1(f)X(f) \tag{16.16}$$

$X_a(f)$ describes the signal on far left hand side of the water (gel). In order to find the signal on the far right side of the water layer, $Z_1(f)$, we need to consider both delay and attenuation along the water interface with the thickness l_{W1}, i.e.,

$$Z_1(f) = e^{-j\beta_W(f)l_{W1}}e^{-\alpha_W(f)l_{W1}}X_a(f) \tag{16.17}$$

In the interface of the water layer and the tissue, only a portion of the signal energy gets to enter the tissue. This portion of the signal, $Z_2(f)$, can be calculated using the transmittance factor between water and tissue, A_{WT}, as follows:

$$Z_2(f) = A_{WT} Z_1(f) \tag{16.18}$$

Now the pulse that has entered the tissue gets attenuated and delayed throughout the tissue. Since we are not assuming that the tissue is a homogeneous environment, the values of attenuation and delay must be calculated for each point and then integrated over the entire linear path to provide the total attenuation and delay across the tissue. This means that the signal at the far right side of the tissue, $Z_3(f)$, can be calculated as follows:

$$Z_3(f) = e^{-j\int_0^l \beta(x,y,f)dx} e^{-\int_0^l \alpha(x,y,f)dx} Z_2(f) \tag{16.19}$$

As can be seen in Equation 16.19, $\alpha(x, y, f)$ and $\beta(x, y, f)$ are assumed to depend on the exact location of the point as well as the exact frequency. The next step is the transmittance of the signal from the far right side of the tissue to the water on the receiver side of the system, which can be represented by the following:

$$Z_4(f) = A_{TW} Z_3(f) \tag{16.20}$$

where A_{TW} is the transmittance factor from the tissue to water. As in the transmitter side, the signal is both attenuated and delayed while passing through the water interface with thickness l_{W2}, i.e., the pressure signal on the far right hand side of the water interface, $Y_a(f)$, will be as follows:

$$Y_a(f) = e^{-j\beta_W(f) l_{W2}} e^{-\alpha_W(f) l_{W2}} Z_4(f) \tag{16.21}$$

Finally, the conversion of the mechanical pressure $Y_a(f)$ to electric signal $Y(f)$, as shown in Figure 16.5, can be formulated as another linear system with an impulse function $H_2(f)$ as follows:

$$Y(f) = H_2(f) Y_a(f) \tag{16.22}$$

The overall relationship between the input $X(f)$ and the output $Y(f)$ of the tissue reduces to the following:

$$\begin{aligned} Y(f) = H_1(f) \\ &\times e^{-j\beta_W(f) l_{W1}} e^{-\alpha_W(f) l_{W1}} \\ &\times A_{WT} e^{-j\int_0^l \beta(x,y,f)dx} e^{-\int_0^l \alpha(x,y,f)dx} \\ &\times A_{TW} e^{-j\beta_W(f) l_{W2}} e^{-\alpha_W(f) l_{W2}} \\ &\times H_2(f) X(f) \end{aligned} \tag{16.23}$$

Next we define the following simplifying notations:

$$l_W = l_{W_1} + l_{W_2} \tag{16.24}$$

and

$$A = A_{TW} \cdot A_{WT} \tag{16.25}$$

Using the previous notation, Equation 16.23 can be rewritten as follows:

$$Y(f) = AH_1(f)H_2(f)e^{-j\beta_W(f)l_W}e^{-\alpha_W(f)l_W}e^{-j\int_0^l \beta(x,y,f)dx}e^{-\int_0^l \alpha(x,y,f)dx}X(f) \tag{16.26}$$

Next we separate the elements in Equation 16.26 that are not tissue dependent and therefore stay the same in all measurements from the parts of the equation that are tissue dependent. In order to do so, we define the variable $Y_W(f)$ as follows:

$$Y_W(f) = AH_1(f)H_2(f)e^{-\alpha_W(f)l_W}X(f) \tag{16.27}$$

Note that $Y_W(f)$ is known for a given frequency, a given drive signal $X(f)$, and a given device with fixed physical properties. Using this definition, Equation 16.26 can be rewritten as follows:

$$Y(f) = Y_W(f)e^{-j\left[\beta_W(f)l_W + \int_0^l \beta(x,y,f)dx\right]}e^{-\int_0^l \alpha(x,y,f)dx} \tag{16.28}$$

Rearranging Equation 16.28 will give

$$e^{-\int_0^l \alpha(x,y,f)dx} = \frac{Y(f)}{Y_W(f)e^{-j\left[\beta_W(f)l_W + \int_0^l \beta(x,y,f)dx\right]}} \tag{16.29}$$

Taking the absolute value of both sides results in the following:

$$e^{-\int_0^l \alpha(x,y,f)dx} = \frac{|Y(f)|}{|Y_W(f)|} \tag{16.30}$$

Now, all we need to do to obtain a tomographic equation is taking the logarithm of both sides of Equation 16.30, i.e.,

$$\int_0^l \alpha(x,y,f)dx = -\ln\left(\frac{|Y(f)|}{|Y_W(f)|}\right) = \ln\left(\frac{|Y_W(f)|}{|Y(f)|}\right) \tag{16.31}$$

As discussed in Chapter 13, Equation 16.31 constitutes a tomographic equation. If several scans are taken in several directions, the process described earlier will reduce to a standard nondiffracting tomography problem that was discussed in Chapter 13. This shows how different ultrasound attenuation characteristics of tissues can be used to form an image of the biological systems.

Next, we discuss a similar ultrasound tomographic system called TOF tomography whose setup is essentially the same as that of the attenuation tomography. However, TOF tomography is based on a set of completely different characteristics of the tissues, which make the resulting images very different from those of attenuation tomography.

16.6.2 Ultrasound Time-of-Flight Tomography

Additional information is retrieved from the TOF of each transmission to obtain details on the speed of sound in the region the sound traverses through. The speed of sound gives details on either the density of the medium or the elastic modulus of the medium, thus providing additional secondary anatomical details. Based on the measurement of the TOF, the time "t_d" is defined as the total time it takes the signal to travel from the transmitter to the receiver and is measured to perform TOF tomography as describe later.

In order to describe TOF tomography, we start by reconsidering Equation 16.26:

$$Y(f) = AH_1(f)H_2(f)e^{-j\beta_W(f)l_W}e^{-\alpha_W(f)l_W}e^{-j\int_0^l \beta(x,y,f)dx}e^{-\int_0^l \alpha(x,y,f)dx}X(f) \tag{16.32}$$

From this relationship, the terms describing the delay from the output to the input are $e^{-\alpha_W(f)l_W}$ (cause by water on both sides) and $e^{-j\int_0^l \beta(x,y,f)dx}$ (caused by the biological tissues). This means that the total delay measured from the source to the receiver can be related to these terms as follows:

$$e^{-j\left[\beta_W(f)l_W+\int_0^l \beta(x,y,f)dx\right]} = e^{-j2\pi f t_d} \tag{16.33}$$

Taking the logarithm of both sides of Equation 16.32,

$$\beta_W(f)l_W + \int_0^l \beta(x,y,f)dx = 2\pi f t_d \tag{16.34}$$

or

$$\int_0^l \beta(x,y,f)dx = 2\pi f t_d - \beta_W(f)l_W \tag{16.35}$$

Equation 16.35 is the tomographic equation that allows forming images of the biological systems based on different speeds of sound waves in different biological tissues. Note that t_d and l_w are measured, and $\beta_w(f)$ is known for all frequencies. Taking several such measurements in several directions provides the measurements for solving the previous tomographic equation.

As mentioned earlier, in some cases, the line of sight access to the biological organs to be imaged may not be possible. In such cases, neither attenuation tomography nor the TOF tomography that requires the transmitter and receiver on different sides of the object may be a suitable solution. For such very important imaging scenario, ultrasound reflection tomography, as introduced later, is used.

16.6.3 Reflection Tomography

Almost all commercial ultrasound imaging systems rely on the principle of sound-echo detection for ultrasound image formation. This process of reflection tomography is illustrated in Figure 16.6. Figure 16.6a shows the physical setup, and Figure 16.6b shows the mathematical model of the system. Short pulse trains, $p(t)$, having a single frequency are transmitted into the biological medium under study. The returning sound waves, $\psi(t)$, are collected in the interval between the emitted bursts of sound. The echo will require a specific amount of time to travel to the point where the direction is reversed, and return back to the probe for detection. In reflection tomography, the reflection index $n(x, y)$ is a function of the biological medium and is utilized to form an image. In the modeling of reflection tomography, we ignore the reflections formed by the interface of water (gel) and the skin. In our first formulation of the system, we also ignore attenuation of the ultrasound wave; however, later on, we will include attenuation in our final formulation of reflection tomography.

As shown in Figure 16.6a, the surface causing the reflection at coordinates (x, y) receives the pulse, $p_1(t)$, which is the delayed version of the emitted pulse, $p(t)$. The transmitted pulse that passes through the separation surface, $z_1(t)$, can then be calculated as follows:

$$z_1(t) = p_1(t)(1 - n(x, y)) \tag{16.36}$$

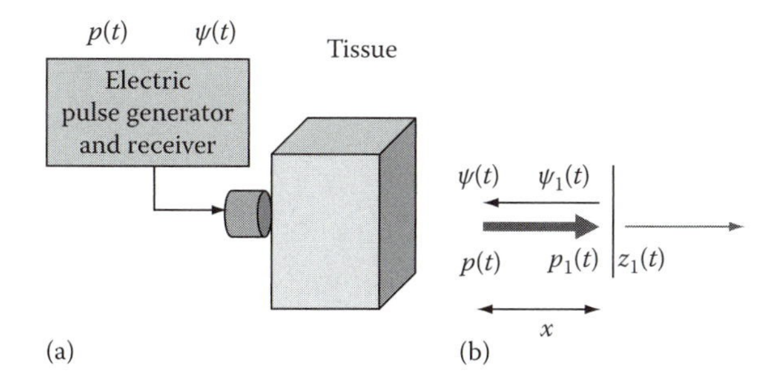

FIGURE 16.6 Diagram of setup (a) and mathematical methodology (b) for ultrasound reflection tomography.

Similarly, we can calculate the reflected wave front at the separation surface as follows:

$$\psi_1(t) = p_1(t)n(x, y) \tag{16.37}$$

Assuming the delay in $p_1(t)$ relative to $p(t)$, $\psi_1(t)$ can be rewritten as follows:

$$\psi_1(t) = p\left(t - \frac{x}{V}\right)n(x, y) \tag{16.38}$$

Now, knowing that $\psi(t)$ is indeed the delayed version of $\psi_1(t)$, we can express the mathematical formulation of the returned pulse as follows:

$$\psi(t) = p\left(t - 2\frac{x}{V}\right)n(x, y) \tag{16.39}$$

In the preceding formulation, we assumed no attenuation throughout the process. Now, in order to have a more accurate formulation of the system, we modify the preceding equations to incorporate attenuation. In formulation reflection tomography, the attenuation effect is often modeled using an experimental rule. This rule states that ultrasound waves traveling a given distance x are attenuated proportional to $\frac{1}{\sqrt{x}}$. This reciprocal of square root law simplifies the formulation and is known to be accurate assumption in almost all biological tissues. Using this rule and assuming that the wave is traveling in x direction, Equations 16.38 and 16.39 can be rewritten as follows:

$$\psi_1(t) = p\left(t - \frac{x}{V}\right) \cdot \frac{n(x, y)}{\sqrt{x}} \tag{16.40}$$

$$\psi(t) = p\left(t - 2\frac{x}{V}\right) \cdot \frac{n(x, y)}{\sqrt{x}} \tag{16.41}$$

In the preceding formulation, we assumed only one reflecting surface, while, in reality, biological tissues at any location inside the body create an echo. This means that what receiver collects is an integral of all these echoes. In other words, the true $\psi(t)$ can be modeled as follows:

$$\psi(t) = \int_{ray} p\left(t - \frac{x}{2c}\right) \frac{n(x, y)}{\sqrt{x}} dx \tag{16.42}$$

The preceding equation is again a tomographic equation that can be solved for its integrand using the tomographic techniques discussed in Chapter 3. Since the value of $p(t)$ is known, once the integrand is estimated, one can easily find $n(x, y)$. As mentioned before, in all tomographic systems, one needs to create several scans in different directions to solve for the integrand. Figure 16.7 shows the ultrasound

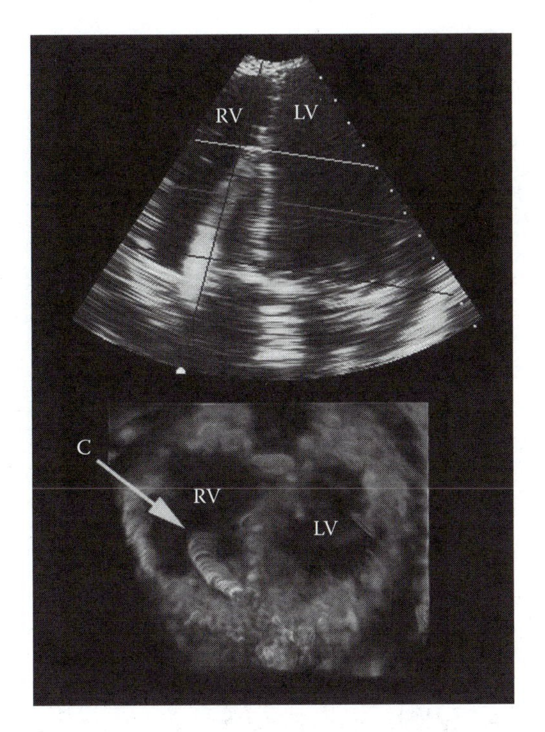

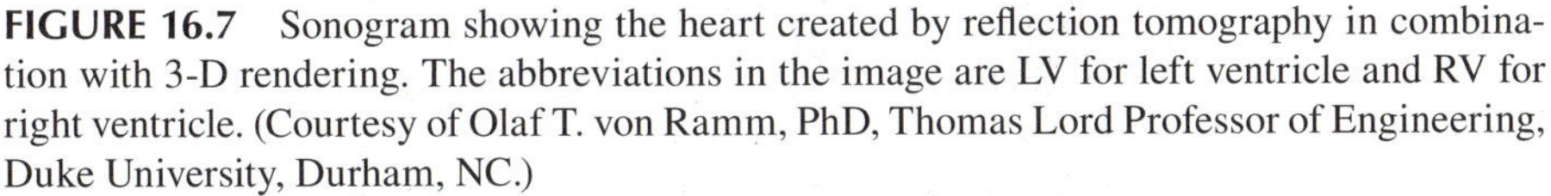

FIGURE 16.7 Sonogram showing the heart created by reflection tomography in combination with 3-D rendering. The abbreviations in the image are LV for left ventricle and RV for right ventricle. (Courtesy of Olaf T. von Ramm, PhD, Thomas Lord Professor of Engineering, Duke University, Durham, NC.)

tomographic images of the heart created by a commercial reflection tomographic system. This is a typical sonogram commonly used for an accurate diagnosis of the heart and its valves.

One specific type of reflection tomography deals with the reflection tomography of moving particles in the plane of view. This specific tomographic system is called Doppler ultrasound imaging as discussed next.

16.6.3.1 Doppler Ultrasound Imaging

The Doppler effect is a phenomenon in which an observer perceives a change in the frequency of the sound emitted by a source when the source or the observer is moving or both are moving. More specifically, the Doppler effect states that changes in the distance beam receptor will affect the frequency of the wave perceived by the receptor. Assuming the frequency of the pressure wave at source as f_0, the frequency perceived by the receptor as f, the velocity of sound emitted by the source as V_{source}, and the velocity of the moving beam or object as V, the perceived frequency is related to the source frequency as follows:

$$f = f_0 \frac{V}{V - V_{source}} \tag{16.43}$$

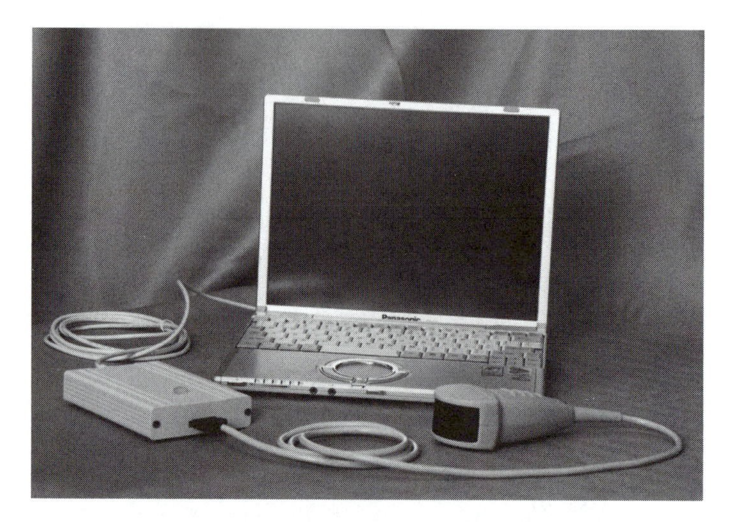

FIGURE 16.8 State-of-the-art portable ultrasound imaging device manufactured by Ardent Sound, Inc., Guided Therapy Systems, Inc., Mesa, AZ.

This effect, i.e., the shift in frequency, is used to register the motion of the moving acoustic scatters within the human body. For scattering material velocities in the 0–1 m/s range, at ultrasound frequencies of 1 and 6 MHz, the Doppler shift frequencies are in the 0–1.3 and 0–8 kHz ranges.

Doppler imaging measures blood velocity and detects blood flow direction. In commercial Doppler systems, the increase in frequency, i.e., flow toward the detector, is colored blue while the decrease in frequency, i.e., movement away from the detector, is illustrated by red.

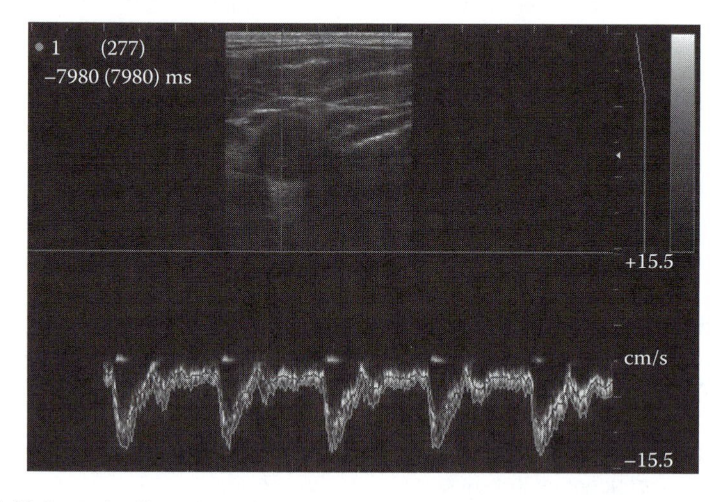

FIGURE 16.9 Pulsatile blood flow captured in a time sequence by Doppler ultrasound imaging. The blood vessel is shown in the upper section of the image, while the bottom half displays the Doppler signal as a function of time. (Courtesy of Ardent Sound, Inc., Guided Therapy Systems, Inc., Mesa, AZ.)

In Figure 16.8, a state-of-the-art portable ultrasound imaging device manufactured by Ardent Sound Therapy, Inc., Mesa, AZ, operating in reflection mode is shown.

Figure 16.9 shows the pulsating characteristics of flow, and the direction of flow is exhibited by the deflection of the Doppler signal (positive or negative).

16.7 MODES OF ULTRASOUND IMAGE REPRESENTATION

Some of the main commercial modes of ultrasound imaging that are used in medical imaging applications are B-mode, M-mode, and TM-modes. These imaging modes are essentially the methods of showing the measures data in the form of images. In B-mode imaging, the amplitude of the collected electronic signal is represented by a relative brightness of the tracking dot on the screen. Figure 16.10 gives a representative B-mode image of a heart in the chest. B-mode is the commonly used way of 2-D image representation.

In M-mode, which is often used for imaging of motion in biological systems, the display keeps track of each B-mode scan by the transducer, while adding subsequent scans as a function of time and position to the same display. While an artifact that provides a reflection remains in one place, the brightness spot does not move in each subsequent scan line; when there is movement, the data created by the moving reflection will change position on the screen as well. Similarly, if the transducer probe is moved and the interface at a given depth increases or decreases in depth with respect to the location of the probe on the outer surface, the inner topography can be performed. The imaging system will record the position or direction of the probe and store this together with the brightness data in a memory bank. With this technique, the adjacent brightness points can be seen as if they are connected, and

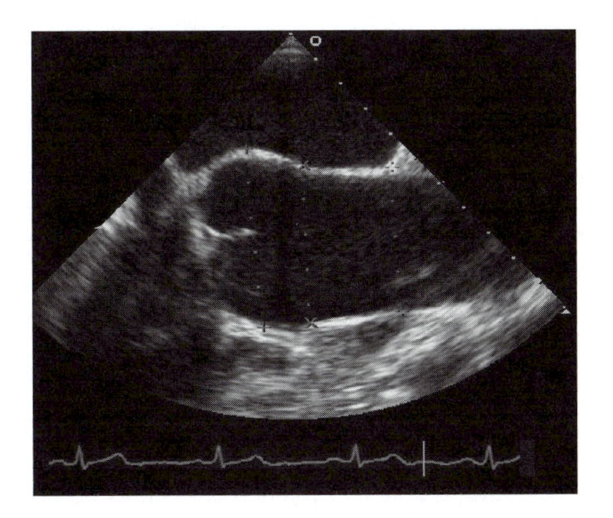

FIGURE 16.10 Sonogram showing a cross section of the heart created by reflection tomography in B-mode. (Courtesy of Brett Fowler, Heineman Research Laboratory, Carolinas Medical Center, Charlotte, NC.)

contour images can be revealed from various depths. M-mode is also frequently used to image movement such as a fetus in the womb, but it is also used to reconstruct an image by moving the transducer itself to compile the image in summation. Heart valve diagnosis applies M-mode imaging, and, in other cardiovascular applications, M-mode is used to analyze deformations in pumping motion of the heart.

16.8 ULTRASOUND IMAGE ARTIFACTS

As with any diagnostic tool, there are limitations to the accuracy of images that are produced. Many of the artifacts seen in ultrasound images are due to the reflective properties of the tissues being analyzed. One artifact arises when two reflective surfaces are close to each other and the sound wave bounces between them. In this case, each time the sound reverberates, some of the sound will transmit through the proximal interface, and an echo will reach the transducer. Consequently, apparent structures are seen in the image at regular intervals descending down into the tissue although there may be no structures there at all. This causes a "comet tail" effect in the image.

Another artifact can be seen behind any highly reflective interface that only transmits a small amount of ultrasound. In such cases, there is not enough sound energy to reach deeper tissues to produce echoes that are received by the transducer. Consequently, there is tissue beyond the highly reflective surface that the device cannot register. The resulting areas appear dark on the image and are called reflective shadows. Echoes reaching the transducer that do not come from the opposite direction of the incident ultrasound beam cause another artifact, called displacement. This can occur when a beam of ultrasound is reflected off two or more reflective surfaces at angles that cause the echo to return to the transducer. In this case, an apparent structure will appear to be in a place where, perhaps, no structure exists.

16.9 THREE-DIMENSIONAL ULTRASOUND IMAGE RECONSTRUCTION

When considering the 2-D ultrasound imaging as a diagnostic tool, some of the limitations of the 2-D systems can be noticed. In 2-D imaging, only one thin slice of the patient can be viewed at any time, and the location of this image plane is controlled by physically manipulating the transducer orientation. Consequently, the technician or the therapist/surgeon must mentally integrate many 2-D images to form an impression of the 3-D anatomy and pathology. This process is time consuming and inefficient, but more importantly rather subjective. In addition, due to the patient's anatomy or position, it is sometimes impossible to orient the 2-D ultrasound transducer to obtain the optimal image plane. Three-dimensional imaging will allow arbitrary orientation of the image viewing plane within the data volume.

Three-dimensional reconstruction of volumes of tissue using ultrasound imaging is one of the most recent advances in ultrasound technology. In order to form 3-D images, one must take consecutive scans of the tissue using normal 2-D techniques and store them in a computer. Then the computer system stacks those images and interpolates the space between the stacked images to create a virtual 3-D model of the tissue. In order to perform this, one must know exactly how far the ultrasound sensor or beam has moved between sequential scans. Unlike computed tomography (CT) and magnetic resonance (MR) imaging, in which 2-D images are usually acquired at a slow rate as a stack of parallel slices, in a fixed orientation, ultrasound provides topographic images at a high rate, and in arbitrary orientations. The high acquisition rate and arbitrary orientation of the images provide unique problems to overcome and opportunities to exploit in extending 2-D ultrasound imaging to 3-D visualization.

There are four typical techniques to view the 3-D image: surface rendering (SR), multiplanar reformatting (MPR), volume rendering (VR), and maximum intensity projection (MIP). SR is based on visualization of surfaces of structures or organs and has been used successfully in rendering of echocardiographic images obtained in obstetrics (Figure 16.11).

The MPR approach is a technique in which computer user interface allows selection of single or multiple planes, including oblique viewing of the 3-D image. The 3-D image is usually presented as a polyhedron representing the boundaries of the reconstructed volumes; the faces of the polyhedron can be moved in or out, parallel to the original or obliquely.

VR displays the entire 3-D image after it has been projected onto a 2-D plane and is used particularly in displaying fetal and vascular anatomy. Figure 16.12 shows an MIP of a 3-D power Doppler image of a finger. The image has been sliced to demonstrate that excellent 3-D images of vascular structures can be obtained.

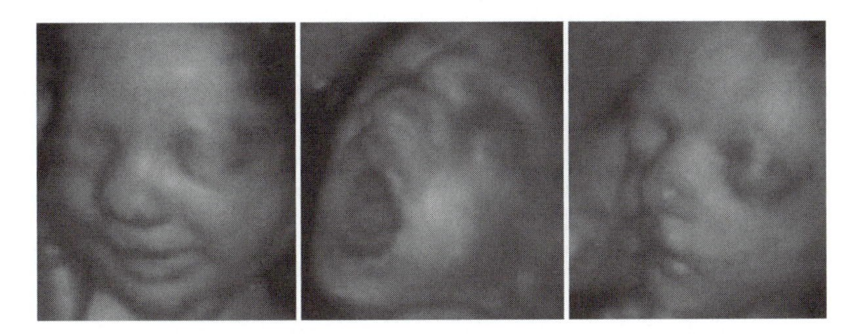

FIGURE 16.11 SR and VR of an exceptional view of a fetus at 24 weeks with enhancement of surfaces of the face of a fetus. (Courtesy of Philips Medical Systems.)

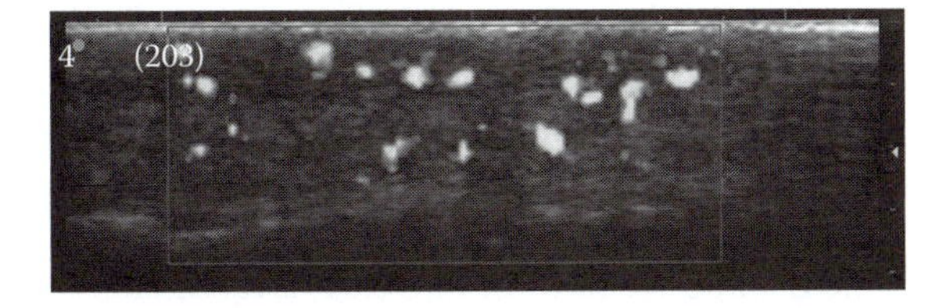

FIGURE 16.12 MIP of a 3-D power Doppler image of a finger. The image has been "sliced" to demonstrate that excellent 3-D images of vascular structures can be obtained. (Courtesy of Ardent Sound, Inc., Guided Therapy Systems, Inc., Mesa, AZ.)

16.10 APPLICATIONS OF ULTRASOUND IMAGING

Ultrasound imaging is often used to provide the bearings for invasive and noninvasive surgery. One of the most well-known applications of ultrasound imaging is monitoring the development of a baby (fetus) in the womb. The same system is sometimes used to determine the sex of the fetus.

A major application of Doppler ultrasound is the study of the heart and human carotid artery disease wherein imaging and frequency shift are combined to produce images of artery and ventricle lumens. As explained earlier, the frequency shift data are used to color code the image, showing direction of flow. Analogous to optical Doppler imaging, flow toward the ultrasound probe is represented in blue due to the shift toward a higher frequency, and flow away from the probe is represented in red (e.g., carotid arteries in red and veins in blue). Obstructions to blood flow are readily evaluated by this method using handheld scanning devices.

Some ultrasound imaging devices provide a virtual reality images on a visor display for image-guided surgeries such as laparoscopic surgery. The virtual reality image can be linked to the position and direction of the surgeon's head to correlate the previously recorded ultrasound images to the corresponding position the operator is looking.

Three-dimensional ultrasound images are sometimes used in vascular surgery. By placing a miniature ultrasound probe in a catheter, the probe can be inserted into the lumen of blood vessels, in particular, the coronary arteries. When a 3-D image of the lumen of the artery can be attained, surgeons obtain more preintervention information on the extent of stenosis, or blockage, and these data could affect the type of intervention chosen. The process also allows pre- and postintervention characterization of vessels to show the effectiveness of the chosen intervention.

Techniques that allow real-time guidance of the needle/fiber into the tissue using ultrasound imaging are currently used for some medical diagnostics applications. In addition to imaging heart valves and blood vessels, ultrasound is the most convenient and inexpensive method for medical evaluations such as gallbladder stones. Ultrasound imaging is also being used for monitoring therapy methods, such as hyperthermia, cryosurgery, drug injections, and as a guide during biopsies and catheter placements.

16.11 PROCESSING AND FEATURE EXTRACTION OF ULTRASONIC IMAGES

Almost all image analysis techniques described in Chapters 4 and 5 are used to trace the outline of organs and other anatomical features and extract features such as volume of the objects. Further image signal and processing can yield tissue discrimination based on the measured frequency spectrum and the localization of these frequency characteristics in the imaging field.

Since there are no definite regularities in the acoustic signals collected from the various impedance discontinuities at the interface of different organ media, there is no clear spatial frequency information on the noise. However, there is a certain degree of omnipresent noise with undetermined frequency content. This noise will need to be eliminated to increase the contrast and resolution obtained from true discrete discontinuities. Because of this noise, it is almost impossible to detect any activation or image feature without resorting to statistical analysis. This analysis requires a model of noise usually assuming a Gaussian distribution.

The noise often comes from discontinuities at angles with the sonic beam, from gradient differences, and from thermal and other motion artifacts. All these suggest that in the analysis of ultrasound images in the frequency domain, the high-frequency contents could be often attributed to noise, and, therefore, the filters can be designed to filter these high-frequency noises out.

Wavelet-based filters are essentially based on an approach that aims at obtaining an optimal trade-off between good signal averaging over homogeneous regions and minimal resolution degradation of image details. Similar to the use of wavelets in other imaging techniques, the wavelet transform has a compression effect since, as mentioned before, it has the tendency to bundle the signal of interest into a significantly fewer number of identifiers with respectively large coefficients. On the other hand, noise can be reduced evenly in the wavelet domain. This in turn results in an enhanced signal-to-noise ratio for those coefficients where the signal is concentrated and hence improves the detection rate. This allows the use of a conservative decision strategy to keep the false-detection rate to a minimum.

A crucial point in the selection of wavelet transforms is the appropriate choice of the wavelet base form, the order of the transform and the iteration depth. Different basis functions offer different compromises. The iteration depth controls the accuracy and the sensitivity. The order, depending on the basis functions, has a great influence on the number of detected coefficients and consequently on the sensitivity and specificity. According to the literature, the Daubechies wavelet analysis seems to be the best fit for most ultrasound image processing applications since the reflection is a more or less binary event, which matches the Daubechie mother wavelet. However, other wavelet analysis may fit the gradient response of inhomogeneous reflection conditions.

The wavelet coefficients, area, volume or size of the object, intensity, eccentricity, elongation, and Fourier coefficients are among the most popular features used in the analysis of ultrasound images.

16.12 IMAGE REGISTRATION

Image registration in ultrasound is used to combine images from an array of transducers to present a single image slice. In most cases, the direction of the beam is used as a reference with respect to the adjacent ray. In other cases, specific landmarks need to be identified to correlate the separately acquired images to form a continuous image. In general, the feedback mechanism of the ultrasound device gives the location and direction of each ray of ultrasound, and the Cartesian representation of the rays serves as the map to reconstruct the image with.

If an ultrasound pulse strikes a tissue interface at an oblique angle, the direction of travel will be changed if the speed of sound is different on either side of the interface. For most soft-tissue interfaces, the effect is small. However, if the propagation path includes fluid (such as in pelvic scans by the transabdominal route), the effect can be significant. The effect of refraction is to diverge the path of the ultrasound beam.

Since the ultrasound image is built up by assuming that sound travels in straight lines, regions of tissue that are affected by refraction will be displayed incorrectly.

A different class of registration problems is concerned with registration of image sequences that follow a process that changes with time. Acquisition of images over time and subsequent registration can be used to study dynamic processes such as tissue perfusion, blood flow, and metabolic or physiological processes. One example of such a process is imaging of the heart where images are acquired in synchrony with the heartbeat, synchronized to the ECG or blood pressure waveform. Synchronized or "gated" acquisitions allow averaging of images over multiple cardiac cycles to reduce image noise in nuclear medicine and MR imaging. In a similar way, temporal registration of x-ray images of the heart before and after injection of contrast material allows synchronous subtraction of mask images. These types of image registration methods assume that the imaging cycle does not change between periods, or for the heart, from beat to beat. A similar principle applies to images acquired at different stages of the breathing cycle, although the breathing cycle is less reproducible, and therefore registration errors will be greater.

One serious consideration in image registration is the use of nonguided freehand imaging. The interpretation of the acquired image relies solely on the anatomical knowledge of the operator, and the mental interpretation of the angle and position of the transducer by the clinician. Most other ultrasound imaging modalities have a built-in feedback mechanism that relates each scan with respect to the previous scan by mechanical and/or electronic feedback.

16.13 COMPARISON OF CT, MRI, AND ULTRASONIC IMAGES

Ultrasonic imaging has many overlaps with x-ray CT imaging as far as the one-to-one image formation is concerned; both mechanisms assume rectilinear propagation of the image carrier. However, ultrasound does not have the same penetration capabilities as the x-ray used in CT scanning, and ultrasound is less harmful than x-ray.

On the other hand, MRI, due to its very high resolution and image quality, provides detailed physiological information, while ultrasound only gives flow feedback. Compared to MRI, the main advantage of ultrasound is the low cost and portability of ultrasound machines. In addition, as will be discussed later, the presence of iron-based or other ferromagnetic materials is prohibited in the MRI room, which calls for the use of often costly tools such as titanium-based surgical tools in the MRI room. No such restriction is applied to ultrasound. Moreover, to ease of conducting ultrasound imaging allows using the machine for imaging of almost all types of patients without the use of sedatives. However, in order to perform MRI on some children and even adults with claustrophobia, the patients need to be sedated or even put to sleep to allow image acquisition.

16.14 BIOEFFECTS OF ULTRASOUND

The following bioeffects of ultrasonic imaging deserve attention: thermal effects, mechanical and cavitational effects, cellular and subcellular effects, biochemical effects, and finally the effects of ultrasound on organs and systems.

Ultrasound waves contain mechanical energy that can be transformed into heat; in which case, an increase in the temperature of the exposed tissues and cells will result. The temperature increase depends on the energy exposure (power and time frame) and the tissue characteristics. In specific therapeutic cases, this temperature effect is desired for destruction of kidney and gallstones; however, for imaging purposes, no harmful temperature increase is recorded at the customary relatively low power density levels.

Two different types of mechanical and cavitational effects can be distinguished. The first-order effect is accomplished by strain and shear stress induced by out-of-phase acceleration of components of the same biological structure. In certain cases, the local particle acceleration can exceed 25,000 times the gravitational acceleration. In such cases, when the focal point is relatively small compared to the structure size, the ultrasound causes tear-and-twist effects. Examples are cellular membrane fatigue, mostly observed in red blood cells, resulting in autolysis of the erythrocytes. Additionally ultrasound may liquefy thixotropic structures, including mitotic and meiotic spindles. Cavitation is the oscillatory activity of highly compressible bodies such as gas bubbles or cavities. This feature depends largely on the pulse duration and can disrupt white and red blood cells and epithelial cells, and may additionally cause blood coagulation dysfunction.

On the cellular and subcellular level, cells may get disrupted by the cavitation process, which produces shear stresses. Some of the reported cellular consequences are swelling of the mitochondria and enlargement of the endoplasmic reticulum. However, no direct effects on the functionality of the mitochondria have been observed, although increased membrane permeability to water has been detected. Due to the relatively long wavelength, no atomic or molecular (DNA) influence has been found.

On the biochemical level, the influence of ultrasound energy has been known to decrease glutathione levels and increases in alanine aminotransferase (ALT) and aspartate aminotransferase (AST) levels in the blood. Additionally an increase in collagen synthesis has also been observed.

In terms of the influence of ultrasound on the developmental stages or organs and systems, there is no conclusive evidence on any effects on fetal growth; however, wound healing seems to be accelerated. Ultrasound has been shown to produce retinal damage and affect the cornea, but, at the same time, ultrasound can also be used to treat mild cases of myopia. One significant risk is damage to the inner ear.

Despite all the evidence cited earlier, no epidemiological data can support any seriously harmful side effect due to ultrasound exposure. This makes ultrasound the most used diagnostic technique in hospitals.

16.15 SUMMARY

Ultrasound imaging uses a rather simple mechanism of acoustic generation by electric transducers that can produce and acquire mechanical displacement. The principle of image formation is based on the detection of attenuation, reflection, and TOF for reflected and transmitted pressure. There are three distinct methods of imaging in use, attenuation tomography, reflection tomography, and TOF tomography. Each of these methods targets a specific anatomical contrast feature. Ultrasound is used in many diagnostics and therapeutic applications due to its harmless effects on the biological tissues.

PROBLEMS

16.1 Intensity of ultrasound is defined as the pressure per unit of area. An ultrasound wave with a frequency of 5 MHz and an intensity of 20 mW/cm^2 traverses a medium with an acoustic discontinuity at 5 mm depth. Assume there is no attenuation in either medium. The power collected by the transducer is 0.2 mW over an aperture of 0.15 cm^2.

a. Calculate the transmitted intensity.

b. Assuming $Z_1 = 1.65 \times 10^6$ kg/m^2 s, calculate Z_2.

c. Calculate the reflected pressure and show that the reflected and transmitted pressure combined would yield the incident pressure.

16.2 The standard deviation of the collected signal for aortic wall divided by the mean signal comes close to 1.91 in all four cases. The ratio for muscle tissue will be less than 1.91. By changing the angle of incidence of the ultrasound beam and recording two new images at that angle and average them out will give a new value for each of the tissues that can be used to discriminate between the lipid, the muscle, the aorta, and aortic wall with plaque. Explain how adipose tissue (lipids) adjacent to muscle tissue can be distinguished from aortic wall and from aortic wall with plaque, respectively (*Hint:* the solution lies in the scattering properties of the tissues).

16.3 A train of ultrasound pulses is bombarding a slab of medium and is described by an intensity profile function of time, $x(t)$. The Fourier transform of this periodic phenomenon is $X(f)$. The transmitted ultrasound wave front is $y(t)$ with Fourier transform, $Y(f)$. The transmitted Fourier transformed wave front is the characteristic transfer function of the medium, $H(f)$, applied to the incident Fourier wave front described by the following equation: $Y(f) = H(f)X(f)$. The transfer function is the Fourier transform of the impulse response function in the time domain for the tissue slab, $h(t)$. The transmitted ultrasound signal is collected on the opposite side of the slab after attenuation over the thickness of the slab.

a. Derive the transfer function when the attenuation coefficient of the tissue is proportional to the frequency for the frequency range used in this experiment, $\alpha_t = \alpha_0 f$, where α_0 is the attenuation coefficient at 1 MHz.

b. Show that the attenuation coefficient can be estimated from the root-mean-square duration of the impulse response. The duration of the impulse response, $D(t)$, is defined as follows:

$$D_t = \left[\frac{\int_{-\infty}^{\infty} (t - t_c)^2 \left| h(t) \right|^2 dt}{\int_{-\infty}^{\infty} \left| h(t) \right|^2 dt} \right]^{1/2} \tag{16.44}$$

where $t_c = l/c$, with c the speed of sound in the tissue and l the thickness of the slab.

16.4 Since the attenuation coefficient of ultrasound waves generally increases with increasing frequency (see Problem 16.3), explain how second harmonic imaging, i.e., using $f_1 = 2 \cdot f$ as the detected frequency, increases the image information.

16.5 Load file "p_16_5.jpg" and display. A blood vessel is imaged by intravascular ultrasound showing the inside wall and the outside wall surrounded by mostly fat. Using MATLAB® and file p_16_5.jpg representing the clinical data, perform the following.*

a. Calculate the relative thickness of the vessel wall with respect to the vessel diameter.

b. Using the fact that the vessel will be pressed against the catheter and that the catheter has a diameter of 5 mm, calculate the thickness of the vessel wall.

16.6 In laser photocoagulation of ventricular tachycardia, diseased heart muscle is denatured with the energy of laser light to destroy the electric activity of a section of the heart wall that is no longer conducting properly because of cell death resulting from a heart attack. Load file "p_16_6.jpg" and display. Figure "p_16_6" shows an ultrasound image of a laser photocoagulated section of the left ventricular wall of a heart seen through the tissue in the fifth intracostal space of the chest. The heated and coagulated tissue is significantly denser than the healthy heart muscle. The transducer operated at 10 MHz. Use the seed growing algorithm to find the outline of the coagulation lesion. Visually choose suitable seed points to start the segmentation process.

16.7 In Doppler flow measurement using ultrasound, the blood flowing toward the transducer will result in a higher frequency than was originally sent in, while blood flowing away from the transducer will give a decrease in ultrasound frequency. Load file "p_16_7.jpg" and display. The blood flow in "p_16_7.jpg" toward the transducer has the increase in frequency colored as blue, while the flow away from the ultrasound transducer decreases the frequency and is illustrated by red. Use the seed growing algorithm to find the perimeter of the left ventricle, and the fraction of turbulent flow using seed and region growing techniques described in Section 4.3. Visually choose some suitable seed points to start the process.†

16.8 Read image "p_16_8.jpg" and show the image. One of the critical assessments to identify the healthy growth of the baby is measuring the diameter of the baby's head. In this problem, we write MATLAB codes to perform this automatically.

a. Apply Laplacian of Gaussian method to detect the edge of the skull of the baby.

b. Once, the baby's head is detected, write the codes to find the diameter of the head. Here, we define the diameter as the largest distance between two points located on the head's contour.

---

* Courtesy of Brett Fowler, Heineman Research Laboratory, Carolinas Medical Center, Charlotte, NC.

† Courtesy of Ardent Sound, Inc., Guided Therapy Systems, Inc., Mesa, AZ.

16.9 Load file "p_16_9.jpg" and display. Figure "p_16_9" shows a combined M-mode and Doppler image of venous blood flow. The blood flow in "p_16_7.jpg" is shown in blue in the upper half of the image, while the bottom section displays the flow velocity characteristics as a function of time.*

a. Use the seed growing algorithm to find the perimeter of the vein using seed and region growing techniques described in Section 4.3. Visually choose some suitable seed points to start the process.

* Courtesy of Ardent Sound, Inc., Guided Therapy Systems, Inc., Mesa, AZ.

17 Positron Emission Tomography

17.1 INTRODUCTION AND OVERVIEW

Positron emission tomography (PET) is a noninvasive nuclear imaging technique that produces images of the metabolic activity of living organisms on the biochemical level. These physiological images are detected by introducing a short-lived positron-emitting radioactive tracer, or radiopharmaceutical, by either intravenous injection or inhalation. Images are created using a process called radioactive labeling in which one atom in a molecule is replaced by a radioactive radionucleotide.

The PET images produced help physicians identify normal and abnormal activity in living tissue. Unlike computed tomography (CT) that primarily provides anatomical images, PET measures functional chemical changes in the tissue. Some of these chemical changes that are typically metabolic activities occur before the resulting abnormalities are visible on other functional imaging modalities such a regular functional magnetic resonance imaging (*f*MRI). The resolution of PET is far less than that of CT and MRI, and, as a result, PET images are often registered with CT or MRI images to superimpose the anatomical details of CT and MRI on the functional information of PET.

Informally speaking, PET recognizes these metabolic changes by measuring the amount of radioactive tracers distributed throughout the body. This information is subsequently used to create a three-dimensional (3-D) image of tissue function from the acquired decay matrix. Due to the availability of various types of radioactive isotopes, the specific metabolic changes resulting from assorted diseases make PET imaging particularly useful in the detection of malignancy in tumors.

In this chapter, we first describe the physical and physiological principles of PET and then describe applications of PET in medical imaging and diagnostics. A closely related imaging technology called single photon emission computed tomography (SPECT) will be discussed briefly as well toward the end of the chapter. Even though SPECT is briefly described in this chapter, this technology will be separately discussed in Chapter 18, which is dedicated to more specialized imaging technologies.

17.2 PHYSICAL AND PHYSIOLOGICAL PRINCIPLES OF PET

The radionucleotide that is administered in the body during PET imaging contains a specified quantity of short-lived radioactively labeled chemical substances that are identical or closely analogous to naturally occurring substances in the body. The radioactive substances used in PET are nucleotides in which some atoms are replaced by their radioisotopes.

After entering the body, the radioactive substance circulates through the bloodstream to reach the organ or tumor of interest. The radionucleotide then emits positrons as part of the natural disintegration process of the unstable isotopes. A positron is the atomic equivalent of a positive electron, both in mass and in charge, except the charge is opposite to that of the electron's charge.

Once the radioactively labeled substance has been absorbed, it keeps emitting positrons. The imaging is made possible by the positron annihilation with an electron, emitting two gamma rays that are sensed by the detectors outside the body. The measured gamma rays are then processed using tomographic methods to identify the location and quantity of the radioactive uptake at each location inside the body. The resulting image provides functional analysis of the organ in question since, as discussed later, the amount of uptake is related to the metabolic functions of the tissues.

In order to better understand the full use of the radioactive isotopes in PET and the incorporation of each radioactive substance in the cellular metabolism, next the production of the isotopes will be further described.

17.2.1 Production of Radionucleotides

The first stage in the development of a radioactive pharmacologic entity is the production of the radionuclide. As mentioned earlier, the radionucleotides administered in the body are in principle very similar to the material abundantly available in biological tissues, except that in the radionucleotides certain atoms are substituted by their short-lived radioactive isotopes. Such radioactively labeled chemical substances are unstable and emit positrons when in the body. The atoms that are replaced by their isotopes are the main elements abundantly found in biological tissues, i.e., ^{11}C, ^{18}F, ^{13}N, and ^{15}O. The radionucleotide can be produced in many different ways; the most prominent method is the use of an on-site cyclotron. Particle bombardment will produce the needed radionuclides.

Fluorodeoxyglucose (FDG) is the most commonly used radioisotope. The production and chemical interactions of the fluoride isotope with other elements will be described briefly. Other radioactive isotopes follow a similar process. FDG is produced by proton bombardment of ^{18}O enriched water, as shown in Figure 17.1,

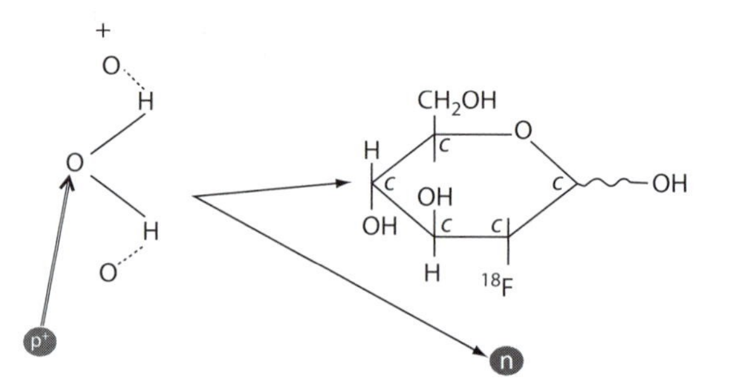

FIGURE 17.1 FDG is produced by proton bombardment of ^{18}O-enriched water and is bound to 1,3,4,6-tetra-O-acetyl-2-O-trifluoromethanesulfonyl-β together with mannose triflate.

causing the $^{18}O(p, n)^{18}F$ reaction. FDG can consequently be recovered as an aqueous solution of ^{18}fluoride and can then be extracted by ion-exchange chromatography. One hour of cyclotron irradiation can produce approximately 800 mCi of ^{18}F. The nomenclatures of related chemicals involved in the production of ^{18}F are $H^{18}F$, $F^{18}F$, and $^{18}F^-$.

It is important to note that ^{18}F can also be produced as a radioactive gas through the deuteron bombardment of neon (^{20}Ne) to produce ^{18}F and an alpha particle. The gaseous state is currently not a popular mechanism and is overall considered a less preferred method.

Now that we have briefly discussed the production of the radioisotopes, next we discuss the degeneration of these substances.

17.2.2 Degeneration Process

The engineered radiopharmaceuticals used in PET have unstable nuclei that degenerate to lower energy states. The decay process is demarcated by a time constant of the decay called the radioactive half-life. The end product of the decay process is generally a stable element that emits no radiation.

The half-life of a radioactive isotope is based on the fact that not all radioactive nuclei decay simultaneously. The decay process is more a probability-determined process, in which the exact isotope that decays cannot be identified with complete certainty. However, the probability of any number of isotopes decaying within a certain interval of time is well known and can be established by empirical methods. The fact that the decay process is irreversible means that the quantity of radioactive isotopes will continuously decline over time. Certain radionucleotides are more stable than others and therefore will take a longer time to produce one single decay event.

The radioactive half-life is formally defined as the time interval in which the atomic count of the isotope has dropped to half the initial quantity as a result of radioactive decay. The half-lives of the main radioisotopes used in PET imaging span a range of almost 100 s to almost 100 min. Specifically, for ^{18}F, as found in an FDG, the half-life is 109.7 min. A shorter half-life is that of the carbon isotope, ^{11}C, which is only 20 min. The other two main isotopes are the nitrogen isotope, ^{13}N, with a half-life of 10 min and the oxygen isotope, ^{15}O, with the half-life of only 124 s.

Out of the four main radioisotopes used in PET scans, the nucleotide fluoride, ^{18}F, is the most commonly used. The fluoride isotope is almost always incorporated into FDG, which is essentially a radioactive equivalent of glucose. Because of its similarity to glucose, FDG is used to measure the glucose metabolic rate in a number of body organ systems. Monitoring the consumption of glucose is therefore measuring the metabolism of the cells. This is why PET is a functional imaging. As shown earlier, the fluoride isotope has a relatively slow decay, which means that it can be shipped after production in the cyclotron and still have ample useable molecular weight left at the time it reaches the hospital that can be as far away as 100 km. This is the main reason for the popularity of FDG.

The next issue that needs to be addressed is the detection of the radionucleotides.

17.3 PET SIGNAL ACQUISITION

All short-lived radioisotopes used in PET imaging decay by positron emission. Positrons (β+) are emitted from the nucleus of radioisotopes that are unstable because they have an excessive number of protons and a positive charge. The positron emission is different from the free proton or odd proton count utilized in NMR imaging as described in Chapter 15.

Positron emission stabilizes the nucleus by removing a positive charge through the conversion of a proton and a neutron, as shown in the following chemical reaction describing the fluoride decay:

$$ {}^{18}_{9}F \rightarrow {}^{0}_{+1}e + {}^{18}_{8}O \tag{17.1}$$

As can be seen in the chemical reaction shown earlier, during the decay process, the radionucleotide is converted into an element whose atomic number is one less than the isotope's atomic number. For radioisotopes used in PET scans, the element formed from positron decay is stable and will not have any remaining decay mechanisms.

The distance an emitted positron travels depends on the rest energy of the positron. Typically, the positron travel distance is limited to approximately 1 mm. The positron combines with an ordinary electron of a nearby atom in an annihilation reaction, forming positronium as an intermediate reaction product. The positron will virtually immediately annihilate after the collision with free electrons abundantly available in the biological tissues. When a positron comes in contact with an electron, the annihilation process releases energy greater than 1 MeV. This reaction is governed by conservation of energy. This energy, which is in the form of gamma rays, is then measured by the detectors in the PET system.

The mass of the positron and the electron combined has enough energy to produce a pair of gamma photons. The merging energy is released as two gamma quanta with 511 keV are emitted at 180° to each other. The positron-electron annihilation process is outlined in Figure 17.2. These photons easily escape from the living tissues and

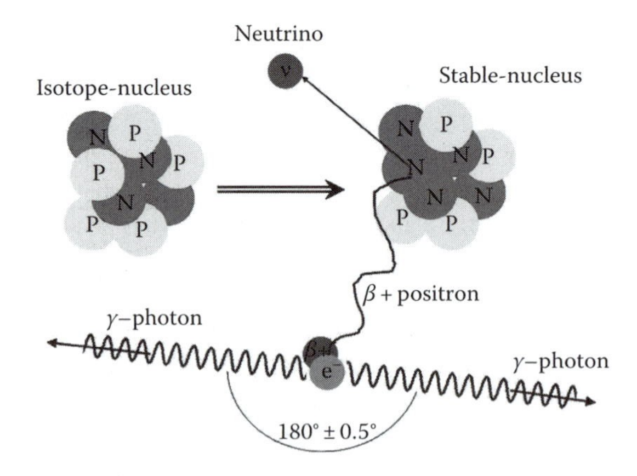

FIGURE 17.2 Positron emission, annihilation as a result of interaction with electron, and gamma pair emission.

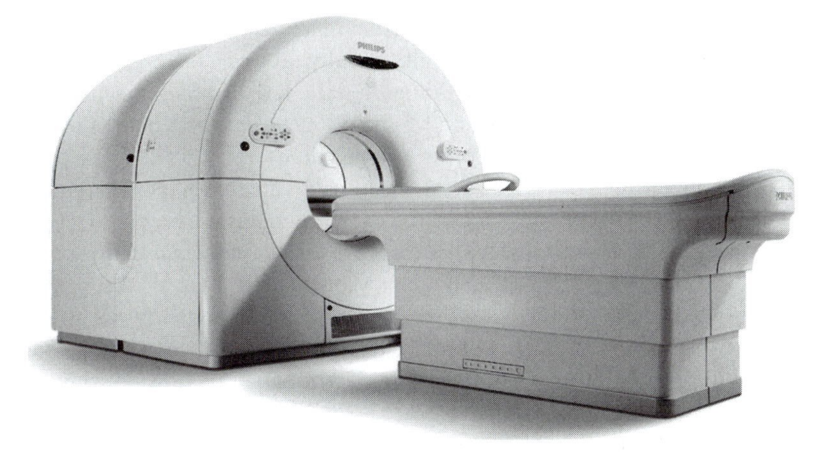

FIGURE 17.3 Philips Medical Systems Gemini CT_PET combo scanner. The rear section of the Gemini is the CT scanner while the front section has the PET scanner. This system allows registration of CT anatomical images with PET physiological information. (Courtesy of Philips Medical Systems, Amsterdam, the Netherlands.)

can be recorded by external detectors. The perpendicular emission of the gamma photons falls on a line of coincidence. The coincidence lines provide a unique detection scheme for forming tomographic images with PET.

Informally speaking, the time-resolved detection of two simultaneous gamma photons on the connecting line of coincidence establishes 1-D indicator of the location of the concentration of the radioisotopes. Additional emissions from the same location will not follow the exact same path, and lines of intersect can be established to yield the second dimension of the isotopes. Detections along the lines of coincidence for all emitted gamma rays are then used in a standard tomographic procedure to produce an image of the tissue based on the nucleotide concentrations.

The layout of a PET imaging device has multiple rings with detectors specifically designed to capture simultaneous occurrences of gamma photon emissions. A diagram of the configuration of a PET imager is shown in Figure 17.3. These detectors are further described in the following.

17.3.1 Radioactive Detection in PET

When the 511 keV gamma rays interact with scintillation such as crystals composed of bismuth germanate (BGO), they are converted into light photons in the crystals. The visible light photons are collected by photosensor arrays, such as charged coupled detection (CCD) elements, and are subsequently converted to electric signals. This conversion and recording process happens almost instantly, and as a result, the scintillation events can be compared among all opposing detectors (along numerous coincidence lines). The distribution of the positron emitting radioisotope depends on the biochemical composition as well as the physiological activities of the tissue being scanned.

PET scanning is invasive, in that radioactive material is injected into the patient. However, the total dose of radiation is small, usually around 7 mSv. This can be compared to 2.2 mSv average annual background radiation, 0.02 mSv for a chest x-ray, up to 8 mSv for a CT scan of the chest, and 2–6 mSv per year for a person that travels frequently on planes (especially the crew of an airplane).

A PET detector ring has several sections called gantry buckets. The buckets are divided even further into blocks. Generally, each block has a detector array with an 8 × 8 configuration of detectors. The detectors are also called bins. In this configuration, each block has 64 detectors. Each gantry bucket has four blocks, providing a subtotal of 256 detectors. Completing the total circumference requires 16 buckets, adding up to 4096 detectors. Most commercial PET systems have two rings, yielding a total of 8192 detectors that all need to be operational at all times during a single scan. Considering that the detector arrays are 8 × 8, and there are two rings, the axial plane is divided into 16 sections for simultaneous scans.

The detectors are closely spaced and have a relatively wide acceptance angle. Based on this fact, the gamma rays from a single positron can be detected by more than one perfectly opposite pair of detectors. The crossover detection between neighboring detectors introduces a slight inaccuracy and distortion in the detection accuracy.

When one detector is matched with a range of detectors at various angles (i.e., not just the one directly across the ring), the system provides a platform for multiple angle of coincidence sampling. This configuration is outlined in Figure 17.4. In this method, the emissions at oblique angles can be detected in multiple pairs for greater accuracy.

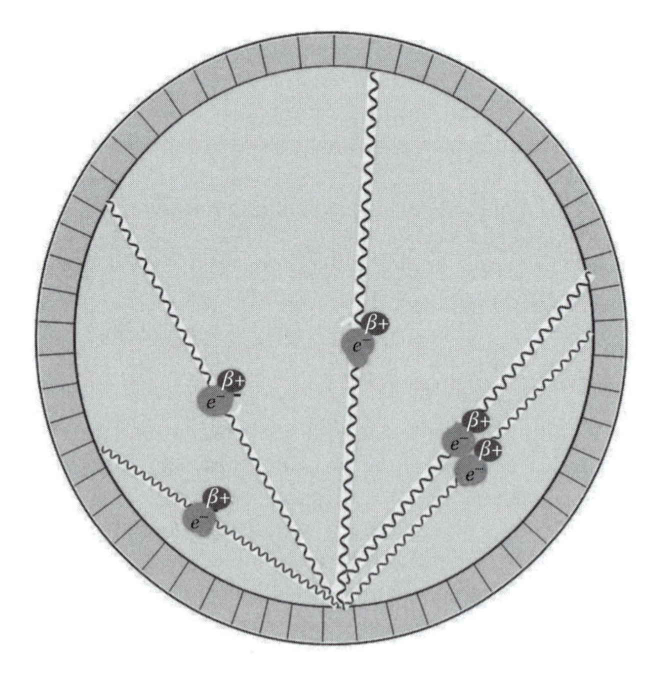

FIGURE 17.4 Coincidence sampling; schematic diagram of fan-beam detection.

Each detector will operate in multiple coincidence sampling mode, interacting with multiple detectors at a range of angles. As discussed in Chapter 11, this method of detector configuration is called fan-beam response.

Another mode of operation collects at perpendicular incidence only and is called coincidence sampling in linear mode. In this configuration, the detectors collect parallel to each other. The parallel mode of detection is illustrated in Figure 17.5. Each mode of operation has its own advantages and disadvantages. For example, the maximum error in location detection often occurs under fan-beam detection, while the crossover differences are relatively limited under parallel ray detection.

Before discussing the significance of the PET modality in medical diagnostics, we briefly review an alternative method of radioactive detection in PET called scintigraphy. In scintigraphy, instead of converting the gamma photons to visible light detection, the high-energy gamma radiation is used to directly detect the gamma photon. The gamma radiation excites a medium in a container with a window that is transparent to gamma radiation. The excited medium (solid, liquid, or gas) degenerates back to its ground state and emits a photon in the visible spectrum in the process. The induced fluorescence is then used to induce a photoelectric effect in the metal wall of the detector to produce a corresponding electric current. This method constitutes an alternative to the CCD mentioned earlier.

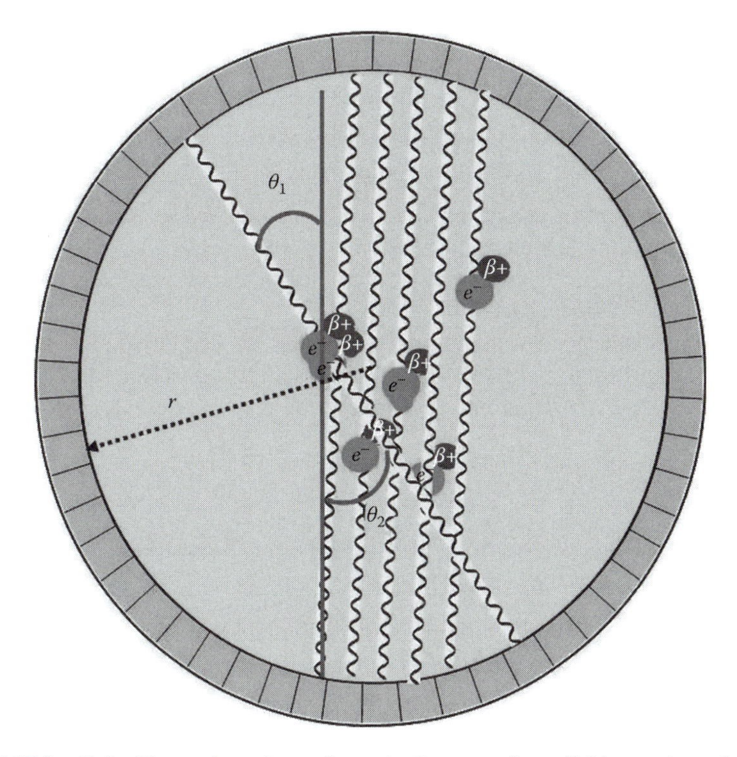

FIGURE 17.5 Coincidence detection; schematic diagram of parallel beam detection.

17.4 PET IMAGE FORMATION

The PET's tomographic reconstruction algorithm uses the coinciding events measured at all angular and linear positions and reconstructs an image that depicts the localization and concentration of the positron-emitting radioisotope within a plane of the organ that was scanned. These sampling features all have an effect on the final image quality.

For a given pair of gamma rays at angles with a conveniently chosen coordinate system (θ_1, θ_2) the detector counts $n(\theta_1, \theta_2)$ coincidence events (see Figure 17.5). The detector ring has a radius r, which places the location of each annihilation event at the respective locations with regard to the detectors as $r\theta_1$ and $r\theta_2$, which are joined by a line segment l_{θ_1,θ_2}.

The detected number of annihilations is proportional to the integrated intensity of the source of radioisotopes in the body, I_n, ignoring attenuation for now. The intensity of the source along the line segment l_{θ_1,θ_2} is represented as follows:

$$I_n \propto r\int_0^l \rho_\gamma[sr\theta_1 + (1-s)r\theta_2]ds \tag{17.2}$$

where ρ_γ is the distribution function of the radioisotopes in the biological volume.

The boundary conditions are given by the fact that the number of decays in a volume element V_{xy} has a Poison distribution with an intensity proportional to

$$I_{n_j} \propto \iint_{V_j} \rho_\gamma(x,y)\,dxdy \tag{17.3}$$

Nonetheless, the gamma radiation pairs will be attenuated as a result of scattering and absorption before reaching the detectors.

The two gamma rays released from the annihilation will be attenuated independently and will be detected independently.

Assuming a universal attenuation coefficient α_γ, the detected decay events will be described by the convolution of the respective gamma pair rays, providing an expression for the gamma rays that make it to the detectors in the following form:

$$I_n = I_0 r\iint_{V_j} \rho_\gamma[sr\theta_1 + (1-s)r\theta_2]e^{-\alpha_\gamma s}ds \tag{17.4}$$

The concentration of isotopes will result in a cumulative recording in various directions of gamma pairs from different locations within the organ over the half-life of the radionucleotide. A concurrent limitation in the time domain is the half-life of the radioisotope itself. The repetition rate of the detections is directly linked to the half-life of the remaining isotopes. The more isotopes are active in an organ, the greater the likelihood that any one of them will decay to a lower energy state, thus providing a higher frequency of detections.

The preceding equations form a topographic problem in which the set of equations must be solved for the integrand. The details on how these tomographic equations are solved using methods such as Fourier slice theorem have been provided in the previous chapters.

17.5 SIGNIFICANCE OF PET

Despite its relatively low resolution, PET imaging has many advantages in imaging and detection of physiological characteristics that are still being explored and expanded. The main significance of PET in biomedical diagnostics lies in the fact that direct metabolic activity can be imaged often on a significantly finer levels than what can be detected using other technologies such as *f*MRI described in Chapter 15.

The applications of PET imaging are significantly more limited than other scintigraphy-based imaging methods due to the extremely short half-lives of the radioisotopes used in PET imaging. A more detailed comparison of the PET with more aggressive nucleotide used in other scintigraphy-based imaging systems will be discussed in Chapter 18.

The medical significance of the PET modality will become more evident in our discussion of the applications of the PET imaging given in the following.

17.6 APPLICATIONS OF PET

PET is an invaluable technique for diagnosing specific diseases and disorders, because it is possible to target the radiochemicals used for particular bodily functions.

17.6.1 Cancer Tumor Detection

The functional imaging features of PET are most prominent in the diagnosis of cancer. Healthy tissue replenishes its cells by continuous regeneration, while old cells gradually die off. Both malignant and benign cancer cells divide more rapidly than normal healthy cells. This process by itself will be identified under PET imaging due to the increased cellular metabolic rate. In cancer detection using PET, the tracer FDG is used because it mimics glucose in its metabolic stage and is avidly taken up and retained by most tumors. As a result, this technique can be used for the diagnosis and monitoring of the treatment of various cancer tumors. Due to its specific sensitivity, PET is mostly used to diagnose brain tumors. Other PET applications in cancer diagnosis are in detection of the breast tumors, lung tumors, and colorectal tumors.

The difference between malignant and benign tumor growth is the fact that in malignant cancer cells the surrounding tissue is destroyed as well. The amount of ^{18}F that accumulates in a tissue over a specific period of time makes it possible to calculate the rate of glucose uptake in that tissue. An accelerated glucose metabolism

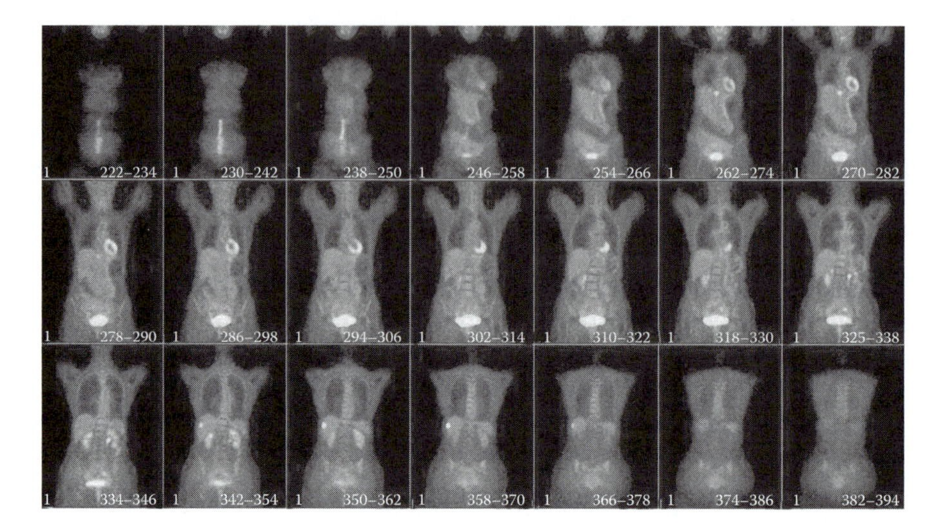

FIGURE 17.6 Selected whole-body PET images of a person with suspected colorectal cancer. (Courtesy of Philips Medical Systems, Amsterdam, the Netherlands.)

and a decreased ability to make energy through aerobic processes are established features of malignant tumor cells. The combination of these features results in a high glucose uptake to maintain the cell metabolism.

In malignant tumors, the cancer also migrates away from the organ in which the tumor is initially formed and starts infiltrating surrounding tissues and organs. This process is called metastasis. Some of these features can be registered in PET imaging. PET imaging is particularly useful in providing whole-body survey to identify widespread tumor infiltration. An additional feature of malignant cells is an increase in glucose (or FDG) transporter molecules at the membrane surface of tumor cells. This is in contrast to benign tumor cells. Since PET scans are typically more expensive than some of the more widely used imaging modalities such as CT, the clinical use of PET for tumor diagnosis is very limited. Figure 17.6 shows a whole-body PET scan of a person with a suspected rectal cancer.

17.6.2 Functional Brain Mapping

Another application of PET imaging is in imaging and diagnosis of the brain. This usage is based on an assumption that areas of high radioactivity are associated with brain activity. What is actually measured indirectly is the flow of blood to different parts of the brain, which is correlated to the level of activity of the neurons. In PET of the brain, the tracer oxygen (^{15}O) is usually used as the radioisotope. In the brain images created using this technology, the areas of the brain that are active, i.e., using a significant level of oxygen, are illuminated. This is why the brain tumors are represented as very bright regions in PET images.

PET has been used in many clinical diagnostic applications such as detection of brain disorders. Specifically, the determination of Alzheimer's disease and other dementia forms the justification for the use of PET imaging. PET imaging shows the metabolic degeneration of the neurotransmitters in the brain of an Alzheimer patient. PET can track the different stages of reduced brain function. While in the early stages of Alzheimer's disease, only limited areas of the brain will be detected to have a lower level of function, in the later stages of Alzheimer's disease, the metabolic activity of larger areas of the brain will progressively appear affected. Particularly, in Alzheimer's disease, the disease follows a certain pattern in affecting the brain under PET imaging. The disease pattern can often be recognized several years in advance of the manifestation of episodes of confusion and recognizable category of dementia or depression.

Other brain disorders that can be located by PET scans are Parkinson's disease and schizophrenia. Other neurological diagnoses that can be performed using PET include the diagnostics and study of the brain activities in epilepsy and stroke. For instance, PET can be used to determine the location of epileptic seizures prior to surgery to develop a road map for the procedure.

Considering the imaging of the neural structures, the pivotal advantage of PET over many of the other available imaging modalities is the ability to reveal activity of neuroreceptors such as the ones that use the neurotransmitters serotonin, dopamine, and noradrenaline. Typical MRI imaging systems are unable to identify neurochemical sites due to the low neurotransmitter concentrations involved (in the order of micromolar concentrations).

17.6.3 Functional Heart Imaging

For diagnostic applications in cardiology, PET with FDG is used to functionally image the heart tissue after a heart attack and determine if there is any latent damage in the heart muscle. In the diagnosis of heart disease, the dead tissue can be separated from the living tissue in a PET scan based on the oxygen isotope interaction. PET imaging is also useful in predicting the success of angioplasty or even bypass surgery. In another cardiovascular application, PET scanning is used to determine blockage of coronary arteries. A PET image of the heart and attached vasculature is illustrated in Figure 17.7.

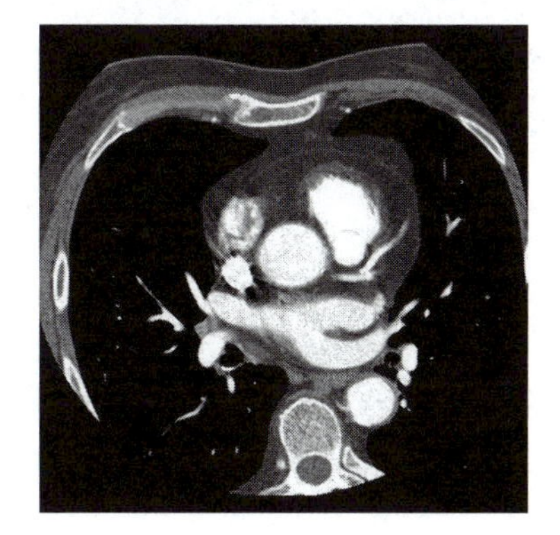

FIGURE 17.7 PET image of the heart and attached vasculature. (Courtesy of Philips Medical Systems, Amsterdam, the Netherlands.)

Despite the numerous benefits of PET for cardiovascular imaging, often the relatively inexpensive SPECT is used for this purpose. SPECT, like PET, acquires the concentration distribution of radionucleotides in a patient's body. The major differences between PET and SPECT are in the choice of radioisotopes and hence the energy of the emission. In PET, two gamma photons are created from the emitted positron particle, while, in SPECT, only one single photon is emitted without a go-between with considerably less energy, approximately 140 keV compared to 511 keV. Due to the nature and configuration of the single photon emitted from the radionucleotides in SPECT, special collimators are required to acquire an image from multiple angles. The use of collimators dramatically reduces the detection efficiency in comparison with PET. This is in sharp contrast with PET imaging, which relies on the perpendicular nature of the emitted gamma photons of annihilation of the positron emitted from the isotope.

Generally, PET has two orders of magnitude greater number of detectors than SPECT, giving PET imaging a much higher resolution. The advantage of SPECT is the wide variety of radionucleotides that are available and the resulting bigger range of detection of diseases. The cost of SPECT imaging is approximately one-third that of PET, which gives it an advantage over PET in certain cases. However, the lower resolution remains an obstacle. SPECT will be described in more detail in Chapter 18.

17.6.4 Anatomical Imaging

As previously discussed, PET provides no significant anatomical information primarily due to the fact that the uptake of radioisotopes in some tissues such as bone is too slow to be recorded. For instance, due to the half-life of the isotopes and the assembly time for bone tissue, the radioactivity has dropped below the detection level at the time of incorporation in the skeletal system.

The anatomical features that can be recognized in PET are mainly due to the a priori metabolic activities that are well known for certain organs such as in the brain and the heart. Other anatomical features will need to be resolved by registering

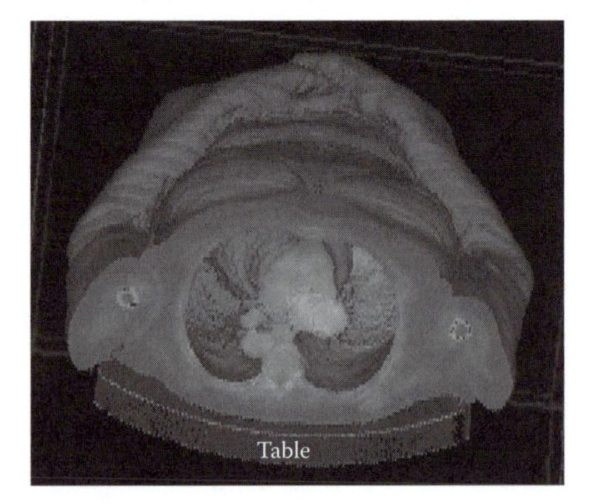

FIGURE 17.8 A 3-D rendering of PET whole-body scan image. (Courtesy of Philips Medical Systems, Amsterdam, the Netherlands.)

the PET images with other scanning techniques that will provide better anatomical details of the biological tissues. In this case, external markers are often needed. These makers are used as tie points to register the two images with each other.

In Figure 17.8, a whole-body PET scan in 3-D rendering shows the anatomical details that can be revealed by PET imaging; note, however, the unevenness in the body surface as acquired by PET imaging.

17.7 PROCESSING AND FEATURE EXTRACTION OF PET IMAGES

Now that we are familiar with the physics of PET and its applications in biomedical diagnostics, we briefly review the computational methods specialized for processing of PET images.

17.7.1 Sources of Noise and Blurring in PET

The fact that two gamma quanta need to be detected simultaneously and the gamma quanta have distinct energy content makes the detection method very precise. There is no significant noise in this energy spectrum, nor is there any background radiation that fits the criteria for detection. Emission from outside the slice of interest is also negligible since such an emission is never registered by both detectors in the plane of observation. The uptake of FDG, and thus ^{18}F, is enhanced during any type of inflammatory process, which can result in false-positive recordings. This reduces the overall accuracy of PET in certain types of diagnostic applications.

While external sources of noise are practically nonexistent in PET, three main sources of blurring contribute in the visible blurring of the PET image. The main source of misreading the location of the source of the positron emission is attributed to the fact that the positron will travel some distance before it interacts with an electron and is annihilated. The two photons that are emitted will be recorded as being displaced from the true location of the isotope by less than 1 mm.

A second source of blurring roots in a 0.5° spread in both the positive and the negative arc from the 180° dual gamma quanta emission. This is another systematic cause of blurring that typically cannot be overcome with the current state of the PET technology.

The third cause of blurring and loss of details is a machine artifact that is a direct result of the spacing of the detectors in the tomographic ring. This last issue also introduces an axial point-spread resulting from the width of the detector, or the thickness of the ring of detectors. The pixel size is the total area of the detector.

While none of these blurring effects can be practically avoided, image processing filters can be used to somehow sharpen the images before processing. All filtering techniques described in Chapter 4, especially the high-boost filter, can be used to address the blurring nature of the PET images.

17.7.2 Image Registration with PET

Since the resolution of PET is very low, it is often required that before any specific image classification decision can be made, the PET image must be registered and superimposed by CT or MR images of the same entity. Combining x-ray tomography with PET is

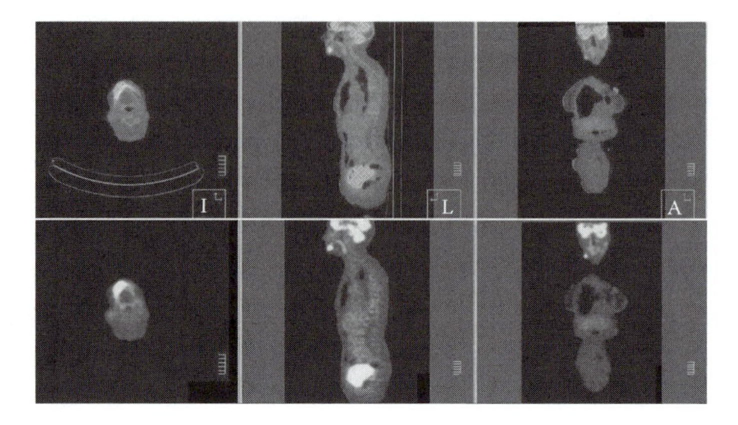

FIGURE 17.9 Registered CT and PET image of a person with details of the head and neck, bottom section PET only. (Courtesy of Philips Medical Systems, Amsterdam, the Netherlands.)

gaining popularity since it can provide both anatomical and physiological images in one session without the need for extensive registration algorithms. The PET/CT combination provides a high-quality diagnostic scanning modality. Figure 17.9 shows a registered CT–PET whole-body scan made by the Philips Gemini imaging device, with specific details on the head and neck area.

As a result, the majority of the image processing methods specialized belong to one of the following two categories. The first group of PET processing techniques includes the registration methods devised to superimpose PET on MR and CT images. The methods in the second category are the segmentation methods that separate and identify the tumor regions from the normal tissues. All the registration methods as well as the segmentation algorithms discussed in Part I of the book are heavily popular in processing of PET images.

In general, in all PET image processing methods, especially in PET wavelet analysis, the performance of the analysis can be significantly enhanced when time dependency and causality of the train of PET images is incorporated in the algorithm. This is particularly significant because the PET images are not static anatomical images, rather physiological information that is continuously changing. In addition, many of the observations made from single PET images can be caused by more than one single phenomenon. For instance, both a tumor and an infection will have similar effects on cellular processes that PET targets for imaging. The only approach that can make a reliable distinction among different possible causes is the time nature of the PET images.

17.8 COMPARISON OF CT, MRI, ULTRASONIC, AND PET IMAGES

Alternative methods of scanning are SPECT, CT, MRI, and *f*MRI. The spatial and temporal resolution of images developed using PET may not be as good as with some of the other techniques. Figure 17.10 illustrates the combination of NMR and PET imaging to reveal baffling details of a tumor scan of the neck after registering the two modalities.

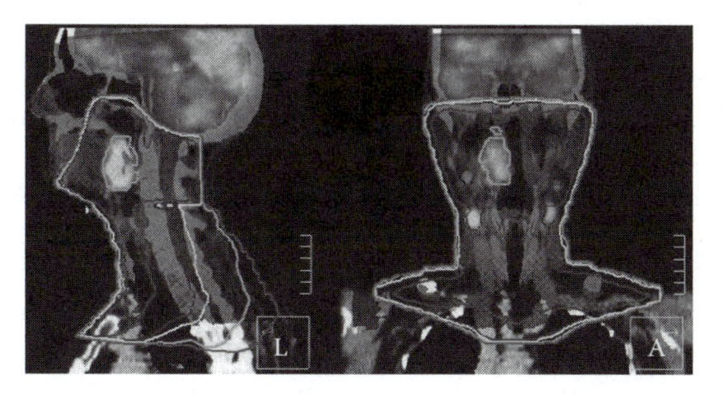

FIGURE 17.10 Registered MRI and PET image of the head and neck. (Courtesy of Philips Medical Systems, Amsterdam, the Netherlands.)

PET scan can detect abnormalities in cellular activity, generally before there is any anatomical change, while other imaging scans, such as CT and MRI, isolate organic anatomical changes in the body.

17.9 SUMMARY

PET scanners are capable of detecting areas of molecular biology detail via the use of radioisotopes that have different rates of uptake depending on the type of tissue involved. In many cases, the PET features will allow to identify diseases earlier and more specifically than ultrasound, x-rays, CT, or MRI. Some of the useful applications of PET scanning over scintillation imaging are examination of brain blood flow and local metabolism of specific organs. PET can also help physicians monitor the treatment of disease. For example, chemotherapy leads to changes in cellular activity, and that is observable by PET long before structural changes can be measured by ultrasound, x-ray CT, and MRI. A typical PET scan gives physicians another tool to evaluate treatments, perhaps even leading to a modification in treatment, before an evaluation could be made using other imaging technologies.

PROBLEMS

17.1 Read the image in file "p_17_1.jpg" and display the image. This is an axial view of a PET scan of the chest showing a section of the heart. The heart is indicated by an arrow. Choose a convenient pixel in the heart region and use seed growing to find the outline of the heart.*

17.2 Read the image in file "p_17_2.jpg" and display the image. This is an axial view of a PET scan of the chest showing a section of the heart. The heart is indicated by an arrow.*

---

* Courtesy of General Electric Healthcare; GEhealthcare.com

a. Register figure "p_17_2.jpg" with respect to image "p_17_1.jpg." Choose as many tie points as you need.
b. Use seed growing to outline the bone structures in both images. Start with a seed in the center of the supposed bone structure.

17.3 Read the image in file "p_17_3.jpg" and display it. This is a combination image of the brain with a suspected brain tumor imaged by CT, PET, and MRI. Each row represents one of the respective imaging modalities.*
a. Use seed growing to identify the location of a suspected tumor in all three imaging techniques.
b. Use Laplacian of Gaussian edge detection methods to find the boundaries of the tumor in the brain. Compare the results with those of Part "a."

17.4 Read the image in file "p_17_4.jpg" and display it. This is a PET image of the kidneys.†
a. Apply seed growing to identify the kidneys.
b. Use Laplacian of Gaussian edge detection methods to find the boundaries of both kidneys. Compare the results with those of Part "a."

17.5 Read images "p_17_5a.jpg" and "p_17_5b.jpg" and display them. Image "p_17_5a.jpg" is an axial view of a whole-body PET image of a person, and image "p_17_5b.jpg" is a CT image of the same section of the body.*
a. Use image registration techniques to find the outline of the lung in both pictures. The right lung is indicated by red arrows.
b. Use image registration techniques to find the outline of the heart in both pictures. The heart is indicated by blue arrows.
c. Use thresholding and registration techniques to determine the outlines of the chest.
d. Perform seed growing methods to identify the outline of the heart in both images.

---

* Courtesy of Philips Medical Systems. http://www.medical.philips.com/main/products/pet/

† Courtesy of General Electric Healthcare. GEhealthcare.com

18 Other Biomedical Imaging Techniques

18.1 INTRODUCTION AND OVERVIEW

From our discussion in previous chapters, it will have become evident that the discipline of biomedical imaging has two main fields of application: anatomical imaging and functional imaging. Even though the distinction between anatomical and functional imaging is sometimes somewhat arbitrary, these two categories discriminate the overall capabilities of the imaging modalities.

Another group of biomedical imaging system, which is not particularly relevant in diagnostics and treatment planning, has become widely used. This group of imaging, commonly referred to as biometrics, falls in the category of methods for personal identification.

Several imaging techniques that can provide near-real-time and three-dimensional (3-D) imaging of biological samples have been described in the previous chapters. Examples are magnetic resonance imaging, x-ray computed tomography, and ultrasound. Each methodology has certain applicability for specific imaging problems. However, while diagnosis of many diseases in their early stages requires a cellular level of resolution, none of these techniques is capable of achieving a reasonable resolution on the cellular level. Cellular imaging requires spatial resolution of less than 10 microns.

In this chapter, we first briefly describe anatomical imaging methods, not covered in previous chapters. The majority of these methods have cellular resolution. Under anatomical imaging category, the imaging techniques on regular optical microscopy, fluorescent microscopy, confocal microscopy, near-field scanning optical microscopy (NSOM), electrical impedance imaging, and electron microscopy are described briefly. Out of these methods, the first four imaging modalities can provide cellular resolution and are mainly used in vitro. Electrical impedance imaging, although not providing cellular resolution, is applied in vivo. Imaging methods such as optical microscopy depend on having access to a sample of the biological tissue under study. A biopsy is often performed to provide the sample.

The functional imaging method covered in this chapter is medical infrared imaging. Under biometrics, the use of fingerprint, retina, and iris recognition for identification purposes is outlined.

18.2 OPTICAL MICROSCOPY

The common microscope is probably the most well-known biomedical imaging device. Apart from some technical limitations, microscopes show the detail on small biological structures up to the smallest building block of life, the cell.

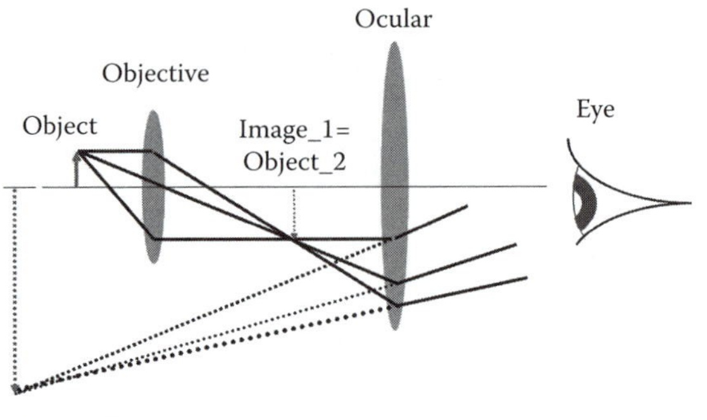

FIGURE 18.1 Basic geometry of the optical microscope.

Basic optical magnification is readily obtained by microscopic imaging. An objective is placed at a distance slightly farther than the focal length of a converging lens to form an image on the opposite side of this lens. The design of the microscope is such that the resulting real image is closer to the next converging lens than its focal lens. As a result of the position of the objective's image, the ocular produces a virtual image that is in fact behind the biological sample. The eye will be positioned in front of a lens, the ocular, and the eye will observe an objective that is apparently in the near point of vision. A real image is formed on the retina of the eye. The basic geometry of the optical microscope is shown in Figure 18.1.

In the projection of the virtual image by the ocular, the image is magnified in the new proportion. This new proportion forms the ration of the second objective distance, d_o, over the virtual image distance, d_i. Through basic geometry, it is evident without derivation that the magnification of the ocular is also equal to the image height, h_i, over the object height, h_o. The standard definition of magnification is given in Equation 18.1:

$$M_{ocular} = \frac{h_i}{h_o} = \frac{d_i}{d_o} \tag{18.1}$$

The objective magnifies the sample in a similar fashion; however, it is often more convenient to express the objective's magnification as an angular magnification. The objective magnification is the ratio of the angle that the image is projected with, θ', over the angle with which the object in the slide is viewed, θ. The angular magnification is then defined as in Equation 18.2:

$$M_{objective} = \frac{\theta'}{\theta} \tag{18.2}$$

The combined magnification is defined as the ocular magnification times the magnification of the objective.

There is a limit to the magnification level that can be achieved by an optical microscope. The size of the lenses and apertures in the construction of the microscope produces diffraction patterns that result in blurring of each demarcated item in the field of view. When the diffraction patterns of two adjacent items overlap, the items cannot be distinguished with any reasonable accuracy. This limitation is called the Rayleigh criterion (also referred to as the Abbe criterion). The Rayleigh criterion gives the boundary conditions for the smallest angle that separates two objects that can be observed clearly for a round aperture/lens as a function of wavelength, λ, and aperture diameter, D, as shown in Equation 18.3:

$$\theta_{\min} = 1.22\frac{\lambda}{D} \tag{18.3}$$

This equation states that the resolution of the optical microscopes is restricted by the wavelength of the light. In addition, since the images created by microscopes need to be perceived and interpreted by the human eyes, the resolution of this technology is also limited by the limitations of the human eyes. Specifically, due to the spacing of the rods and cones in the retina of the eye, the maximum useful magnification of the optical microscope is only 600 times. Despite these limitations, the compound microscope has allowed biologists to examine specimens and objects whose sizes are within micrometer range. Such objects include cells and some of their organelles.

One of the main disadvantages of optical microscopy is the fact that a tissue slice is needed. This requires biopsy, i.e., removal of a sample from the biological medium, which is an invasive process.

Nowadays, virtually every professional microscope has an accessory that will provide a mounting alternative for a camera to record the histology image for filing and image processing. All image processing techniques discussed in the previous chapters are used to improve the quality of the captured images. A representative image of an optical microscope with camera attached is shown in Figure 18.2. A histology image of an aneurysm in heart muscle captured by an optical microscope is shown in Figure 18.3.

The demand for increased detail and resolution has led to the development of several other imaging techniques, mainly initially based on the principle of optical microscopy. Next, we discuss one of these technologies called fluorescent microscopy.

18.3 FLUORESCENT MICROSCOPY

The phenomenon of fluorescence was discovered by the end of nineteenth century by the British scientist George G. Stokes (1819–1903). Stokes observed that several chromophores emit light after illumination. Specifically, he noted that the emitted light from some biological samples after illumination has a longer wavelength than the irradiation source. This observation led to a new generation of microscopes that allow imaging of biological tissues based on the fluoresce emission of the objects in the sample.

Several biological molecules and objects, such as pigments, resins, and vitamins, exhibit a phenomenon known as autofluorescence. Other tissues may not be

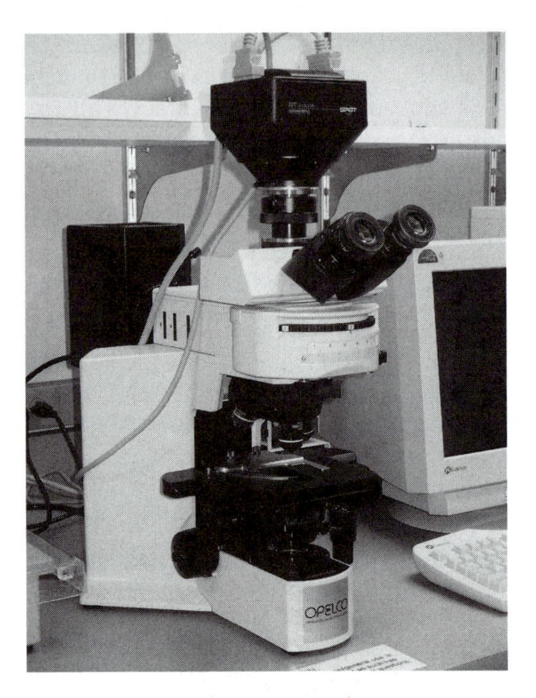

FIGURE 18.2 Representative image of an optical microscope with camera attached on top.

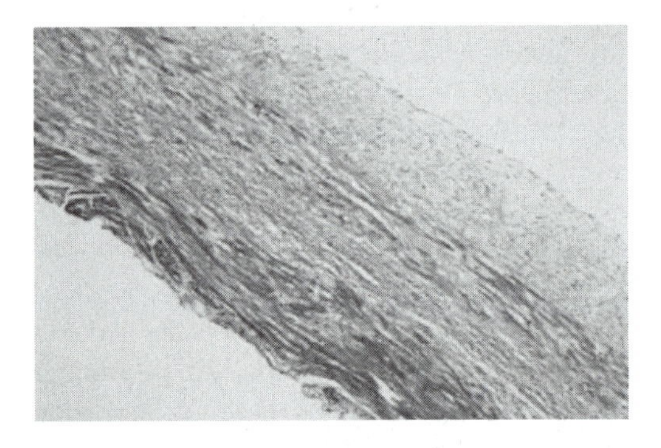

FIGURE 18.3 Histology slide of an aneurysm in a heart obtained by optical microscopy.

fluorescent, and as a result, artificial fluorophores were developed to stain particular tissues for specific recognition and registration purposes. This fluorescence tagging is the main method used in fluorescent microscopy.

The application of fluorescence microscopy is mostly in the detection of specific proteins or other molecules in cells and tissues. The mechanism of fluorescent imaging often relies on attaching specific fluorescent dyes to the molecules that serve as highly specific staining reagents. These tag molecules selectively bind to specific macromolecules in cells or nestle themselves in the extracellular matrix. Figure 18.4 shows a fluorescent microscope with three laser wavelengths.

Two commonly used fluorescent dyes used in biological research are fluorescence and rhodamine. Fluorescence glows with intense green under blue light excitation

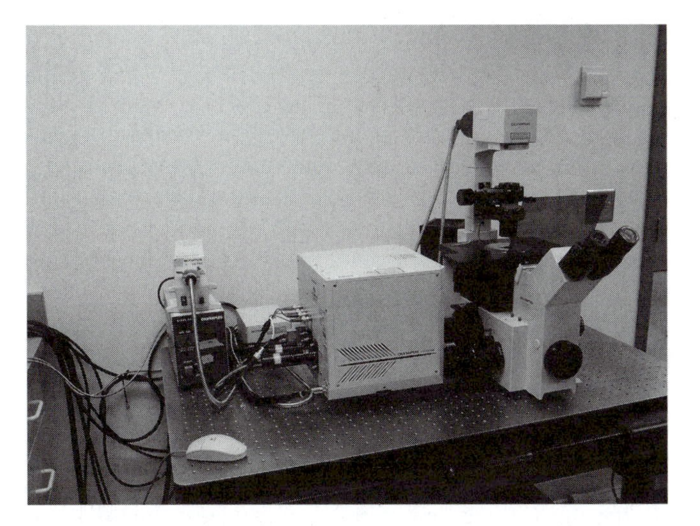

FIGURE 18.4 Picture of a fluorescent microscope with red, green, and blue lasers attached.

and rhodamine when excited by green–yellow light emits deep red. The distribution of different molecules within one single cell can be visualized by coupling one tag molecule to fluorescence and another to rhodamine. The two tags can be identified by switching the optical filters that are transparent at the respective fluorescent wavelengths. Figure 18.5 shows the histology of a mouse uterus stained by the stain phycoerythrin (PE) that emits red light under green illumination.

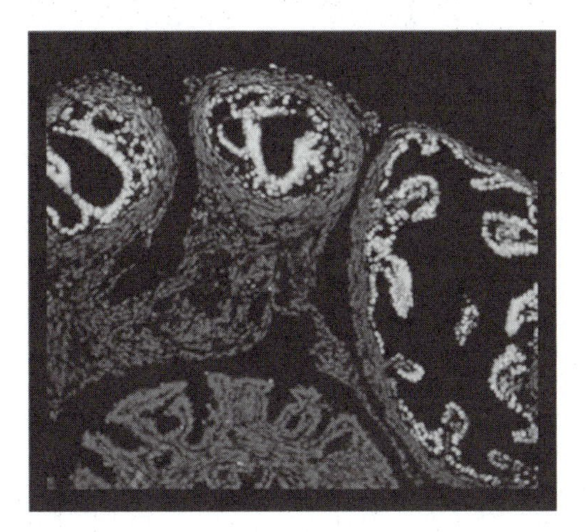

FIGURE 18.5 Representative fluorescent microscopy image of TUNEL assay of normal cycling mouse ovary with AKR strain. Two stains were used in this image, PI for the nuclear staining and FITC for the TUNEL-positive cell staining. The PI fluoresces red and the TRITC fluoresces green; the combined effect produces yellow color in the image. (Courtesy of Elizabeth Jablonski, Department of Biology, University of North Carolina at Charlotte, Charlotte, NC.)

Indirect functional imaging of the cell is possible using fluorescent microscopy. This is done by monitoring the oxygen level in different parts of a sample. In order to do so, an oxygen-quenching fluorescent dye, tris (1,10-phenanthroline) ruthenium (II) chloral hydrate, incorporated in a silicone rubber membrane is attached to an excised portion of the circulation system. The contact between the membrane and the vasculature then indicates the oxygen concentration and therefore the distribution of the blood flowing through the respective blood vessels. The membrane fluoresces proportional to the oxygen concentration of the blood in contact with the membrane.

The image acquisition for the fluorescent microscopy will be identical to that for the standard optical microscope. The only difference will be the lack of specific anatomical details due to the optical filtering. It is therefore customary to combine standard optical microscopy with fluorescent microscopy.

Images created by regular optical as well as fluorescent microscopy are two-dimensional (2-D) and therefore miss the details on the third dimension. The need for examining the third dimension of the samples led to the development of yet another imaging technique based on the principles of the fluorescent microscope. The next section describes this technology that is called confocal microscopy.

18.4 CONFOCAL MICROSCOPY

Confocal microscopy is a "stereo" version of fluoroscopic microscopy with the important advantages of performing 3-D imaging. Confocal microscopy uses a scanning laser beam that is focused to a point inside the tissue sample. An illustration of the focusing mechanism is illustrated in Figure 18.6. The backscattered light that is collected by a lens and a pinhole only allows the light coming from the exact focal point of the lens to pass the pinhole. This light comes from the same location that the laser beam was initially focused.

The laser beam passes through a set of scanning mirrors that provide three degrees of freedom for motion. The laser wavelength matches the excitation wavelength of the particular fluorochrome that is most appropriate for the imaging needs. Most frequently, multiple laser wavelengths are available to excite several fluorescent dyes for added contrast and information.

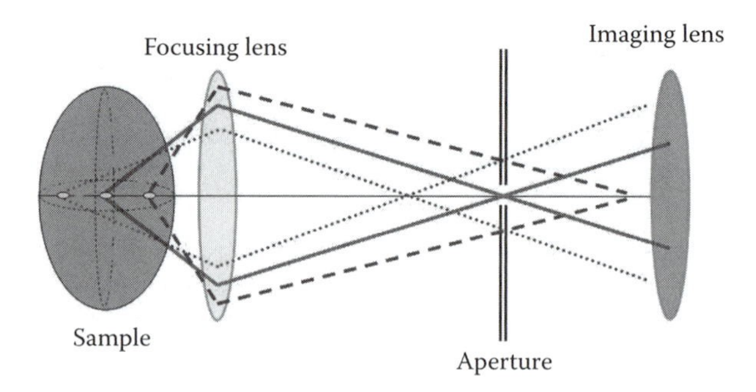

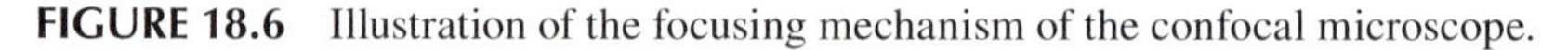
FIGURE 18.6 Illustration of the focusing mechanism of the confocal microscope.

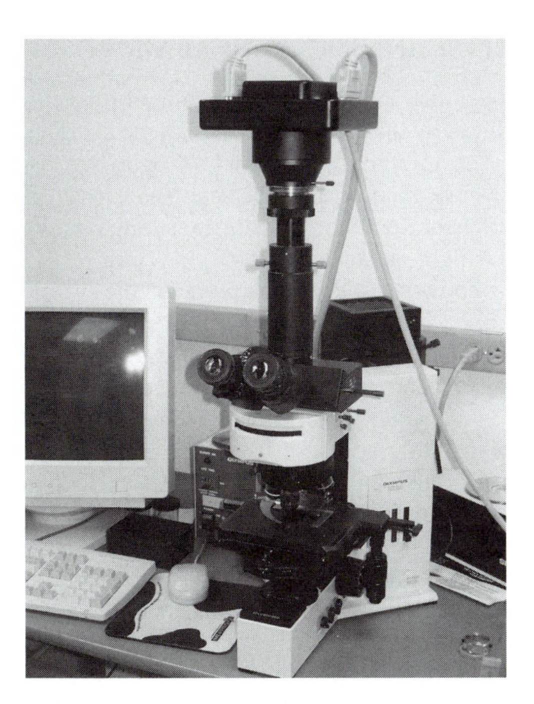

FIGURE 18.7 Representative image of a confocal microscope.

The specimen needs to be labeled with a fluorescent probe. Both the reflected light and emitted fluorescent light from the specimen is captured by the objective lens. A beam splitter separates the fluorescent light from the laser light. A photomultiplier positioned behind the analyzing pinhole produces a video signal during the scanning process. A series of confocal images at successive planes into the specimen are acquired and used in a 3-D image reconstruction algorithm. Figure 18.7 gives a representative image of a confocal microscope.

Laser scanning confocal microscopy offers the following four major advantages over standard microscopy. The generation of 3-D images is the primary significant improvement. Another advantage is the fact that a greater image resolution can be achieved. Additionally, higher magnification is possible by avoiding some of the diffraction limited imaging restrictions. Finally, stray light aberrations are limited due to the small dimension of the illuminating light spot in the focal plane.

Although confocal microscopy provides higher resolution than standard optical microscopy, it still has inherent limitations in resolution due to the properties of the light such as the wavelength. Specifically, any optical microscopy, including confocal imaging, has a fundamental drawback as the maximum attainable resolution is limited by the wavelength of the illuminating source. This limitation, imposed by the Rayleigh criterion, significantly restricts the potentials of these technologies for subcellular imaging. An attempt to have both high-resolution and 3-D imaging capabilities has resulted in the near-field scanning optical microscope, which will be discussed next.

18.5 NEAR-FIELD SCANNING OPTICAL MICROSCOPY

NSOM circumvents the diffraction-limited imaging of the entire sample caused by the lens. This is achieved by the scanning of the sample using a subwavelength aperture. The subwavelength aperture is usually a fiber optic that has been stretched and etched to form a tip whose diameter is in the nanometer range. This fiber optic functions as the point source for scanning with the transmitted or reflected light captured with a highly sensitive light radiance detector.

The sample is moved with respect to the probe on the x–y plane while maintaining a constant distance with the surface of the sample. The NSOM measures the attenuation or reflection of each data point to perform either a density measurement or a reflectivity measurement. The transmission density measurement is similar to basic x-ray imaging in many ways, while the reflection NSOM resembles ultrasound density imaging. The NSOM, as described earlier, gives an intensity profile that is representative of the local tissue density combined with a topographic profile.

In addition to collecting the intensity of the detected light, the scanning stage also has a feedback mechanism that measures the force between the fiber-optic probe and the sample. This principle is known as atomic force microscopy, which is not very useful in biological imaging on its own generally. In the case of the NSOM, the fiber-optic probe is within nanometers from the surface of the sample, hence the name near field. Due to the close proximity of the probe to the sample, great care needs to be taken not to disturb the sample itself. The sample will have a topography of its own that has greater variations than the separation between the sample and the probe. The feedback mechanism applies a voltage to a motor to maintain the exact same distance between the sample and the probe during the entire planar scan by adjusting the position of the probe until the force has returned to the default value. The distance is logged for the entire scan by means of the feedback voltage for height adjustment, and the sample height distribution can be plotted from these data.

The most common imaging mode of NSOM is the transmission mode. In this mode, the light launched through the probe is transmitted through the sample and detected by a detector. The detector records the intensity variations over the sample as it is raster scanned. These are converted into voltage values and a 2-D intensity image is built up in addition to the topography image from the "atomic force" microscope.

A third and rather novel measurement mode of NSOM has been inspired by a more general imaging technique called phase-contrast microscopy. In the phase mode of NSOM, by measuring the phase delay in transmission at each (x, y) coordinates, the optical density can be analyzed with greater detail than based on attenuation only. The optical phase is an indication of the local index of refraction and can thus reveal details about the chemical composition of the sample. The phase information is obtained with the use of interferometry.

As any other microscopic imaging discussed so far, the resolution of the NSOM is restricted by the wavelength used for imaging. Specifically, the resolution of an NSOM is identified by the size of the point light source used, which is typically in the order of 50–100 nm. Figure 18.8 shows the NSOM image of a red blood cell.

Standard microscopy has the disadvantage of giving only a view of the contents of a slide averaged over the thickness of the slide. Furthermore, almost all the

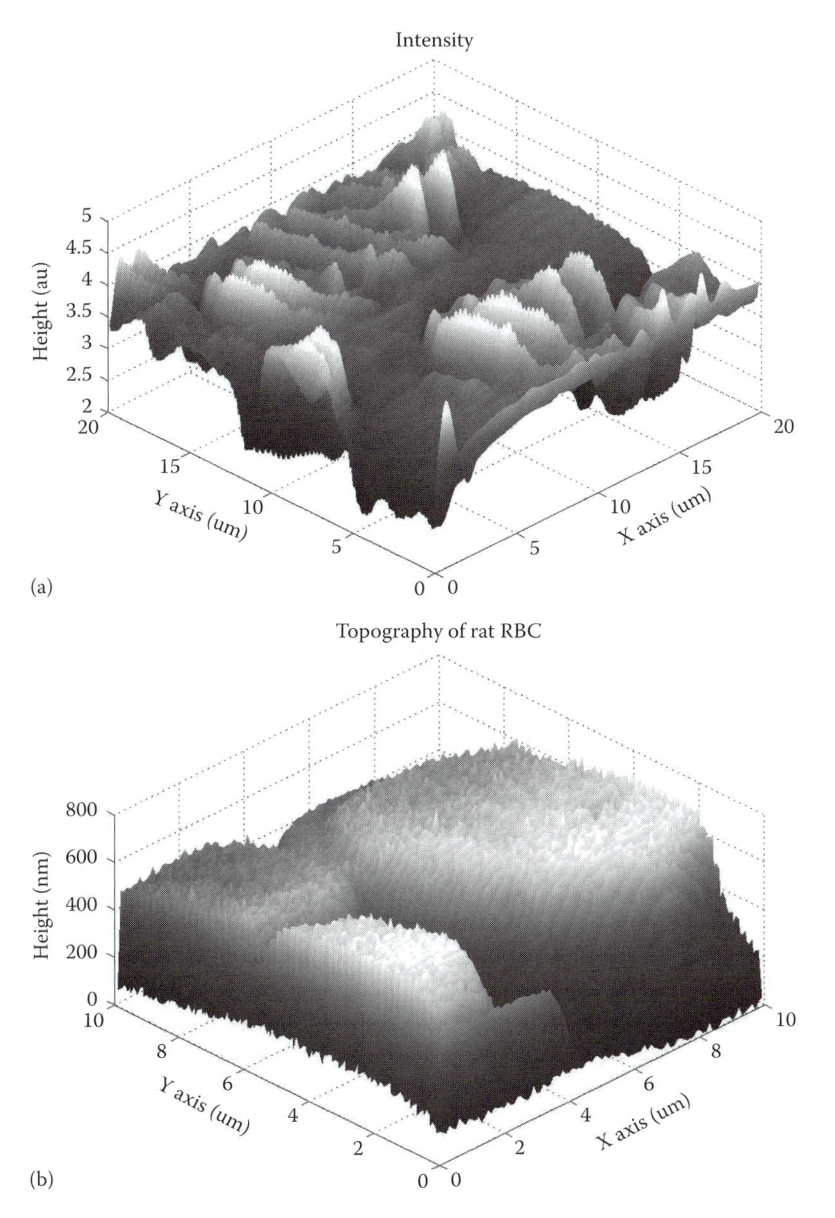

FIGURE 18.8 Imaging modalities of NSOM applied to a red blood cell. (a) Intensity profile of red blood cell, (b) topography of red blood cell, and (c) phase image of red blood cell. (Courtesy of Kert Edward, Department of Physics and Optical Science, University of North Carolina at Charlotte, Charlotte, NC.)

(*continued*)

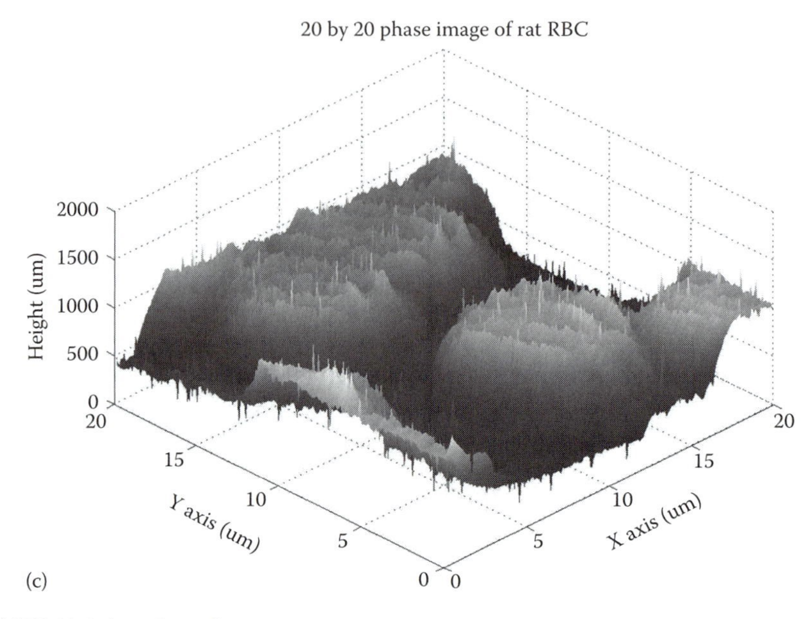

FIGURE 18.8 (continued)

previously described optical microscopy techniques are limited to in vitro imaging. Another optical imaging technique with 3-D capabilities, which will not be discussed in this chapter, is optical coherence tomography (OCT). This technology is an attempt to overcome the limitations of other optical microscopy by incorporating the coherence nature of light in an imaging technique. OCT used interferometry to collect light from a specific depth inside a tissue section only.

18.6 ELECTRICAL IMPEDANCE IMAGING

Electrical impedance imaging is related to EEG, ECG, and EMG measurement through the fact that, in almost all cases, the electrical parameters of an organ are measured by means of electrodes placed on the surface. The major difference of electrical impedance imaging with the aforementioned methods is that instead of action potential measurements, this technology measures the electrical impedance between electrodes.

The real impedance of biological tissues ranges from 0.65 Ω for cerebrospinal fluid to a resistance of 150 Ω for bone tissue. These values compare to a whole body resistance of approximately 500 Ω. Selected dielectric properties are presented in Table 18.1.

Electrical impedance imaging utilizes the differences of electrical impedances across the biological tissues to create an image of the body. In this technology, a weak electrical current in the range of milliamps with DC to several kHz frequencies is applied to the surface of the skin, and using the electrodes positioned in different parts of the body, the drop in electrical potentials at several positions is measured. Based on the injected current and the measured voltages, the electrical impedances in many locations on the skin are measured and used to form an image.

TABLE 18.1
Dielectric Properties of Some Biological Tissues

Tissue	Resistance (Ω)	Speed of Light (m/s) × 10^8
Air	High	2.998
Lung	53	0.4206
Fat	113	0.8958
Muscle	50	0.3978
Heart	49.2	0.3912
Cartilage	58	0.4628

Some electrical impedance imaging systems apply tomographic methods to retrieve depth information from the combined data input from various locations. In certain cases, the electrodes can be placed in hemispherical or cylindrical symmetric configuration to derive the cross-sectional impedance of an organ or body part; however, in nonresearch setups, only 2-D surface imaging is performed. Electrical impedance imaging is an in vivo diagnostic utility. A representative cylindrical electrical impedance imaging method is shown in Figure 18.9; the recordings of this method are illustrated in Figure 18.10.

Electrical impedance imaging can provide a relatively inexpensive methodology for diagnosing specific problems. The electrical impedance imaging can monitor the effects of esophageal reflux and pelvic blood volume. In thoracic medicine, it can be used to quantify the amount of lung water, certain conditions of sleep apnea, and different aspects of ventilation. In neurology, the influence of electrical impedance changes will be most pronounced in epilepsy and cerebral hemorrhage and ischemia.

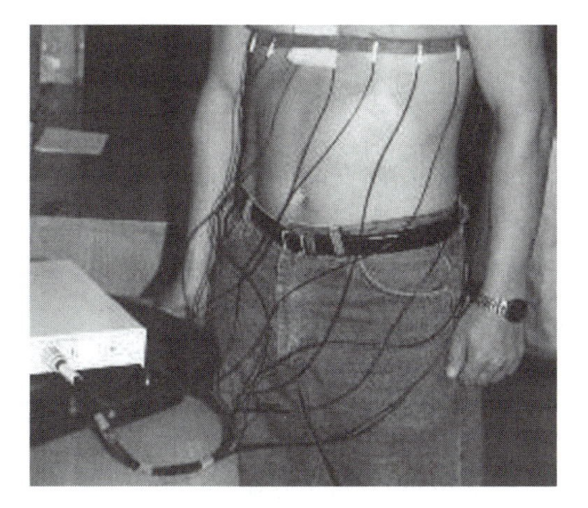

FIGURE 18.9 Representative cylindrical electrical impedance imaging method by means of a strap-on belt. (Courtesy of Dr. Alexander V. Korjenevsky, Institute of Radio-Engineering and Electronics, Russian Academy of Sciences, Moscow, Russia.)

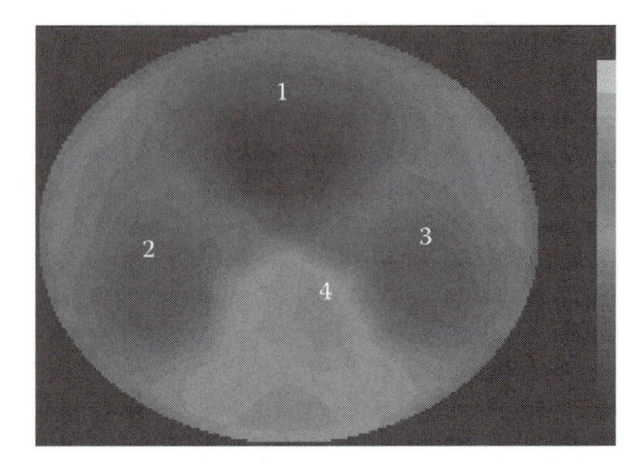

FIGURE 18.10 Representative recordings by the belt method shown in Figure 18.9. (Courtesy of Dr. Alexander V. Korjenevsky, Institute of Radio-Engineering and Electronics, Russian Academy of Sciences, Moscow, Russia.)

The electrical impedance of tissues under hyperthermic and hypothermic conditions is a highly sensitive indicator that is used to locate latent damage regions.

Several tissues have an inherent anisotropy in the impedance tomography, such as muscle tissue. As a result, the tomographic image interpretation depends on the direction in which the measurements are made in combination with the actual measured values. In addition, due to the fact that the measured impedances depend on the frequency of the applied current, additional details can be obtained when multiple frequency measurements are made.

18.7 ELECTRON MICROSCOPY

As mentioned so far, the primary imaging resolution limitation is related to the wavelength of the imaging source. A shorter wavelength will provide better resolution.

After the French physicist Louis de Broglie (1892–1987) defined the wave nature of electrons, a new vehicle for imaging was introduced. The De Broglie postulate links the momentum p of an object to an associated wavelength as outlined in Equation 18.4:

$$p = \frac{KE}{C} = \frac{hf}{C} = \frac{h}{\lambda} \tag{18.4}$$

where

KE is the kinetic energy of the particle
h is Planck's constant
C is the speed of light
f and λ are the respective frequency and wavelength of the moving electron

Using this theoretical description, electron acceleration over a potential difference of 54 V will result in a wavelength of 0.165 nm. This electron wavelength is actually in the same range as x-ray photons. Electrons are detected either by semiconductor material or a panel doped with fluorescent material.

Two types of electron microscopes can be distinguished: the transmission electron microscope and the scanning electron microscope. Both types of electron microscopes require a vacuum to minimize the ionization effects of electrons interacting with air before probing the sample. In addition, the sample preparation will most certainly result in complete cell death. These requirements rule out in vivo imaging.

18.7.1 Transmission Electron Microscopy

The transmission electron microscopy (TEM) produces a 2-D attenuation image. The attenuation images from TEM provide data on the structure of the internal components of the specimen. With special specimen preparation procedures, the TEM can also be used for the localization of elements, enzymes, and proteins.

The transmission electron microscope operates in a magnification range from 10,000 to 100,000 times with a resolution of approximately 2.5 nm.

Figure 18.11 shows a TEM image of a motor neuron, and Figure 18.12 shows a cell in the intermediate stage of mitosis. Figure 18.13 is a TEM image of a nerve axon with Schwan cell.

18.7.2 Scanning Electron Microscopy

The scanning electron microscopy (SEM) uses a 2–3 nm spot of electrons that scans the surface of the specimen. In addition to elastic backscatter, secondary electrons

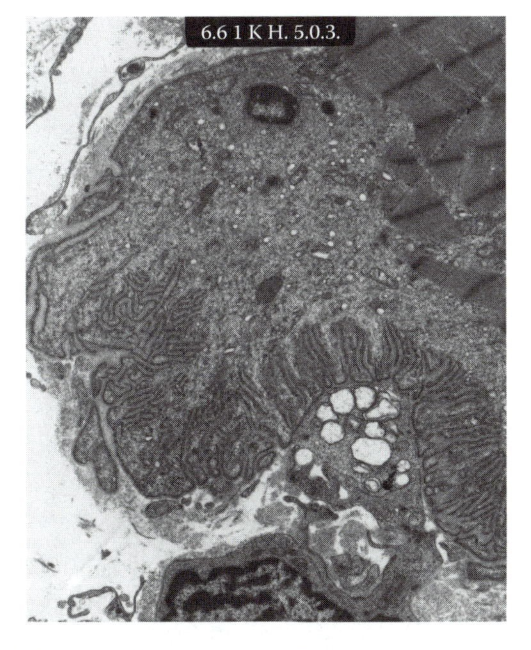

FIGURE 18.11 TEM image of a motor plate. The z-bands of the muscle are clearly visible as well as the impulse transmission by means of pockets of chemicals drifting from the nerve synapse to the muscle. (Courtesy of Winston Wiggins, Daisy Ridings, and Alicia Roh, Carolinas Medical Center, Charlotte, NC.)

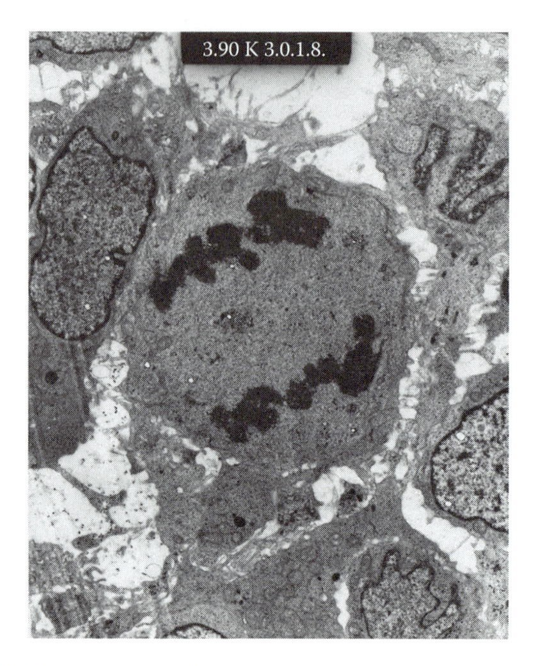

FIGURE 18.12 TEM image of a cell in the intermediate stage of mitosis. (Courtesy of Winston Wiggins, Daisy Ridings, and Alicia Roh, Carolinas Medical Center, Charlotte, NC.)

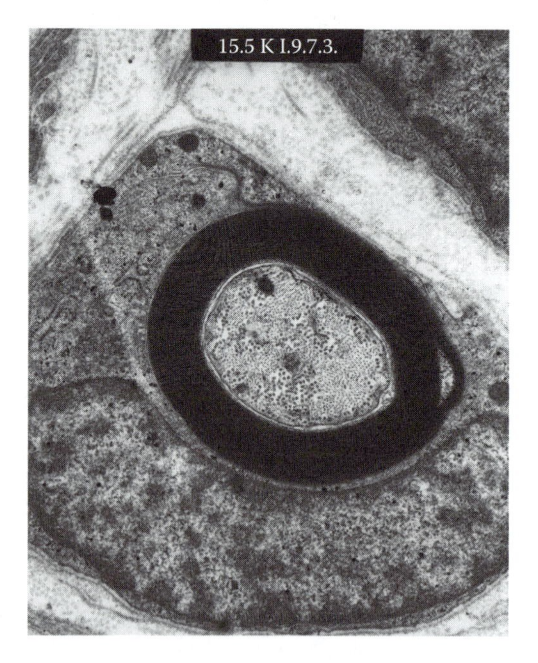

FIGURE 18.13 TEM image of a nerve axon with Schwan cell. (Courtesy of Winston Wiggins, Daisy Ridings and Alicia Roh, Carolinas Medical Center, Charlotte, NC.)

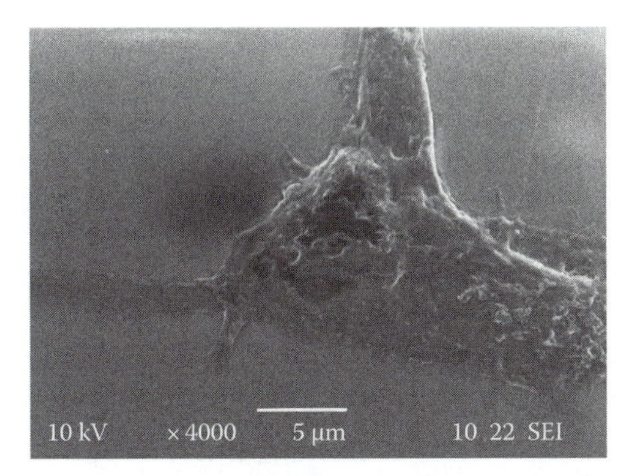

FIGURE 18.14 SEM image of an endothelial cell. (Courtesy of Dr. Mark Clemens, University of North Carolina at Charlotte, Charlotte, NC.)

are the result of inelastic collisions and will thus hold information about the elements the incident electron interacted with. The SEM produces a topographic image of the sample in addition to material characterization resulting from the inelastic scatter.

The SEM provides a 3-D perspective with significant depth of the field and high resolution. The magnification of the SEM ranges from 1,000 to 10,000 times providing a resolution of approximately 20 nm. Figure 18.14 shows an endothelial cell obtained in SEM mode imaging.

18.8 INFRARED IMAGING

Temperature can be defined as the average kinetic energy of all molecules and atoms in motion in an object. It is known that every vibrating object emits an electromagnetic radiation whose frequency is directly proportional to the temperature of the object. The peak emission wavelength emitted by an object can be identified by Wien's displacement law as follows:

$$\lambda = \frac{2.898 \times 10^{-3}}{T} \tag{18.5}$$

This equation indicates that by measuring the peak emission wavelength, the temperature of an object can be determined. Lower energetic electromagnetic radiation will be in the infrared spectrum, while higher energy electromagnetic radiation is in the visible and ultraviolet spectrum. At the room temperature or at the body temperature, objects emit in the near infrared. Only at temperatures exceeding the boiling point of water the emissions will be in the visible spectrum. A thermographic CCD camera that records the infrared emission can then collect detailed temperature measurements of the objects. An example is of a thermographic image obtained during laser irradiation of a heart while eliminating the focal source of an arrhythmia by laser photocoagulation.

The thermographic imaging method uses various size CCD arrays, mostly limited to 8 bit image depth. The temperature display is either in gray scale or pseudocolor.

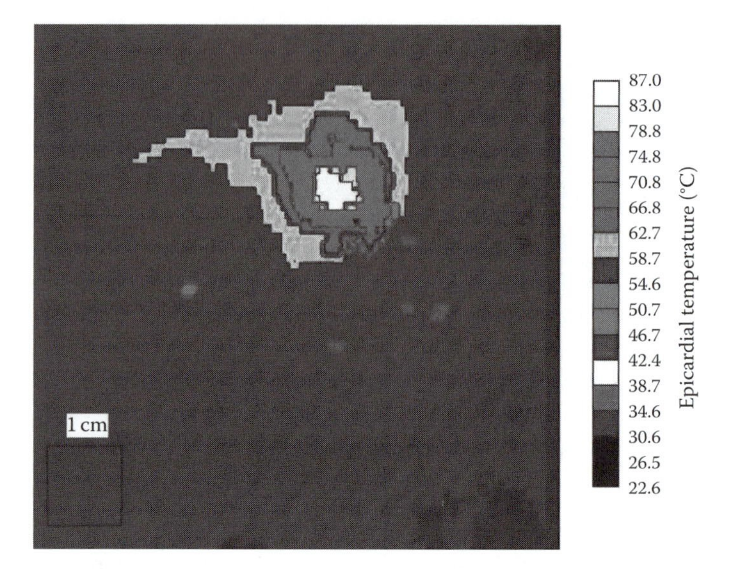

FIGURE 18.15 Example of a thermographic image in false color coding, obtained during laser irradiation of a heart while eliminating the focal source of an arrhythmia by laser photocoagulation.

In gray-scale display, white is the hottest and black is the coldest with the preset range. In false-color mode, the display will have a legend explaining the color coding as shown in Figure 18.15.

Infrared imaging is a functional imaging module. Biological processes such as the cellular metabolism produce heat, and thermographic imaging can thus provide information on local metabolic activities. Infrared thermography offers a significant contribution in imaging postoperative infections. Infrared imaging is also used to detect areas of breast with increased metabolic activity, which can be breast cancer tumors in the early stages of tumor formation. However, this technology is not capable of discriminating between malignant or benign tumors. The typical false alarms in classification of tumors using infrared imaging are often due to other types of tissues with increased metabolic activity such as cysts and tissues under inflammatory reactions.

18.9 BIOMETRICS

Biometrics is the science that uses the unique identifiers each human has for personal identification. Fingerprints, retinal maps, and iris color patterns are significantly unique for each person and are therefore heavily used for personal identification. DNA analysis is another personal identification method that is rather more costly, harder to access, more time consuming, and more complicated than the three methods mentioned earlier. Fingerprint analysis and iris recognition are used in security screenings and criminal identifications on a daily basis.

Voice recognition is also considered to be one of the personal identifiers that is even easier to obtain compared to the three methods discussed in this chapter.

However; voice recognition is subject to change and requires adaptive algorithms that are much more complex than the image recognition algorithms used in fingerprint recognition, iris identification, and retinal scans.

18.9.1 Biometrics Methodology

Regardless of the specific biological images used for biometrics, the process of image registration and classification is a sensitive procedure that is rather different from other biomedical image processing methods. Unlike tracking of the development of one single patient or comparing patients against each other for confirmation or rejection of a diagnosis, the image processing procedure of biometrics recognition is to process a given image and identify one of the individual whose biometric image is previously stored in the dataset. In other words, in biometrics image processing, the method is supposed to match the given image with all those stored in a database and identify the best match.

Biometrics image processing often involves extracting a number of features and characteristics from each image and matching these features with those of the images in the database. The image processing steps involved in all of the three biometrics methods discussed involve noise reduction, image enhancement, and feature extraction. The primary concern with both verification and authentication will be the alignment of the respective scans, i.e., registration. The orientation will rely on certain anatomical features in retinal scans and more on characteristics within the image for the fingerprint analysis and the iris scan. The number of these extracted features that are unique to each particular person range from 400 characteristics in retinal scanning to 90 characteristics in fingerprint analysis. After these characteristics have been extracted, they are matched to the cases in the database.

The methods used for extracting the features are application specific. For instance, in fingerprinting, a typical feature extraction method is based on the estimation of patterns using B-splines. In other words, B-splines that are polynomial approximations are applied to describe the curvy patterns in fingerprint and then the coefficients of these polynomials are used as the features/characteristics. The used feature can also be based on specific subgroups of patterns observed in the fingerprint. These features are described later in this section. As another example of feature extraction for biometrics, consider the processing of iris images. In one particular image processing method specialized for iris matching, first the iris images are decomposed using discrete wavelet transform (DWT) and then the DWT coefficients in particular levels are used as the features.

The algorithms used for matching include Bayesian classification and different families of neural networks. These algorithms are fed with the extracted image processing characteristics and are trained to identify the best match in a very large database. Multilayer sigmoid neural networks are by far the most commonly used algorithms for matching of biometrics.

Due to the sensitive and costly risk of misclassification in biometrics matching, a special attention is given to the error analysis. In the statistical analysis of errors in biometrics matching, the following error concepts are widely used. A type I error represents a false negative, which is a failure to identify the correct person.

A type II error represents a false positive, implying that an impostor or innocent bystander is identified as the correct subject. The false acceptance rate (FAR) stands for the rate at which the algorithm accepts an incorrect subject as true. Another classification error is the false rejection rate (FRR), which stands for the rate at which the algorithm incorrectly discards or rejects a matching subject. The crossover error rate (CER) compares the FAR to the FRR and provides the statistical point where the false rejection rate equals the FAR. Each one of these error types can be measured based on different statistical modeling, which is beyond the scope of this chapter.

Having discussed the general biometrics methodologies, next we discuss the specific types of bioinformatics identification.

18.9.2 Biometrics Using Fingerprints

The use of fingerprints for recognition purposes dates back to the late eighteen hundreds. It is widely assumed that fingerprint of a person does not change over time and therefore is a unique identifier of its owner. The hypothesis that fingerprints are unique has so far not been discarded; however, fingerprints do change as a result of factors such as scars or surgical alterations.

Several reference points used in fingerprint identification are shown in Figure 18.16. The various features that are identified in the fingerprint classification are divided in major and minor features. The main reference points that identify the subpatterns in the fingerprint are outlined in Figure 18.16. These are some additional minor reference features, also shown in Figure 18.16, that are used in the complete fingerprint analysis and recognition.

The major features are the presence of either or any of the following three characteristics in the ridge pattern: an arch, a loop, or a whorl as illustrated in Figure 18.16. Some of the minor features are certain ridge features such as ridge branches (bifurcations) or ridge endings. The minor features are grouped in a category

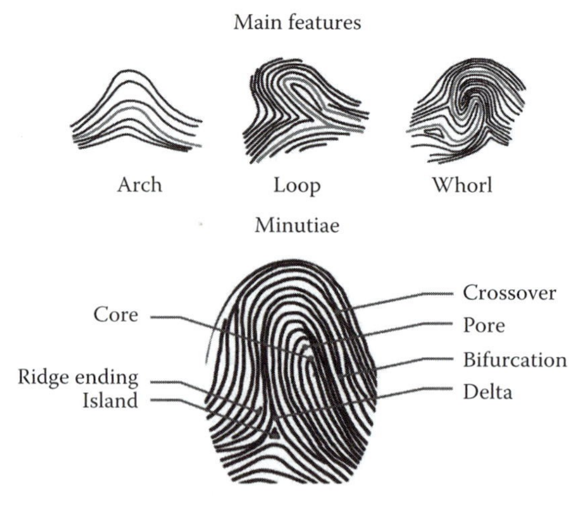

FIGURE 18.16 Characteristic reference points used in fingerprint identification.

called minutiae. The characteristics are organized based on type of formation, orientation, spatial frequency, curvature, and position of arches. Some of the fingerprint minutiae are crossovers in the ridges, the shape of the core of an arch, islands, delta-shaped ridge formations, and seemingly bidirectional deadened ridges.

When these features are captures for a given person, they are matched against the same features captured for all cases in the dataset. Fingerprinting is the most commonly used biometrics method and is heavily used in security applications.

18.9.3 Biometrics Using Retina Scans

Retina scans are invaluable tools for personal identification purposes. A retinal scan analyzes the topographical distribution of blood vessels in the retina, using the fovea and the optic nerve as locations for registration. A diagram outlining the general appearance of the retina is illustrated in Figure 18.17. Even though each person's retina is known to be unique, several diseases can result in retinal damages that alter the retinal pattern and need to be identified and tracked regularly.

Retinal imaging also has several medical and diagnostics applications. The clinical diagnostic value of retinal recognition is evident in the identification of retinal arterial and venous blockage, epiretinal membrane formation, diagnosis of macular degeneration, occurrence of macular edema, macular hole formation, retinal tearing, retinal detachment (often experienced in diabetic patients), and degeneration of the photoreceptor rods in the retina (which is often a hereditary disease). Several of the pathological conditions best identified by retinal scans will eventually result in blindness if not caught in time.

Retinal scan is rather invasive because for an accurate recording a laser or other light source must be used to illuminate the retina, passing through the cornea and

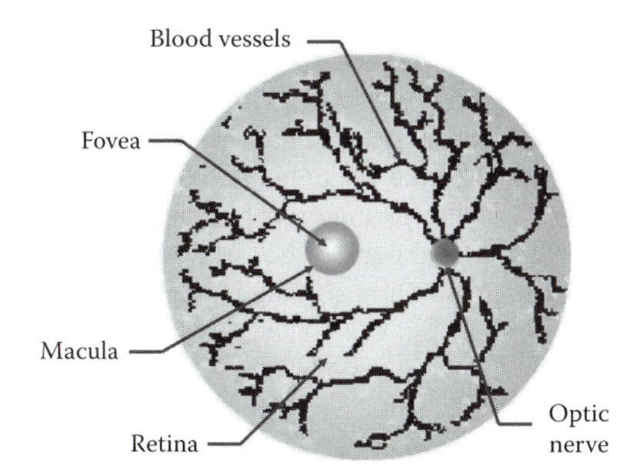

FIGURE 18.17 Diagram outlining the general appearance of the retina. The fovea has the highest concentration of optical receptor and, in particular, the cone needed for color vision. The macula is the region directly surrounding the fovea used for reading and other daily activities. The macula has both cones and rods. The rods are used for black-and-white vision. The entrance of the optic nerve through the retina forms the so-called blind spot, since there is a local absence of optical sensors. The network of blood vessels delivers nutrients and oxygen to the optical sensors.

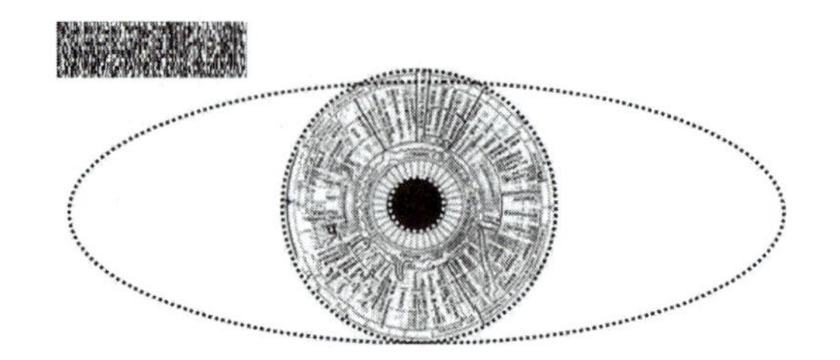

FIGURE 18.18 Diagram of the iris and the position of the iris with respect to the eyelid used for authentication and identification. Since the iris identification uses a binary data format, a bar code is often sufficient to represent the characteristics of the iris as illustrated in the top left corner.

pupil of the eye. The scan is usually performed by infrared illumination to highlight the blood vessels in the background. Infrared light provides a natural contrast medium.

18.9.4 Biometrics Using Iris Scans

The iris is the part of the eye that forms an aperture in response to different levels of illumination. The iris is fully formed before birth and does not change unless affected by trauma or disease throughout the life of the individual.

The iris can be captured with a camera and stored in a database for comparison and recognition purposes. Iris scans read between 266 and 400 different characteristics and will require the matches of approximately 200–300 characteristics to produce a significant match for authentication. The iris has chromophores imbedded that provide a distinctive coloration in combination with additional anatomical features such as color patterns and topographical configurations (such as rifts, rings, coronas, and furrows) that can be traced. A general diagram of the points of interest in iris recognition is illustrated in Figure 18.18.

The main complication with iris scanning for personal identification is the pathological conditions that can alter the appearance of the iris, as mentioned earlier. Additional complications are the formation of pigment on the inside of the iris (nevus) and neovascularization of the iris (rubeosis), which dramatically changes the reference points used in iris recognition although it is not directly a clinical concern.

18.10 SUMMARY

In this chapter, we have seen that there are several other imaging modalities that are currently being used in medicine or are in the developmental stages of eventually becoming diagnostic tools. The anatomical imaging methods we discussed in this chapter include several optical microscopy techniques, fluorescent microscope, confocal microscope, NSOM, electrical impedance imaging, and electron microscopy. In the category of functional imaging, the methodology of infrared thermographic imaging was discussed. We also described the three main practical identification techniques used in biometrics.

PROBLEMS

18.1 Read the image in file "p_18_1.jpg" and display the image. The image contains a SEM image of an endothelial cell.*

a. Choose a convenient seed point in the region of the endothelial cell and use seed growing to find the outline of the cell.
b. Find the counter of the cell and mark it in the image.
c. Calculate the length of the major and minor axes.
d. Use Fourier descriptors to compress the size of the counter information.

18.2 Collect the fingerprints of the index finger and thumb of three friends and\or family members.

a. Orient each of the fingerprints to have greater orientation accuracy.
b. Collect as many features and minutiae on each of the fingerprints.
c. Compare the fingerprints of the individuals comparing one of the main features and three of the minutiae.

18.3 Read file "p_18_3.jpg" and display the image. Image "p_18_3.jpg" is an electrical impedance image of a human chest.† In this image, the gray scale signifies the relative magnitude of the electrical impedance. Use histogram-based thresholding to outline the regions of equivalent impedance. Choose a mid-range gray-scale level to find the regions that correspond to each other in the four sections of the chest.

18.4 Read file "p_18_4.jpg" and display. Image "p_18_4.jpg" is a histology slide of a disease call ragged red fiber, which is a genetic mitochondrial defect related to the disease called MERRF syndrome (myoclonus epilepsy associated with ragged red fibers).‡ MERRF syndrome is a muscular disorder that falls in the category called mitochondrial encephalomyopathies. (Courtesy of Winston Wiggins, Daisy Ridings and Alicia Roh, Carolinas Medical Center, Charlotte, NC.)

a. Use a high-boost filter to improve the quality of the image.
b. Use segmentation methods to identify the z-band in the muscle fibers (one z-band is indicated by a blue arrow).
c. Isolate the muscle cells that have clear normal muscle structure (well-defined z-bands, etc.) from muscle cell that are deviating in structure. For this, calculate suitable image processing features for each cell and perform a K-means clustering. Then, identify the cluster that best represent normal cells.

---

* Courtesy of Mark G. Clemens, University of North Carolina at Charlotte, Charlotte, NC.

† Courtesy of Dr. Alexander V. Korjenevsky, Institute of Radio-Engineering and Electronics, Russian Academy of Sciences, Moscow, Russia.

‡ Courtesy of Winston Wiggins, Daisy Ridings and Alicia Roh of Carolinas Medical Center, Charlotte, NC.

Index

A

B

C

D

E

H

I

K

L

M

N

O

P

Q

R

S

V

W

X

Z